T0342514

Dictionary
of
Nutrition and
Dietetics

Karen Eich Drummond,
M.S., R.D., F.A.D.A., F.M.P

JOHN WILEY & SONS, INC.

New York • Chichester • Weinheim • Brisbane • Singapore • Toronto

Library of Congress Cataloging-in-Publication Data:

ISBN 0-471-29370-9

10 9 8 7 6 5 4 3 2

Dedicated to today's and tomorrow's
dietetic students.

PREFACE

The Dictionary of Nutrition & Dietetics is a comprehensive, understandable resource for anyone looking for nutrition information, as well as for undergraduate nutrition and dietetics students looking for a dictionary that pulls together much of their diverse education. The terms selected for this dictionary come from many areas.

- Nutrition

- Lifespan nutrition

- Medical nutrition therapy

- Human anatomy and physiology

- Nutritional biochemistry

- Medical diagnosis and treatment

- Management of clinical dietetics

- Research

- Communications

- Community nutrition

- Nutrition education

One difference you will find with definitions in this dictionary is that they are rarely one sentence long. A dictionary should tell you what you need to know, not confuse you, so definitions in this dictionary are purposely longer and use easy-to-understand language. In addition to longer definitions, this dictionary uses a multitude of charts, tables, and illustrations to increase understanding and give additional information in a format that is quick and easy-to-use.

Definitions for terms that encompass practical nutrition topics (such as The Food Guide Pyramid), nutrients (such as fat), and nutrition and disease (such as cardiovascular disease) are given in special feature boxes. Here is a listing of the topics you will find covered in each of these three areas.

Practical Nutrition Focus

Dietary Guidelines for Americans

Five-A-Day

Hypertension

Inflammatory Bowel Disease

Iron-Deficiency Anemia

Osteoporosis

Peptic Ulcer Disease

Renal Failure

Stroke

Ulcerative Colitis and Crohn's Disease

As a supplement to the dictionary, four appendices give you details on where to get nutrition information (including Internet sites) and professional associations (including publications and certifications), and additional information on the Recommended Dietary Allowances and nutrition labels.

I hope this dictionary gets put to good use in the years to follow! In the meantime, please direct any comments and suggestions for me to Van Nostrand Reinhold.

Karen Drummond,
M.S., R.D., F.A.D.A., F.M.P.

TABLE OF CONTENTS

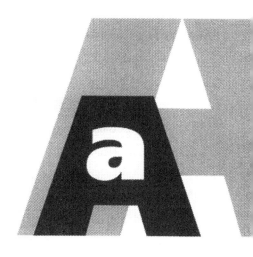

Abbreviations, Medical Chart Shortened forms of terms commonly used in the medical chart (see Table A.1).

Table A.1 Medical Chart Abbreviations

abd	Abdomen	CHD	Coronary heart disease
ADL	Activities of daily living	chem	Chemotherapy
ad lib	As desired	CHF	Congestive heart failure
alb	Albumin	c/o	Complains of
ALL	Acute lymphocytic leukemia	COPD	Chronic obstructive pulmonary disease
AML	Acute myelogenous leukemia		
ARDS	Adult respiratory distress syndrome	CRF	Chronic renal failure
		CV	Cardiovascular
ASHD	Arteriosclerotic heart disease	DOE	Dysnea on exertion
b.i.d.	Two times daily	DBW	Desirable body weight
BM	Bowel movement	DM	Diabetes mellitus
BMR	Basal metabolic rate	Dx	Diagnosis
BP	Blood pressure	ECG, EKG	Electrocardiogram
BUN	Blood urea nitrogen		
c	With	EEG	Electroencephalogram
Ca	Cancer	FBS	Fasting blood sugar
CBC	Complete blood count	GI	Gastrointestinal
cc	Milliliter (cubic centimeter)	gm	Gram

1

Table A.1 Medical Chart Abbreviations (continued)

GTT	Glucose tolerance test	qh	Every hour
Hb/ Hgb	Hemoglobin	qid	Four times a day
Hct	Hematocrit	RBC	Red blood cell, red blood cell count
h.s.	Bedtime	Rx	Treatment
IM	Intramuscular	$\bar{s}$	Without
IV	Intravenous	SOB	Shortness of breath
IVP	Intravenous pyelogram	stat	Immediately
K	Potassium	tab	Tablet
Meq.	Milliequivalent	TIA	Transcient ischemic attack
mets	Metastases	tid	Three times a day
mg	Milligram	TP	Total protein
ml	Milliliter	TPR	Temperature, pulse, and respiration
MOM	Milk of Magnesia		
Na	Sodium	UGI	Upper gastrointestinal
NIDDM	Non-insulin-dependent diabetes mellitus	URI	Upper respiratory infection
		UTI	Urinary tract infection
NPO	Nothing by mouth	vs	Vital signs
NTG	Nitroglycerin	WBC	White blood cell, white blood cell count
OOB	Out of bed		
OT	Occupational therapy	WNL	Within normal limits
PH	Past history	wt	Weight
po	By mouth	x	Times
prn	As necessary	♂	Male
PT	Physical therapy	♀	Female
pt	Patient	+	Positive
PUD	Peptic ulcer disease	−	Negative
qd	Every day	≥	Greater than
q	Every	<	Less than

Abdomen Also called the *abdominal cavity*, the space below the chest on the front side of the body. It contains the **stomach, small** and **large intestine, liver, gallbladder, spleen,** and **pancreas.** The membrane surrounding the abdominal cavity is the peritoneum. Above the abdominal cavity is the thoracic cavity and below it is the pelvic cavity.

Abetalipoproteinemia A rare, inherited disorder in which the failure of the intestinal mucosa to make **apoprotein** B causes defective formation of **chylomicrons, very low-density lipoproteins** (VLDL), and **low-density lipoproteins** (LDL). The disease is characterized by **fat** malabsorption, growth retardation, and neurologic and visual abnormalities.

Abscess A localized inflammation with pus in any part of the body. For example, a pulmonary abscess is a large collection of pus in the lungs.

Absorption The passage of nutrients after digestion through the walls of the **intestines** into the intestinal cells. Nutrients are then transferred into the **blood** or **lymph** and transported through the body via these systems. A few **nutrients** are absorbed elsewhere in the **gastrointestinal tract.**

Abstract A brief written summary of research or presentations, such as oral or poster presentations. Abstracts commonly appear at the beginning of a research paper but they can also stand alone.

Acceptable Daily Intake (ADI) The amount of sweetener an individual can consume on a daily basis over a lifetime without ill effect. ADIs are set by the **Food and Drug Administration.**

Accountability The responsibility for performing a task or producing a result.

Acesulfame-Potassium or **Acesulfame-K** An artificial sweetener marketed under the trade names Sunette and Sweet One. It is used as a table-top sweetener and to sweeten chewing gums, candies, baked goods, desserts, and beverages. Acesulfame-K is 200 times sweeter than **sucrose** and is stable in cooking and baking. It is an organic **salt** consisting of carbon, nitrogen, **oxygen,** hydrogen, **sulphur,** and **potassium** atoms, and is excreted unchanged so it contains no **calories.**

Acetaldehyde Also called **ethanal,** a simple **aldehyde** formed from the oxidation or breakdown of **ethanol,** or ethyl **alcohol.** Acetaldehyde is what causes the "hangover" after drinking. Ethanol is primarily oxidized or broken down in **liver** cells where alcohol dehydrogenase and NAD+ catalyze the reaction. Acetaldehyde is converted to **acetic acid** and then **acetyl coA** (see Figure A.1).

Acetaminophen A common analgesic (pain-killing) and antipyretic (fever-reducing) medication sold under the trade name Tylenol®. It does not have the anti-inflammatory properties of other similar products.

Figure A.1 Acetaldehyde

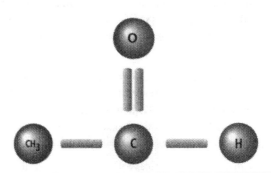

Acetic Acid The acid in vinegar that gives it its sour taste.

Acetoacetic Acid A **ketone body** (along with **acetone** and B-hydroxybutyric acid). See also **ketone bodies.**

Acetone The simplest **ketone** that is one of the **ketone bodies** (along with **acetoacetic acid** and B-hydroxybutyric acid). See also **ketone bodies.** (See Figure A.2)

Figure A.2 Acetone

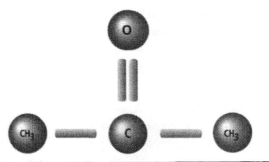

Acetylcholine A major body **neurotransmitter** released at the ends of some **nerve** cells. Acetylcholine is a quaternary ammonium **salt** present in an inactive form in nerve cells. The arrival of a nerve impulse leads to its release into the synaptic cleft, the gap between nerve cells. The acetylcholine molecules diffuse across the synapse where they combine with receptor molecules on the adjacent nerve cell or **muscle** cell, causing the signal to be passed along.

Acetyl Coenzyme A A coenzyme, derived from an acetyl group attaching itself to Coenzyme A (which contains **pantothenic acid**), that has important roles in the metabolism of **glucose** and **fatty acids**. Commonly called **acetyl coA**, it is the common compound formed from glucose, fatty acids, and **amino acids**. Acetyl coA starts off the **tricarboxylic acid cycle** and also provides the carbon atoms for fatty acid synthesis.

Achalasia When the smooth **muscles** along the **gastrointestinal tract**, especially where two parts join, fail to relax. Most commonly, the lower esophageal **sphincter** has trouble relaxing during swallowing, causing **dysphagia** (difficulty in swallowing), a feeling of fullness, and vomiting. Treatment includes small and frequent meals, moderate **protein** and **carbohydrate**, low **fiber**, omission of foods that might irritate the **esophagus** such as citrus juices or highly spiced foods, and dilating or widening the lower esophageal **sphincter** surgically.

Achlorhydria Absence or reduced amount of **hydrochloric acid** in the stomach. Hydrochloric acid helps denature ingested **proteins** and the **stomach enzyme pepsin** is more active under acidic conditions. In achlorhydria, protein digestion may be affected.

Acid A molecule or ion that gives up one or more of its hydrogen atoms when it ionizes in solution. **Acids** neutralize **bases** by donating hydrogen ions.

Acid-Base Balance The process in which the body buffers the **acids** and **bases** normally produced in the body so the **blood** is neither too acidic or basic. Acid-base balance is critical to life. The respiratory system, renal system, and **buffers** found in the blood all contribute to maintaining acid-base balance.

Acidosis A condition in which the pH of the **blood** decreases or becomes more acidic. In metabolic acidosis, there are changes in the bicarbonate level in the blood **plasma** that could be due to **dehydration** or **ketosis**. In respiratory acidosis, **carbon dioxide** is retained in the body which can cause a drop in blood pH. See also **ketosis**.

Accountability The obligation of a worker to the supervisor to carry out the responsibilities delegated and to produce the results expected.

Acquired Immunodeficiency Syndrome (AIDS) A serious illness that harms the body's ability to fight infection. A virus called HIV (human immunodeficiency virus) causes AIDS and affects people in different ways. Some infected individuals show no signs of infection, whereas others start to develop signs of HIV infection, which are usually less severe than found in individuals with full-blown AIDS. HIV is spread primarily through sexual intercourse with an HIV-infected person or by sharing a needle with an HIV-infected person.

Action Research Disciplined inquiry in an organization to improve the quality of the organization and its performance. Action research is popular in education where it takes the following steps.

1. Select area of inquiry.
2. Collect data
3. Organize data.
4. Analyze and interpret data.
5. Take action.

A teacher in a classroom may do action research to see which teaching method is most effective.

Active Listening The most effective level of listening that is possible. Active listening does not come naturally; rather it is a learned skill requiring much concentration and sensitivity. The active listener has three important skills: attending, sensing, and responding skills (see Table A.2).

Table A.2 Active Listening Skills

1. The active listener uses attending skills, which include giving both appropriate verbal and nonverbal messages to indicate attentiveness. Examples of attending behaviors include making eye contact, nodding the head, or using expressions such as "Go on," and creating a private atmosphere in which to talk.

2. The active listener uses sensing skills to examine the nonverbal behaviors or messages of the speaker. Nonverbal communication includes thoughts and ideas that an individual communicates, not only through the voice, but also through the body, physical distance, or dress. The active listener attends to body language—specifically to body posture, facial expressions, vocal inflections, and gestures that are used to communicate attitudes and feelings.

3. Responding skills are used to understand the speaker's message to the fullest. These include asking questions to get more information or clarify feelings, trying to get the speaker to say more, or helping the speaker toward greater understanding.

Active Site The site on an **enzyme** where the **substrate** binds and the catalytic reaction occurs.

Active Transport When substances travel across the cell membrane, like swimming upstream, and they require energy from the cell to do so.

Acylation The process of attaching **fatty acids** to **glycerol** to make a **triglyceride**.

Acyl Carrier Protein (ACP) In **lipogenesis** (fat synthesis), a structure that carries the acetyl group and growing **fatty acid**. ACP contains **pantothenic acid**, a **vitamin**.

Adequate Diet A diet that provides enough of the essential nutrients and **calories**.

Additives See **food additives**.

Adenocarcinoma A tumor of a gland.

Adenoids Lymphoid tissue found in the **pharynx**. Also called **tonsils**.

Adenosine   A **nucleoside** made of adenine (a **purine**) and **ribose**.

Adenosine Diphosphate (ADP)   A dephosphorylated form of **adenosine triphosphate (ATP)** that accepts a phosphate group in the ATP energy cycle.

Adenosine Triphosphate (ATP)   A high-energy phosphate compound that is the immediate storage form for energy in **cells**. ATP contains **adenosine** (a **nucleotide**) and three phosphoric acid groups. ATP is the universal energy carrier of the cell. By splitting the terminal phosphate bond of ATP to make **ADP**, energy is released for cellular work.

Adherence   The degree to which a **client** follows a prescribed dietary regimen.

Adipocytes   Adipose (**fat**) **cells**.

Adipose Tissue   Loose fibrous connective tissue that contains many adipose **cells**. Adipose tissue is abundant just under the **skin** and around the **organs** where it helps maintain warmth and provides protection. Adipose tissue also represents a reservoir of extra energy.

Adrenal Glands   Two small glands, each located on top of each **kidney**. Each adrenal gland has two parts: the **cortex** (outer part) and the **medulla** (middle part). The cortex secretes a group of **hormones** known as **corticosteroids**, **steroid hormones**, or **corticoids**. The steroid hormones are made from **cholesterol**. The medulla secretes a group of hormones known as **catecholamines**.

The corticosteroids secreted by the cortex are of three types.

1. **Mineralocorticoids**—These hormones regulate the balance of **sodium** and **potassium** in the **blood**. The most important mineralocorticoid is **aldosterone**. Aldosterone increases sodium **reabsorption** and potassium excretion by the kidney. Aldosterone is secreted in response to high blood potassium levels.

2. **Glucocorticoids**—The glucocorticoids regulate the **metabolism** of **glucose, fat,** and **protein** and suppress the inflammatory response. The most important glucocorticoid is **hydrocortisone**, also called **cortisol**. Hydrocortisone suppresses the **immune system** and has an anti-inflammatory effect. Hydrocortisone also stimulates the breakdown of protein to **amino acids** in the **skeletal muscle** and increases **gluconeogenesis** in the **liver**. Cortisone is a synthetic hormone similar to cortisol. When the body is stressed, **corticotropin-releasing factor** (CRF) is made by the **hypothalamus** and travels to the **pituitary** where it causes the production and secretion of **adrenocorticotropic hormone** (ACTH). ACTH, the stress hormone, causes the adrenal cortex to make and secrete cortisol.

3. Sex Steroids—Sex hormones, such as **estrogens** and **androgens**, supplement the sex steroids secreted by the reproductive organs.

The catecholamine hormones secreted by the medulla are of two types.

1. **Epinephrine or adrenaline**—Epinephrine stimulates increased cardiac output, dilates respiratory passageways, increases the respiratory rate, and increases glycogenolysis (breakdown of glycogen to glucose) and lipolysis (breakdown of triglycerides into glycerol and fatty acids) so that blood sugar and fatty acid levels rise.

2. **Norepinephrine** or **noradrenaline**—Norepinephrine increases **blood pressure** because it constricts blood vessels. It also dilates respiratory passageways, increases the respiratory rate, and increases glycogenolysis and lipolysis, like epinephrine but to a lesser degree.

The catecholamines mimic the actions of the **sympathetic nervous system** by increasing the heartbeat, respiratory rate, blood pressure, and blood sugar levels during stress (see Table A.3).

Table A.3 Adrenal Hormones

Adrenal Cortex	Adrenal Medulla
Corticosteroids or Steroid Hormones	Catecholamines
1. Mineralocorticoids— Aldosterone	1. Epinephrine or adrenaline
2. Glucocorticoids— Cortisol or hydrocortisone	2. Norepinephrine or noradrenaline
3. Sex Steroids— Estrogen, androgens	

Adrenaline See **epinephrine.**

Adrenocorticotropic Hormone (ACTH) An anterior **pituitary hormone** that causes the adrenal cortex to make and secrete the glucocorticoids. The **glucocorticoids** suppress the **immune response** and increase **blood glucose levels.**

Aerobic Requiring **oxygen.**

Aerobic Cellular Respiration See **respiration.**

Afferent Transporting or conveying towards the center.

Afferent Nerves **Neurons** that conduct impulses from sensory receptors into the **central nervous system** (brain and spinal cord). Also called **sensory nerves.** See also **neuron.**

Affirmative Action A federal policy that requires organizations to correct past discriminatory practices by making extra efforts to recruit, hire, and promote qualified members of protected groups. This is implemented by having organizations set up affirmative action programs to ensure a balanced and representative work force. Affirmative action programs are required for employers with federal contracts over a certain amount, as well as employers who have been found guilty of discriminatory employment practices. See also **equal employment opportunity.**

Agenda Setting The process by which issues, such as **nutrition education** for school-age children, compete successfully for the U.S. government's attention and action.

Agglutination A fatal reaction during a **blood** transfusion due to mismatch of **antigens** and **antibodies.** During a blood transfusion, if the antigens of the donor's blood are incompatible with recipient's antibodies, the recipient's blood will clump. See also **blood types.**

Agreement Exchanges of promises between two parties. Agreements may be verbal or written as a letter of agreement or contract. A letter of agreement is less formal than a contract but both are legally binding. A letter of agreement should specify what the agreement is for, who is providing it, when, where, and how. Payment fees and schedules of payment should also be included as well the term, or length, of the agreement and how it can be terminated. Contracts need legal advice; therefore, they are used if more risk is involved or more control is needed.

Alanine Aminotransferase (ALT) See SGPT (**serum glutamic pyruvic transaminase**).

Albumin A **blood plasma protein** that accounts for about 60 percent of the plasma proteins. Albumins are made in the **liver.** They perform the important job of providing the osmotic pressure needed to draw water from the surrounding tissue fluid into the **capillaries.** By fighting water's tendency to leave the **blood** and leak into the tissue spaces, albumins maintain normal blood volume and **blood pressure.**

Alcohol Ethanol Current evidence suggests that moderate drinking of alcoholic beverages is associated with a lower risk for **coronary heart disease** in some individuals. However, higher levels of alcohol intake raise the risk for **high blood pressure, stroke, heart disease,** certain **cancers,** accidents, violence, suicides, birth defects, and overall **mortality.**

Moderate drinking is defined as no more than one drink per day for women and no more than two drinks per day for men. Count as one drink:

- 12 ounces of regular beer (150 calories)

- 5 ounces of wine (100 calories)

- 1.5 ounces of 80-proof distilled spirits (100 calories)

Some people should not drink alcoholic beverages at all. These include:

- Children and adolescents.

- Individuals of any age who cannot restrict their drinking to moderate levels. This is a special concern for recovering alcoholics and people whose family members have alcohol problems.

- Women who are trying to conceive or who are pregnant. Major birth defects, including fetal alcohol syndrome, have been attributed to heavy drinking by the mother while pregnant. Although there is no conclusive evidence that an occasional drink is harmful to the fetus or to the pregnant women, a safe level of alcohol intake during pregnancy has not been established.

- Individuals who plan to drive or take part in activities that require attention or skill. Most people retain some alcohol in the blood up to two to three hours after a single drink.

- Individuals using prescription and over-the-counter medications. Alcohol may alter the effectiveness or toxicity of medicines. Also, some medications may increase blood alcohol levels or increase the adverse effect of alcohol on the brain.

If you drink alcoholic beverages, do so in moderation, with meals, and when consumption does not put you or others at risk.

Alcohol Dehydrogenase An **enzyme** that is necessary for **ethanol** to be broken down to **acetaldehyde**.

Aldehyde A group of organic compounds formed when an alkyl group is positioned on one of the two remaining carbon bonds of a carbonyl group and a hydrogen is positioned on the other (see Figure A.3).

Figure A.3 Aldehyde

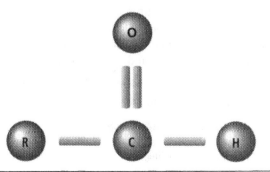

Aldose A **monosaccharide** with an **aldehyde** group.

Aldosterone A **hormone** secreted by the adrenal cortex that increases **sodium reabsorption** and **potassium** excretion by the kidney. Aldosterone is secreted in response to high blood potassium levels.

Alkaline Phosphatase (ALK) A laboratory test done on **blood serum** to determine the level of alkaline phosphatase. In **liver** disease, the level of this **enzyme** is increased.

Alkalosis A dangerous condition in which the **blood** is too basic.

Alimentary Tract The **digestive tract**, also called the **gastrointestinal tract.** See also **gastrointestinal tract.**

Allergy See **food allergy.**

Alopecia Partial or complete loss of hair. Alopecia occurs for reasons such as age and certain anticancer treatments.

Alpha-Tocopherol Equivalents The measure of **vitamin E** in food that takes into account the **vitamin** activity of the different tocopherols (forms of vitamin E).

Alveoli (Singular: alveolus) 1) Air sacs at the end of the **bronchioles** (air passages in the lungs) that have thin walls so **oxygen** and **carbon dioxide** can diffuse into and out of the **blood.** 2) Small sac-like areas in the **mammary glands** that produce and secrete milk.

Amenorrhea No menstrual discharge. Amenorrhea can be due to a number of reasons, such as during extreme weight loss or **malnutrition**, malfunctioning of the **pituitary gland**, or drugs. Amenorrhea is seen in anorexics and athletes undergoing strenuous training.

American Dietetic Association The professional organization of dietitians in the United States. See Also **registered dietitian.**

Americans with Disabilities Act (ADA) Federal legislation that gives civil rights protections to individuals with disabilities similar to those provided to individuals on the basis of race, sex, national origin, age, and religion. It guarantees equal opportunity for individuals with disabilities in employment, transportation, telecommunications, public accommodations, and state and local government services.

Amino Group The nitrogen-containing part of an **amino acid** (the building blocks of **protein**): $-NH_2$.

Amino Acid Pool The overall amount of **amino acids** distributed in the **blood**, the **organs**, and the body's cells. Amino acids from foods stock these pools as well as amino acids from body **proteins** that have been dismantled. (See Figure A.4.)

Amino Acids Organic compounds that function as the building blocks of **proteins**. Chemically, the alpha carbon of an amino acid (first carbon of the chain) is connected to: a hydrogen, an amino group ($-NH_2$), a **carboxyl group** ($-COOH$), and a side chain that varies for each amino acid (see Figure A.4).

Figure A.4 Amino Acid

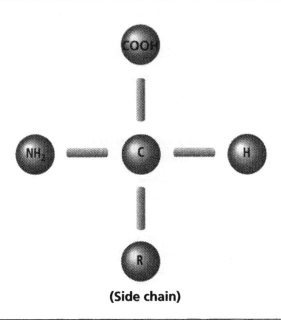

(Side chain)

Aminopeptidase A **digestive enzyme** attached to the cell membrane of microvilli in the **small intestine**. Aminopeptidase is a brush border **enzyme** that cuts the **peptide bonds** from the **amino** ends of **proteins** to produce **amino acids**, **dipeptides**, and **tripeptides**.

Amniocentesis Removal of **amniotic fluid** from a pregnant woman usually between the 16th and 20th weeks of pregnancy. Cells of the **fetus** are found in the **amniotic fluid** and can be tested for abnormalities such as **Down's syndrome**. The sex of the fetus can also be determined.

Amniotic Fluid The liquid that surrounds the **fetus** and protects it during pregnancy.

Amniotic Sac The protected bag or sac that cushions and protects the **fetus** during pregnancy.

Amphipathic Molecules Molecules with one end that is attracted to water (hydrophilic) while the other end is not attracted to water (hydrophobic).

Amphoteric In chemistry, a molecule that acts like an **acid** in the presence of a **base**, and like a base in the presence of an acid.

Amylase A group of **starch**-splitting **enzymes** that aid in digestion. Amylase is produced in the saliva (**ptyalin**) and by the **pancreas** (pancreatic amylase).

Amylopectin One of the two different polymers found in **starch** (the other polymer is **amylose**). Amylopectin is larger than amylose and is branched. Amylopectin is a **polysaccharide**.

Amylose One of the two different polymers found in **starch** (the other polymer is **amylopectin**). Amylose is a linear molecule and a **polysaccharide**.

Amyotrophic Lateral Sclerosis (ALS) A progressive disease in which **motor neurons** in the spinal cord and brain stem degenerate. Also called *Lou Gehrig's disease* after the famous baseball player who died from ALS. **Muscles** slowly become weak and then **atrophy** causing problems such as difficulty in swallowing and talking. There is no cure.

Anabolic Steroids A group of synthetic derivates of testosterone (male sex hormone) that enhance growth and repair of tissue. Athletes sometimes illegally abuse these drugs.

Anabolism The metabolic process in which body tissues and substances are built. In anabolism, larger molecules are made from smaller ones.

Analytical Research See **research**.

Anaerobic Not requiring **oxygen**.

Anaerobic Respiration The **metabolic pathway** in which **glucose** is converted to lactic acid. First, glucose is converted by **glycolysis** to pyruvate. When conditions are **anaerobic**, in other words not enough **oxygen** is present, the **NADH** produced in glycolysis gives up its two hydrogen atoms to **pyruvic acid**, making lactic acid. This reaction regenerates the **NAD+** that is needed by the cell. Anaerobic respiration produces a net gain of two ATP molecules for each glucose molecule. **Red blood cells** respire only anaerobically. However, in other parts of the body, anaerobic respiration is appropriate only for short periods of time when more oxygen is needed than can be supplied (such as during some forms of exercise).

Anastomoses A surgically-created opening between two spaces or **organs**.

Androgens Male **hormones** such as testosterone made primarily by the testes and needed for secondary sex characteristics and reproduction.

Anemia Any condition in which there is a low **hemoglobin** concentration and/or low **erythrocyte** count. The most common type of anemia is **iron-deficiency anemia**, caused by an **iron** deficiency.

Other types of anemia follow.

1. Aplastic anemia—A disorder in which the bone marrow, site of **blood cell** synthesis, does not produce new blood cells. It may be caused by certain antibiotics, radiation, or chemicals such as benzene.

2. **Pernicious anemia**—Lowered numbers of mature **red blood cells** due to an inability to absorb **vitamin B12** into the body. Vitamin B12 is different from other vitamins in that it requires a compound called R-protein (produced in most body fluids) and a compound called intrinsic factor (produced in the **stomach**) to be absorbed. Vitamin B12 attaches to the R-protein in the stomach and is then released in the **small intestine** where it complexes with the intrinsic factor. Vitamin B12 is then carried to the **ileum** (the last segment of the small intestine) where it is absorbed. In pernicious anemia, intrinsic factor is usually missing so vitamin B12 can't be absorbed. Vitamin B12 is necessary for the development of red blood cells. Untreated, pernicious anemia eventually causes damage to the **nervous system**.

3. **Megaloblastic anemia**—A **blood** disorder in which there are abnormally large, immature, red blood cells that don't function properly. Megaloblastic anemia is due to a deficiency of **folate** or vitamin B12.

Anergy A decreased immunological reaction to an **antigen** (a foreign substance such as a virus).

Aneurysm A bulging of a **blood** vessel wall that can lead to hemorrhage and stroke. Aneurysms are often caused by hardening of the **arteries** and **high blood pressure**. See also **stroke.**

Angina Pectoris An episode in which the **heart** muscle doesn't get enough **blood** and **oxygen** such as during exertion, causing chest pain. Angina occurs because of a damaged, closed, or narrowed **coronary artery. Atherosclerosis** is the underlying cause in most cases. Drugs such as nitroglycerine normally are used to treat angina. Angina does not always lead to **heart attacks**. Sometimes **collateral circulation** (opening of smaller **arteries** to supply blood to an area where a larger artery is damaged, closed, or narrowed) develops to relieve angina pain due to coronary artery disease.

Angiography X-ray study of **blood** vessels and the **heart** by first injecting a dye or contrast material. X-rays are then taken of the blood vessels which may show blood clots, narrowing of vessels, cysts, and tumors. This technique often is used to examine the vessels of the heart, **kidney**, and lungs.

Angioplasty A procedure in which a tiny balloon is inserted into blocked **heart arteries** and their branches, and then inflated to compress the **plaque** that is obstructing the flow of blood to the heart.

Angiotensin I See **renin**.

Angiotensin II See **renin**.

Anion A negative ion.

Anomeric Carbon The carbon in organic compounds, such as **amino acids**, that has four different groups attached to it.

Anomers The isomers that form when a **monosaccharide** forms a ring. If the **oxygen** attached to the anomeric carbon is down, it is the alpha isomer. If the oxygen attached to the anomeric carbon is up, it is the beta isomer.

Anorexia Lack of appetite.

Anorexia Nervosa See **eating disorders**.

Antagonist A substance whose action opposes another substance.

Antepartum The period during pregnancy before labor and delivery of the infant.

Anthropometrics The use of tools to measure the size, weight, and proportions of the body. Height and weight measurements are very useful when steps are taken to make sure they are accurate. Adults should be weighed on beam balance scales that are calibrated periodically to ensure accuracy. The best time to weigh patients is in the morning before breakfast and after the **bladder** has been emptied. For consistency, patients should be weighed at the same time of day each time and wear the same amount of clothing. There are specialized scales available to measure bedridden patients. Even when weights are taken correctly, factors such as fluid retention may adversely affect the weight reading.

An accurate measurement for height is also very important yet many health care institutions rely upon the patient's self-reported height, which is often incorrect. Whenever possible, height should be measured with the patient standing straight against a measuring tape or stick on a vertical wall or instrument.

The patient's actual body weight should be compared to **height weight tables**. A simple rule of thumb used often by dietitians to evaluate weight is given below.

Women:	*Medium frame:*	Allow 100 pounds for first 5 feet of height, plus 5 pounds for each additional inch
	Small frame:	Subtract 10 percent
	Large frame:	Add 10 percent
Men:	*Medium frame:*	Allow 106 pounds for first 5 feet of height, plus 6 pounds for each additional inch

Small frame: Subtract 10 percent
Large frame: Add 10 percent

A patient may be at nutritional risk if his or her weight is 80 percent, or less, of the standard weight (sometimes called desirable weight), or 120 percent, or more, of the standard weight. Here is how to calculate percent standard weight.

Percent of Standard Weight $= \dfrac{\textbf{Actual Weight}}{\textbf{Standard Weight}} \times 100$

In addition to getting accurate height and weight measurements, the patient should be asked about his or her usual body weight. A patient may be at nutritional risk if there has been a 5 percent weight loss over the past month, 7.5 percent weight loss during the previous three months, or 10 percent over the previous six months. Here is how to calculate percent weight change.

Percent Weight Change $= \dfrac{\textbf{Usual Weight minus Actual Weight}}{\textbf{Usual Weight}} \times 100$

Other anthropometric measurements include **triceps skin fold** (TSF) and **mid-upper-arm circumference** (MAC). Taking these measurements accurately requires much skill and practice. To take the MAC, find the midpoint of the patient's upper arm (use the nondominant arm) and measure the distance around it in centimeters. To take the TSF, use your thumb and index finger to grab a piece of skin and subcutaneous **fat** just above the mid-upper-arm point on the back of the arm. Maintain your grasp and, using the skinfold caliper, measure the compressed skinfold quickly. Take two or three readings to increase your accuracy. TSF gives an estimation of the amount of subcutaneous fat. By using the following **mid-upper-arm muscle circumference** (MAMC), you can get an estimate of the body's **skeletal muscle** mass.

MAMC (cm) = MAC (cm) – (3.14 x TSF in cm)

Each of these measures (MAC, TSF, and MAMC) can be compared to standards.

Antibodies Proteins that bind foreign molecules called **antigens**. Each antibody can bind to one kind of antigen. All possible antibodies are not in the body at any one time. They are formed by an **immune response** whenever a new antigen enters the body. See also **immune system.**

Antidiuretic Hormone (ADH) A **hormone** made in the **hypothalamus** and secreted from the posterior **pituitary gland**. ADH acts on the distal tubules in the **kidney** to reabsorb water into the bloodstream. Also called **vasopressin.**

Antiemetic A medication that tries to prevent vomiting and nausea.

Antigen Any foreign substance, such as bacteria, viruses, and toxins, that stimulate the production of **antibodies** to fight and destroy them.

Antimetabolite A substance, such as a drug, that resembles an essential **metabolite** in the body and thereby interferes with the normal functioning of this essential metabolite.

Antioxidant A compound that combines with **oxygen** so oxygen is not available to oxidize, or destroy, important substances. Antioxidants prevent the oxidation of **unsaturated fatty acids** in the cell membrane, **DNA** (the genetic code), and other cell parts that substances called free radicals try to destroy. In the absence of antioxidants, free radicals may destroy cells (possibly accelerating the aging process) and alter DNA (possibly increasing the risk for cancerous cells to develop). Free radicals may also contribute to the development of **cardiovascular disease**. In the process of functioning as an antioxidant, the antioxidant is itself oxidized or destroyed. Important antioxidants in the body include beta carotene (a precursor of **vitamin A**), **vitamin E**, and **vitamin C**.

Antrum The lower portion of the **stomach** that empties into the **duodenum** through the pyloric valve.

Anus The opening of the digestive tract through which feces travels to the outside of the body.

Aorta The largest **artery** in the body located at the opening of the **heart's** left ventricle. The aorta receives freshly oxygenated blood from the left ventricle. Branches of the aorta carry the blood to the body's cells. See also **heart**.

Apgar Score A test to determine a newborn's physical health. At one minute of age, the newborn is given a score for heart rate, breathing, muscle tone, reflexes, and color. A doctor, Virginia Apgar, created the scores to tell quickly at birth which babies needed immediate treatment.

Aphasia Speaking or speech loss due to a **nervous system** problem. There are many degrees and forms of aphasia.

Apoenzyme An **enzyme** without its **cofactor**.

Apoprotein A **protein** that links up with specific receptor sites on **lipoproteins** and activates certain lipoprotein functions. See also **lipoprotein**.

Appendix A fingerlike projection attached to the **cecum** that contains lymphatic tissue. If the appendix ruptures, it is surgically removed.

Appetite The psychological desire to eat.

Applied Research Research to give practical applications or solutions to problems.

Appraisal See **performance evaluation.**

Arbitration A means of deciding a dispute in which negotiating parties submit the dispute to a third party (an arbitrator) to make a decision.

Areola The pigmented area around the nipple of the human breast.

Ariboflavinosis Clinical symptoms of **riboflavin** deficiency.

Arrhythmia Abnormal **heart** rhythms such as **bradycardia** (less than 60 beats per minute) or **tachycardia** (faster than 100 beats per minute).

Arterial Blood Pressure The pressure of **blood** within **arteries** as it's pumped through the body by the **heart.**

Arteriole A small **artery.** Arterioles are thinner than arteries and carry **blood** to the **capillaries.**

Arteriosclerosis A disorder of the **arteries** in which the walls become hardened through deposits and lose their elasticity. See **atherosclerosis.**

Artery Large **blood** vessels that take blood with **oxygen** away from the **heart** to the rest of the body. The arterial wall is made of three layers or tunics: the **tunica intima** (this lines the artery), **tunica media** (this is the muscular middle layer), and **tunica externa.** The arterial wall is elastic so it can withstand the high pressure of the pumping heart. Arteries have thicker, more muscular walls than **veins.**

Ascites The abnormal accumulation of fluid in the **abdomen.** Ascites is common in **cirrhosis** (end-stage liver disease).

Ascorbic Acid The chemical name for **vitamin C.**

Aspartame A low-calorie sweetener. Aspartame is marketed in the United States under the brand name NutraSweet [R] and as Equal tabletop sweetener. It is 200 times sweeter than **sucrose** and has an acceptable flavor with no bitter aftertaste to most people.

Aspartame is made by joining two **protein** components, **aspartic acid** and **phenylalanine,** and a small amount of methanol. Aspartic acid and phenylalanine are building blocks of protein. Methanol is found naturally in the body and in many foods such as fruit and vegetable juices. In the intestinal tract, aspartame is broken down into its three components which are metabolized in the same way as if they had come from food. Aspartame contains four **calories**/gram but so little of it is needed to get sweetness that the calorie content is negligible.

Aspartame is used as a tabletop sweetener, to sweeten many prepared foods, and in simple recipes that do not require lengthy heating or baking. Aspartame's components separate when heated over time, resulting in a loss of sweetness. Aspartame is best used at the end of the cooking cycle. Aspartame can be found in diet soft drinks, powdered drink mixes, cocoa mixes, pudding and gelatin mixes, frozen desserts, and fruit spreads and toppings. If you drink canned diet soft drinks, chances are it is sweetened with aspartame. Fountain-made diet soft drinks are more commonly sweetened with a blend of aspartame and **saccharin** because saccharin helps maintain the right amount of sweetness.

The only group of individuals for whom aspartame is a known health hazard is those people who have the disease **phenylketonuria (PKU)** because they are unable to metabolize phenylalanine. For this reason, any product containing aspartame carries a warning label. Some other people also may be sensitive to aspartame and need to limit their intake.

Aspartic Acid Transaminase (AST) See SGOT (**serum glutamic oxalacetic transaminase**).

Aspiration 1) Fluid is withdrawn from a cavity or sac with a suction device, such as a needle. 2) When food, vomit, or other foreign substances accidentally enter the lungs.

Asterixis Flapping of the hands as seen in hepatic coma.

Ataxia Uncoordinated gait when walking. Ataxia may be due to damage to the spinal cord or brain, or could be the result of head injury, tumor, or other causes.

Atheroma In **atherosclerosis**, the fatty **plaque** seen in the inner arterial walls.

Atherosclerosis A type of "hardening of the arteries" in which **cholesterol, fat**, and other substances in the **blood** build up in the walls of the **arteries**. As the process continues, the arteries to the **heart** or brain may narrow, cutting down the flow of oxygen-rich blood and nutrients. If the closed artery is a **coronary artery**, a **heart attack** can result. If the closed artery takes blood to the brain, a **stroke** can occur. Atherosclerosis is a major form of **arteriosclerosis**. See also **myocardial infarction** (heart attack) and **stroke**.

Atony Lack of normal **muscle** strength or tone.

Atria (Singular: atrium) The upper chambers of the **heart**. See also **heart**.

Atrioventricular Node (A-V NODE) A region of the heart at the base of the wall between the two **atria**. The A-V node receives electrical impulses from the **sinoatrial node**, then sends electrical impulses to specialized muscles fibers, called the **bundle of His**. The bundle of His then carries the impulses to the ventricles, causing them to contract. See also **sinoatrial node**.

Atrophy A decrease in the size of **muscle** because of not being used.

Authority The rights and powers to make the necessary decisions and take the necessary actions to get the job done. Formal authority is the authority given to you by virtue of your position within the organization. Real authority is the actual authority given to you by those above and below you in the organization to make the necessary decisions and carry them out.

Autonomic Nervous System (ANS) Nerves that control involuntary body functions such as smooth (visceral) muscle, cardiac muscle, and glands. For the ANS to work, impulses are first conducted from the central nervous system to autonomic neurons (or nerve cells). The ANS is composed of the sympathetic and parasympathetic divisions. The effects of **parasympathetic nerves** are quite often opposite to the effects of sympathetic nerves. See also nervous system, sympathetic nerves, and parasympathetic nerves.

Axillary Nodes **Lymph** nodes under the arm.

Axon The part of a **nerve** cell or **neuron** that carries the nervous impulse along the nerve cell and away from the cell body. See also **neuron**.

Azotemia A toxic state in which excessive amounts of urea and other nitrogenous waste products occur in the blood. Azotemia, also called uremia, occurs in renal failure.

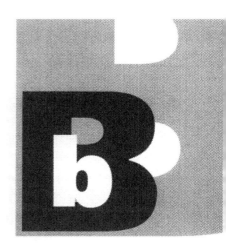

Baby Bottle Tooth Decay Serious tooth decay in babies caused by letting a baby go to bed with a bottle of juice, formula, cow's milk, or breast milk.

Balanced Diet A diet that does not overemphasize certain foods at the expense of other foods. For example, if you drink a lot of soft drinks, you may not be drinking much milk, a rich source of the mineral calcium.

Balance Sheet Statement of assets, liabilities, and owner's equity at a point in time.

Bargaining Unit All employees eligible to choose a **union** to represent and bargain collectively for them.

Barium Enema When barium sulfate is injected by enema into the **rectum**, and x-rays are taken of the rectum and **colon**. Because x-rays cannot penetrate barium sulfate, the x-ray gives a good picture of the colon and rectum.

Basal Energy Expenditure (BEE) Equivalent to **basal metabolic rate**. To calculate BEE, use the following equations.

Men: 66.47 + (13.75 x weight in kilograms) + (5.00 x height in centimeters) – (6.76 x age)

Women: 655.10 + (9.56 x weight in kilograms) + (1.85 x height in centimeters) – (4.68 x age)

Basal Metabolism The minimum amount of energy needed by the body for vital functions (heartbeat, breathing, and so on) when at rest and awake, but not eating.

Basal Metabolic Rate The rate at which the body uses energy to support basal metabolic needs.

Base A chemical substance that accepts hydrogen ions from an **acid**. Also called alkali.

Baseline Data The first set of data collected about a **client** before further data is collected and/or before beginning an **intervention**. For example, the first time a woman has a mammogram, it is considered to be baseline data against which further mammograms will be viewed.

Basophils A type of **leukocyte (white blood cell)** that releases the anticoagulant **heparin**. See also **leukocyte**.

B Cells A type of **lymphocyte (white blood cell)** involved in the **immune system**. B cells are made in the bone marrow stem cells and then travel to **lymph** tissues. When a B cell encounters a specific **antigen**, the B cell transforms into a cell, called a plasma cell, that produces large amounts of antibodies during its brief life span of five to seven days. The **antibodies** made by plasma cells are called **immunoglobulins**, such as IgG and IgE. Immunoglobulins travel in the blood to where they are needed to react with and neutralize **antigens**. The resulting antigen-antibody complexes activate a series of nine **proteins**, called complement, that help the antibody destroy antigens. See also **immune system**.

Benign Not malignant.

Behavioral Objectives A learning objective that states the outcome in terms of an observable and measurable behavior and the conditions under which the behavior should be exhibited.

Behavior Modification A counseling treatment practice that influences behaviors using methods based largely on **operant conditioning** principles. The following operant conditioning concepts help an individual move toward desirable behaviors, also called target behaviors.

- Reinforcement—When a response is followed by a reinforcing stimulus, such as praise or a physical reward, it is more likely to occur again.

- Extinction—When an unwanted behavior is reinforced, the behavior will disappear when the reinforcement stops.

- Shaping—Shaping is a process in which positive reinforcement is used as a learner's behavior approaches the desired behavior.

- Stimulus control—Environmental cues or stimuli can influence eating behaviors for better or worse. Controlling the stimuli is important for eating behaviors to be self-directed.

Behavior modification techniques have been used extensively in weight control programs. Target eating behaviors that discourage overeating, such as eating at certain times and at a specified place, are identified and reinforced. Also called behavior therapy or contingency management. See also **operant conditioning**.

Beikost Solid and semisolid baby foods that infants normally start to eat between five to seven months of age.

Benchmarking Comparing specific measures of performance against data on those measures in "best practice" organizations.

Beriberi A disease of the peripheral nerves caused by a deficiency of the **vitamin thiamin**. Symptoms include weakness, loss of feeling and pain in the extremities (hands and feet), swelling, and abnormal **heart** rhythms. Beriberi may be seen in the United States in individuals addicted to **alcohol**.

Beta-Blocker A class of drugs used to treat **hypertension**, angina, and cardiac arrhythmias. Beta-blockers block the action of **epinephrine** so the **heart** beats more slowly and cardiac output decreases. Beta-blockers also decrease plasma **renin** activity. See also **renin**.

NUTRIENT FOCUS: BETA CAROTENE

A precursor of **vitamin A** that functions as an **antioxidant** in the body. Beta carotene is the most abundant **carotenoid**. Beta carotene is found in dark green vegetables, such as spinach, and deep orange fruits and vegetables, such as apricots, carrots, and sweet potatoes. Beta carotene has an orange color seen in many vitamin A rich fruits and vegetables, but in some cases its orange color is masked by dark green chlorophyll found in vegetables such as broccoli. See also **carotenoid**.

Beta Oxidation A series of reactions in which **fatty acids** are oxidized or catabolized to yield **acetyl coA** and the reduced coenzymes, **NADH** and **FADH$_2$**. Acetyl coA then enters the **tricarboxylic cycle** and the reduced coenzymes enter the electron transport chain to yield energy (**ATP**).

Bicarbonate An alkaline (basic) compound. It is secreted by the **pancreas** to neutralize the acidic **stomach** contents when it enters the **small intestine**.

Bile A yellow-green secretion of the **liver** that is stored in the **gallbladder**. When fat enters the **small intestine**, a **hormone** (**cholecystokinin** or **CCK**) is secreted by the **duodenum**. CCK makes the gallbladder contract. Bile is important because it emulsifies fats. Bile contains **bile salts, bilirubin, cholesterol**, and other substances.

Bile salts, such as taurocholate and chenodeoxycholate, are made from cholesterol. Bile salts are important in the digestion and absorption of fats because they clump together in the duodenum to form micelles which emulsify or break up fat globules. Bilirubin is a pigment produced from the destruction of **hemoglobin** that is secreted via the bile. Bilirubin is partly responsible for the color of feces.

Bile Salts See **bile**.

Biliary Pertaining to **bile** ducts and **organs**. See also **gallbladder** and **bile**.

Bilirubin A pigment that is produced in the **spleen, liver,** and bone marrow from the destruction of the **heme** portion of **hemoglobin.** Bilirubin is excreted by the liver via **bile** and is partly responsible for the color of feces. Also called **bile pigment.** See also **bile.**

Binge Eating Disorder See **eating disorders.**

Bioavailability The amount of a nutrient that is absorbed from foods and therefore able to be used in the body.

Biopsy The removal of a piece of tissue from a living being (such as from the **liver**) for diagnostic study.

Biotechnology The use of genetic engineering to create an abundant supply of better tasting and more nutritious foods. Genetic engineering is a process that allows plant breeders to modify the genetic makeup of a plant species precisely and predictably, creating improved varieties faster and easier than can be done using more traditional plant-breeding techniques.

NUTRIENT FOCUS: BIOTIN

A **water-soluble vitamin** that is involved in the **metabolism** of **carbohydrates, fats,** and **proteins.** No **RDA** is set for biotin because the specific requirement has not been established yet; instead, an **estimated safe and adequate daily dietary intake** has been established.

Biotin is widespread in foods. Good sources of biotin include liver, egg yolk, cheese, and peanuts. Intestinal bacteria make considerable amounts of biotin. Deficiency and toxicity concerns are not known.

Bladder See **urinary bladder.**

Bleeding Time The amount of time it takes for a small puncture wound to stop bleeding (usually, eight minutes or less).

Blood The transport system of the body for foods, gases, wastes, and **hormones** or chemical messengers. Blood is made of **plasma,** a clear liquid, and cells or formed elements. Plasma is made of water, **proteins, sugar, salts,** hormones, and **vitamins.** Blood cells include **erythrocytes (red blood cells), leukocytes (white blood cells),** and platelets or **thrombocytes (clotting** cells). Blood is about 55 percent plasma and 45 percent cells (see Figure B.1).

Blood-Brain Barrier Capillaries in the brain that let certain substances in and keep certain harmful substances out.

Blood Cells The formed elements found in the blood: **erythrocytes, leukocytes,** and **thrombocytes.** See also **erythrocytes, leukocytes,** and **thrombocytes.**

Blood Cholesterol **Cholesterol** circulating in the bloodstream. The **blood** carries it for use by all parts of the body. A high level of blood cholesterol leads

Figure B.1 Composition of Blood

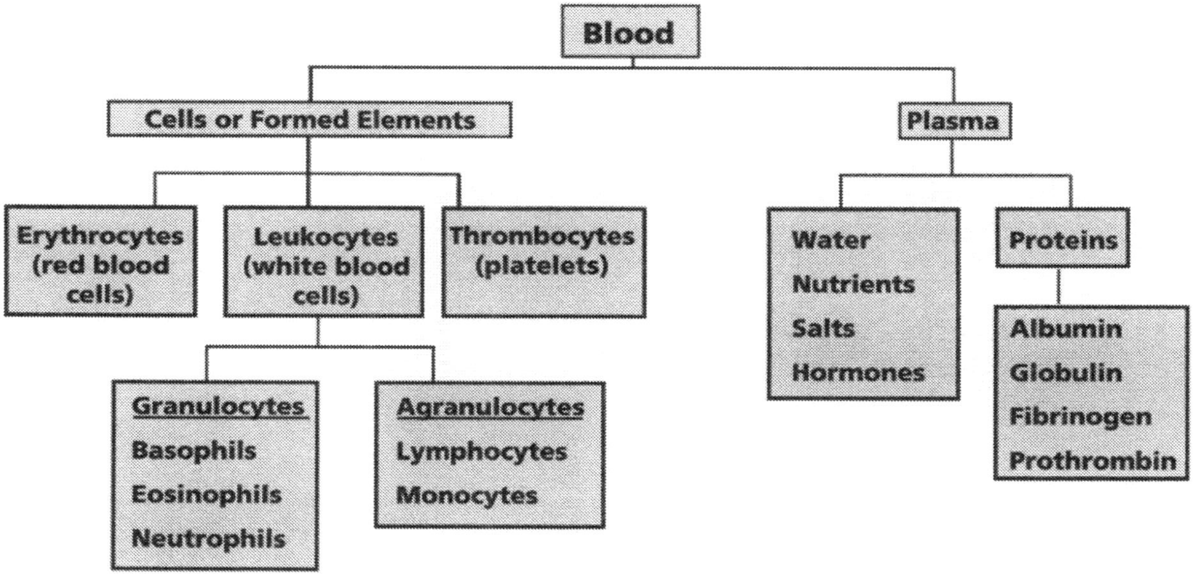

Blood

Plasma

Proteins

Albumin
Globulin
Fibrinogen
Prothrombin

Water
Nutrients
Salts
Hormones

Cells or Formed Elements

Thrombocytes
(platelets)

Leukocytes
(white blood
cells)

Erythrocytes
(red blood
cells)

Agranulocytes
Lymphocytes
Monocytes

Granulocytes
Basophils
Eosinophils
Neutrophils

to **atherosclerosis** and an increased risk of heart disease. See also **cholesterol** and **lipoproteins**.

Blood Clotting A process resulting in the formation of a fibrin clot in damaged **blood** vessels or tissue. Platelets start the process of blood clotting by clumping at the site of injury and releasing **thromboplastin**. In combination with calcium and clotting factors, thromboplastin stimulates the conversion of **prothrombin** to **thrombin**, an **enzyme**. Thrombin converts **fibrinogen** (a **blood plasma protein**) to fibrin, the protein threads that actually form the clot. Fibrin acts like mesh to trap all of the **blood cells**. Clotting can occur in abnormal situations such as an **embolus**. See also **emboli**.

Blood Glucose Level The concentration of **glucose** in the **blood**. Blood glucose level is stated in milligrams of glucose per 100 milliliters (ml) of blood. The normal range varies but is usually about 70 to 120 mg/100ml. **Insulin** and **glucagon** are two major **hormones** that control blood glucose, also called **blood sugar**, levels.

Blood Groups See **blood types**.

Blood Plasma The liquid part of the **blood** that consists of water, nutrients, **salt**, **proteins**, **hormones**, and other substances.

Blood Pressure The force that the **blood** exerts on the arterial walls. Blood pressure is measured using the familiar inflatable cuff, called a sphygmomanometer, and the stethoscope. The blood pressure reading is reported in two numbers such as 120/80. The top number is the systolic blood pressure, which is the pressure exerted against the artery walls when the heart contracts. The bottom number is the diastolic blood pressure, which is the lowest pressure remaining in the **arteries** between heartbeats when the heart is at rest. For adults, normal systolic blood pressure is less than 130 mm Hg, and normal diastolic blood pressure is less than 85 mm Hg. Optimal blood pressure for adults is less than 120/80. See also **hypertension**.

Blood Types Four main groups of human blood based on a specific combination of **antigens** on the surface of the **red blood cell** and **antibody** factors in the **plasma**.

Type A—Type A antigens and anti-B antibody

Type B—Type B antigens and anti-A antibody

Type AB—both Type A and Type B antigens and no anti-A or anti-B antibodies

Type O—neither Type A or Type B antigens and both anti-A and anti-B antibodies

During a blood transfusion, if the antigens of the donor's blood are incompatible with recipient's antibodies, the recipient's blood will clump, which is fatal. The clumping reaction is called **agglutination**.

Blood type is inherited.

Blood Urea Nitrogen (BUN) A laboratory test that measures the amount of **urea** in the **blood**. The normal level for urea is low because it is dangerous at high levels, which can occur in **renal failure** (see **uremia**) and also situations in which excessive amounts of body **protein** are catabolized, such as burns, cancer, or sepsis. Urea results from the breakdown of protein in the body, so it contains nitrogen. After being formed in the **liver**, urea travels through the blood to be excreted in the urine.

Body Composition The relative sizes of the body's four compartments: **fat**, lean body mass (**muscle**), water, and **bone**.

Body Mass Index (BMI) A method used to estimate ideal body weight.

The BMI is calculated as follows (see Figure B.2).

$$\text{BMI} = \frac{\text{body weight (in kilograms)}}{\text{height (in meters)}^2}$$

The BMI has a direct and continuous relationship to **morbidity** (incidence of disease) and **mortality** in studies of large populations; however, it is harder to understand. The BMI is a more sensitive indicator than height/weight tables and can be calculated easily using a nomogram. Each nomogram provides desirable weight and the 20 percent and 40 percent overweight level of men and women of varying heights and weights. These values are read off the central scale after a ruler is placed across the nomogram between the height and weight values. When the BMI exceeds 30, there are increased obesity-related health risks.

Bones **Organs** made of connective tissue and a large supply of **blood vessels** and **nerves**. See also **cortical bone**, **trabecular bone**, **long bones**, and **short bones**.

Bone Deposition The formation of **bone** by **osteoblasts** or bone-forming cells.

Bone Remodeling A continual process during life in which bone is rebuilt. Bone is very dynamic and is being remodeled constantly.

Bone Resorption Dissolution of **bone** produced by the action of **osteoclasts**. Calcium and phosphate from the bone are returned to the blood.

Botulism See **foodborne illness**.

Bowel Intestine. See also **large intestine** and **small intestine**.

Bowman's Capsule A capsule surrounding the **glomerulus** of the **nephron** in the **kidney**. Also called **glomerular capsule**. See also **nephron**.

Figure B.2 Nomograms

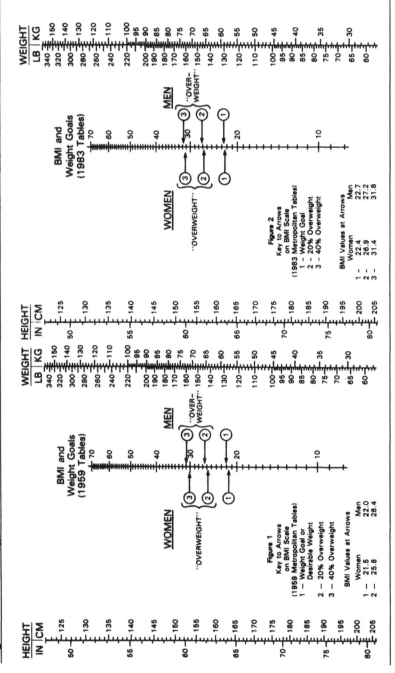

Nomograms for Body Mass Index based on 1959 and 1983 Metropolitan Life
Insurance Company Tables. Weight and heights are without clothes.

Bradycardia An abnormal condition in which the **heart** beats at a rate slower than normal (60 beats per minute). Bradycardia may be due to a brain tumor, malfunctioning of the vagus nerve, or other causes. Bradycardia can occur normally in endurance-trained athletes.

Branched Chain Amino Acids The **amino acids** valine, leucine, and isoleucine. These amino acids are prevalent in skeletal **muscles** and can directly provide energy for muscles.

Bronchi (Singular: bronchus) Large air passages in the lungs in which inhaled air and exhaled air pass. Also called **bronchial tubes**.

Bronchioles Smallest branches of the **bronchi** that end in the **alveoli**. See also **alveoli**.

Brown Fat A specialized form of **adipose tissue** found in infants and adults (to a lesser extent) that has an extensive **blood** supply and is specially equipped to burn energy and create heat. Much of a baby's brown fat disappears as it grows but adults still have some brown fat.

Brush Border The bristle-like covering of microvilli on the villi (fingerlike projections) of the **small intestine's** wall. Each villus in the intestine is in turn covered with smaller projections called microvilli. In the area of the brush border, nutrients are made ready for **absorption**. The terms brush border and microvilli are often used interchangeably.

Budget An operational plan for the income and expenditure of money for a given period.

Buffers Compounds that help maintain the optimum pH of cells and fluids. Examples of buffers include **proteins** and **hemoglobin**.

Bulimia Nervosa See **eating disorders**.

Bundle of His A band of **muscle** fibers in the **heart** that receives electrical impulses from the **atrioventricular node** and then carries the impulses to the ventricles, causing them to contract. See also **atrioventricular node**.

Burns Injury to tissues due to fire, steam, hot liquids, chemicals, lightning, electricity, or radiation. Burns are classified as follows.

First-degree burn—A superficial lesion in the **epidermis**.

Second-degree burn—A lesion cutting through the epidermis and dermis.

Third-degree burn—A lesion that destroys the epidermis and dermis and damages the subcutaneous layer.

Bursae (Singular: bursa) A sac-like structure filled with **synovial fluid** located around **joints**. Bursae lubricate movement in joints, such as the elbow or knee, where friction would normally develop.

Business and Industry Foodservice Foodservice operations feeding people who are working. Business and industry (commonly referred to as *B & I*) foodservices provide meals, for example, in light manufacturing plants, financial and insurance companies, service companies, and high-tech businesses. Foodservices usually are provided using a cafeteria and sometimes also executive dining rooms. Vending and catering are common.

Business Ownership Structures The various ways that a business can be owned and operated (see Table B.1).

Table B.1 Legal and Financial Consequences of Alternative Business Structures

Who owns and operates the business	Legal requirements to establish business	Legal and financial liability	Dissolving the business	Advantages	Disadvantages
Sole proprietorship					
One person owns entirety and makes all decisions.	Minimum. Should register business name; get any licenses required.	Unlimited. No legal distinction between the owner and the business; courts may take personal assets to cover debts.	Simply lock the front door and cleanout the cash box!	Easy to form and dissolve; owner retains all profits; you are your own boss; flexible.	No continuity if owner dies or quits; unlimited legal and financial liability; management and other resources limited to those of owner.
General partnership					
Two or more people, each of whom owns and is responsible for 100% of the business.	Register name. Get licenses. Need formal written agreement. If none, Uniform Partnership Act applies.	Unlimited. Each partner is responsible for 100% of company debts. Court may take personal assets to cover debts. If only one partner has assets, these will be attached to cover joint debt. Court does not divide debts equally.	Complex to dissolve; not unlike a divorce. Assets must be divided, as must debts. If the business is to continue, certain legal requirements to the departing partner must be met.	Easy to form; expands borrowing ability, financial assets and management skills available to the business.	Complex to dissolve; unlimited liability of all partners; potential for management conflicts.

Table B.1 Legal and Financial Consequences of Alternative Business Structures (continued)

Who owns and operates the business	Legal requirements to establish business	Legal and financial liability	Dissolving the business	Advantages	Disadvantages
Limited partnership					
Two or more general and two or more limited partners whose ownership is limited to the amount of their financial investment.	Same as for general partnership, plus written agreement regarding limitations of investments.	Same as general partnership. Liability of limited partners is limited to amount of their investment in the company. Beyond that amount, their personal assets are shielded.	Same as general partnerships.	Same as general partnerships; often the "silent" partners provide needed capital but do not participate in management.	Limited partners have "limited" commitment to the business and may decide to withdraw assets at critical point in business progress.
Joint venture					
Two or more persons joined for a limited time period to perform only a specific business activity.	Same as limited partnerships.	Same as limited partnerships.	Automatically terminates on either expiration of limited period or when activity that was the venture's purpose is completed.	Has limited purpose and existence in time with limited commitment by owners.	Can pursue only those purposes for which venture was formed; to perpetuate self, must change to other business structure.

Table B.1 Legal and Financial Consequences of Alternative Business Structures (continued)

Who owns and operates the business	Legal requirements to establish business	Legal and financial liability	Dissolving the business	Advantages	Disadvantages
Corporation					
Stockholders own a portion of shares of the business according to how much money they have invested in the business. Management is hired by the Board of Directors to oversee business operations.	Created by filing a legal request with the secretary of state. Should be filed by an attorney. State imposes various restrictions on activities and requires various reports to be filed annually. Corporation has separate legal identity from its owners or shareholders.	Corporation is legally and financially liable, its owners or shareholders are not. Courts cannot reach the assets of owners; they are shielded by the corporation.	Difficult to dissolve. Assets of the corporation are apportioned among holders on the basis of number of shares held.	Limited financial liability of owners; expansive borrowing power; expanded management skills available.	Costly to form and dissolve; "double" taxation on profits; various legal restrictions on activities.

Table B.1 Legal and Financial Consequences of Alternative Business Structures (continued)

Who owns and operates the business	Legal requirements to establish business	Legal and financial liability	Dissolving the business	Advantages	Disadvantages
Personal corporation					
Owners must all be dissolve; members of the same profession. Like a corporation can hire a manager or designate one or more owners as managing member.	Same as a corporation. To declare Section 1244 stock, requires separate legal filing with state and Internal Revenue Service.	Same as corporation plus malpractice suits are individual to a member and cannot be assessed against the corporation.	Same as corporation.	Same tax advantages as sole proprietor; share in corporate profits by pre-agreed amounts	Complex to same liability as partnerships.
Subchapter S corporation					
A special category of corporation created for a corporation owned by only one person.	Owner must become a corporation under state law as specified above under corporations.	As with a corporation, the individual owners' assets are shielded; tax filing require-ments arespecific— must fileunder Section S of Internal Revenue Service laws using form.	Same as corporation.	Same tax advantages as sole proprietor— avoids double taxation.	Same as sole proprietor.

Source: Cross, Audrey T: Practical and legal considerations of private nutrition practice. Copyright the American Dietetic Association. Reprinted by permission from JOURNAL OF THE AMERICAN DIETETIC ASSOCIATION, Vol. 95: 23-24.

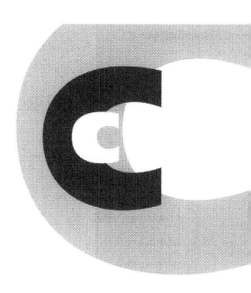

Cachexia A serious state of body wasting and deterioration as seen in starvation and **cancers** marked by **malnutrition** and tremendous weight loss.

Caffeine A stimulant in certain foods and beverages that is the most widely used drug in Western society. Eighty percent of Americans drink at least one caffeine-containing beverage each day, and average caffeine consumption is about 280 milligrams. Caffeine is present in over 60 plant species in various parts of the world, such as the coffee bean in Arabia, the tea leaf in China, the kola nut in West Africa, and the cocoa bean in Mexico. Coffee, tea, cola, and cocoa are the most common sources of caffeine in the American diet, with coffee being the chief source. The caffeine content of coffee or tea depends on the variety of coffee bean or tea leaf, the particle size, the method of brewing, and the amount of time to brew or steep. Brewed coffee always has more caffeine than instant coffee and espresso coffee always has more caffeine than regularly brewed coffee. Espresso is made by forcing hot water under pressure through finely ground, dark-roast beans. Because it is brewed with less water, it contains more caffeine than regular coffee.

In soft drinks caffeine is both a natural and an added ingredient. The **Food and Drug Administration** requires caffeine as an ingredient in colas and pepper-flavored beverages and allows it to be added to other soft drinks as well. About five percent of the caffeine in colas and pepper-flavored soft drinks is obtained naturally from cola nuts; the remaining 95 percent is added caffeine. Caffeine-free soft drinks contain virtually no caffeine and comprise a small part of the soft drink market.

Numerous prescription and nonprescription drugs also contain caffeine. It is often used in alertness or stay-awake tablets, headache and pain relief remedies, cold products, and **diuretics**. When caffeine is an ingredient, it must be listed on the product label (see Table C.1).

Table C.1 Caffeine Content of Beverages, Foods, and Drugs

Item	Milligrams Caffeine	
	Average	Range
Coffee (5-ounce cup)		
Brewed, drip method	115	60–180
Brewed, percolator	80	40–170
Instant	65	30–120
Decaffeinated, brewed	3	2–5
Decaffeinated, instant	2	1–5
Tea (5-ounce cup)		
Brewed, major U.S. brands	40	20–90
Brewed, imported brands	60	25–110
Instant	30	25–50
Iced (12-ounce glass)	70	67–76
Soft drinks (12-ounce can)		
Cola, pepper		30–46
Decaffeinated cola, pepper		0–2
Cherry cola		36–46
Lemon-lime		0
Other citrus		0–64
Root beer		0
Ginger ale		0
Tonic water		0
Other regular soda		0–44
Juice added		0
Diet cola, pepper		0.6
Decaffeinated diet cola, pepper		0–0.2
Diet cherry cola		0–46
Diet lemon-lime, diet root beer		0
Other diets		0–70
Club soda, seltzer, sparkling water		0

Table C.1   Caffeine Content of Beverages, Foods, and Drugs (continued)

Item	Milligrams Caffeine Average	Range
Cocoa		
Cocoa beverage (5-ounce cup)	4	2–20
Chocolate milk beverage (8 ounces)	5	2–7
Milk chocolate (1 ounce)	6	1–15
Dark chocolate, semisweet (1 ounce)	20	5–35
Baker's chocolate (1 ounce)	26	26
Chocolate-flavored syrup (1 ounce)	4	4
Prescription drugs: caffeine per tablet or capsule		
Cafergot (migraine headaches)	100	
Norgesic Forte (muscle relaxant)	60	
Fiorinal (tension headache)	40	
Darvon (pain relief)	32	
Synalogos-DC (pain relief)	30	
Nonprescription drugs: caffeine per tablet or capsule		
Alertness Tablets		
No Doz	100	
Pain relief		
Anacin, Maximum Strength Anacin	32	
Vanquish	33	
Excedrin	65	
Midol	32	
Diuretics		
Aqua-Ban	100	
Cold/Allergy Remedies		
Coryban-D capsules	30	

Source: Lecos, Chris W. 1987–1988. Caffeine jitters: some safety questions remain. *FDA Consumer* 21(10):22-27.

Caffeine is absorbed very well into the body and is rapidly absorbed into the bloodstream. For most people, caffeine increases **blood pressure** and heart rate, increases attentiveness and performance, and gives relief from fatigue. In high doses it can produce insomnia, nervousness, a racing heart, and other troublesome symptoms. Many people build a tolerance to caffeine's effects that may then lead to increased usage.

It is easy to become physically addicted to caffeine. When caffeine is withdrawn, symptoms include headache, fatigue, irritability, depression, and poor concentration. The symptoms peak on day one or two and progressively decrease over the course of a week. It has been shown that moderate consumption—about one or two 10-ounce cups of coffee daily (or the equivalent of caffeine from other sources)—often causes these debilitating symptoms of caffeine withdrawal. To minimize withdrawal symptoms, experts recommend reducing your caffeine intake by about 20 percent a week over four to five weeks.

Calcium Channel Blockers A class of drugs used to treat **hypertension** and angina. Calcium channel blockers dilate **blood** vessels by blocking **calcium** from getting into the **muscles** that line the blood vessels. The muscles relax, causing dilation.

Calcitonin A **hormone** secreted by the **thyroid gland** when **blood** levels of **calcium** are high. Calcitonin lowers blood levels of calcium and phosphate.

Calcitriol The active **hormone** form of **vitamin D** that is also called *1,25-dihydroxy vitamin D*. Calcitriol is produced in the **kidney** in response to an increase in **parathyroid hormone** caused by low **blood calcium** levels. Calcitriol acts like a **steroid** hormone and elevates **plasma** calcium and **phosphorus** by increasing absorption in the intestine, increasing **reabsorption** in the renal tubules, and stimulating the mobilizing of calcium from the **bone** fluid compartment.

NUTRIENT FOCUS: CALCIUM

A major mineral used for building **bones** and teeth. Calcium also circulates in the **blood**, where a constant level is maintained so it is always available for use. Calcium helps blood to clot, muscles to contract (including the **heart** muscle), **nerves** to transmit impulses, and also helps maintain normal blood pressure.

The major sources of calcium are milk and milk products. Not all milk products are as rich in calcium as milk. As a matter of fact, butter, cream, cottage cheese, and cream cheese contain very little calcium. One glass of milk or yogurt or one ounce of cheese each have a little less than half of the **RDA** for most adults (see Table C.2).

About 30 percent of the calcium you eat is absorbed. The body absorbs more calcium (up to 60 percent) during growth and pregnancy when additional calcium is needed. Absorption is higher for younger people than for older people.

Postmenopausal women, who are at high risk of developing **osteoporosis**, often absorb the least calcium. **Vitamin D** helps calcium get absorbed and is added to milk. Certain substances interfere with calcium absorption, such as the tannins in tea and large amounts of phytic acid, a binder found in wheat bran and whole grains. See also **osteoporosis**.

Table C.2 Calcium in Selected Foods

Food	Calcium Content
Milk, skim, 8 ounces	302
Milk, 2%, 8 ounces	297
Milk, whole, 8 ounces	291
Yogurt, low-fat, 1 cup	415
Yogurt, low-fat with fruit, 1 cup	345
Yogurt, frozen, 1 cup	200
Ice cream, 1 cup	176
Cottage cheese, creamed, 1 cup	147
Swiss cheese, 1 ounce	272
Parmesan, 1 ounce	390
Cheddar, 1 ounce	204
Mozzarella, 1 ounce	183
American cheese, 1 ounce	174
Cheese pizza, 1/4 of 14-inch pie	332
Macaroni and cheese, 1/2 cup	181
Orange juice, calcium fortified, 8 ounces	300
Sardines with bones, 3 ounces	372
Oysters, 1 cup	226
Shrimp, 3 ounces	98
Tofu, 3-1/2 ounces	128

Table C.2 Calcium in Selected Foods (continued)

Food	Calcium Content
Dried navy beans, cooked, 1 cup	95
Turnip greens, frozen and cooked, 1 cup	249
Kale, frozen and cooked, 1 cup	179
Mustard greens, 1 cup	104
Broccoli, frozen and cooked, 1 cup	94
Oatmeal, instant, fortified, 1 packet	160
Pancakes, from mix, 1–4 inch pancake	30
Wheat bread, 1 slice	30

Source: *Nutritive Value of Foods*, U.S. Department of Agriculture Home and Garden Bulletin Number 72.

Calculus An abnormal stone that forms in the body. Calculi most often occur in the **kidneys, gallbladder,** and **joints.**

Calorie A unit of energy. One calorie represents the amount of heat needed to raise 1 gram of water 1 degree Celsius. The energy in food is measured in kilocalories. One kilocalorie represents the amount of heat needed to raise 1000 g of water 1 degree Celsius. In nutrition, it is common to shorten the word kilocalorie to calorie.

Calyx The cup-like collecting region of the renal pelvis. Also see **kidney.**

Cancellous Bone See **trabecular bone.**

NUTRITION AND DISEASE FOCUS: CANCER

A group of diseases characterized by unrestrained cell division and growth that can disrupt the normal functioning of an **organ** and also spread beyond the tissue in which it started. Cancer is basically a two-step process. First, a carcinogen, such as an x-ray, starts or initiates the sequence by altering the genetic material of a cell, the **deoxyribonucleic acid (DNA),** causing a mutation. Often these cells are repaired or replaced. When repair or replacement does not occur, however, promoters such as **alcohol** can advance development of the mutated cell into a tumor. Promoters do not initiate cancer but enhance its development once initiation has occurred. The tumor may disrupt normal body functions and leave the tissue for other sites, a process called **metastasis.** (See Figure C.1.)

Figure C.1 Process of Cancer

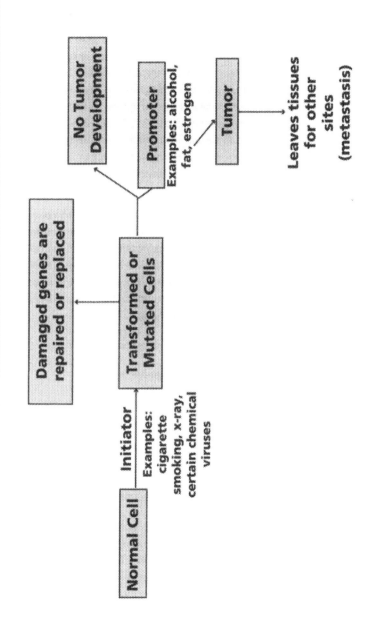

Cancer develops as a result of interactions between environmental factors (such as diet, smoking, alcohol, and radiation) and genetic factors. Research suggests that diet plays a role in the cause of certain cancers. In 1989, the National Academy of Sciences report, *Diet and Health: Implications for Reducing Chronic Disease Risk*, stated that in countries with better diets, cancer rates are about half that of the United States. For example, breast cancer rates are four to seven times higher in the U.S. than in Asia. This difference is not explained by genetics because when Asian women move to the U.S., their risk doubles after 10 years. Estimates of how much cancer is caused by diet varies. In 1986 a National Cancer Institute report estimated that about 35 percent of all cancer deaths are associated with the typical American diet which is high in fat and calories, and low in **fiber**, fruits, and vegetables. The most common cancers are cancer of the lungs, breast, **colon** and **rectum**, prostate, **bladder**, and skin. Of these cancers, all but one (skin cancer) are associated with diet.

So what is wrong with the American diet that seems to enhance certain types of cancer? Basically our diet has: too much fat, too much **saturated fat**, too little fiber, and too few fruits and vegetables. The National Cancer Institute estimates that significant reductions in cancer incidence could be achieved by the year 2000 if all Americans adopted and maintained a low fat, high fiber, and high fruit and vegetable diet. The National Cancer Institute estimates the following reductions in incidence could be achieved by dietary changes.

- 50 percent reduction in colon and rectum cancer cases

- 25 percent reduction in breast cancer cases

- 15 percent reduction in cancers of the prostate, endometrium, and **gallbladder**

- Possibly also reductions in cancers of the **stomach**, esophagus, **pancreas**, ovaries, **liver**, lung, and bladder

Some of the reasons for dietary changes are as follows.

- Dietary fat does not initiate cancer, but promotes its development once started. It may be that certain forms of fat promote cancer more than others. **Monounsaturated fatty acids** (found in olive oil) and **omega-3 fatty acids** (found in fatty fish) may be protective whereas **linoleic acid**, an **omega-6 fatty acid** found in many vegetable oils, may be a promoter.

- Fiber may help prevent certain cancers by:

  - Reducing the amount of time for feces to be formed in the colon and eliminated from the rectum and therefore decreasing the time the bowel is exposed to potential carcinogens

- Holding onto water in the intestinal tract, increasing stool bulk, which may dilute carcinogen concentrations in the colon

- Binding with **bile acids** in the intestinal tract, some of which can be converted by organisms in the colon into cancer-causing compounds

- Fruits and vegetables help reduce the risk of cancer because they are rich sources of **carotenoids, vitamin C**, and fiber. **Beta carotene**, the most abundant carotenoid, may inhibit the initiation and promotion of cancers in the body because it is a powerful antioxidant. **Antioxidants** combine with **oxygen** so oxygen is not available to oxidize, or destroy, important substances. Antioxidants prevent the oxidation of **unsaturated fatty acids** in the cell membrane, **DNA** (the genetic code), and other cell parts that substances called free radicals try to destroy. In the absence of antioxidants, free radicals may destroy cells (possibly accelerating the aging process) and alter DNA (possibly increasing the risk for cancerous cells to develop). Free radicals are produced in the body through normal metabolism or as a result of exposure to cigarette smoke, radiation, ultraviolet light, air pollutants, some pesticides, or alcohol. Vitamin C also acts as an antioxidant by preventing the oxidation of certain chemicals, such as nitrosamines, to active carcinogens. Nitrates and nitrites are used in the curing of cold cuts, frankfurters, bacon, and other cured meats. Nitrates can be converted to nitrites by bacteria in the mouth or **gastrointestinal tract.** Nitrites can then be converted into nitrosamines in the mouth, stomach, and colon. Vitamin C inhibits nitrosamine formation in the gastrointestinal tract.

- Some vegetables, as well as other plant foods (such as fruits, grains, herbs, and spices), contain **phytochemicals**, minute compounds found in plants that fight the formation of cancer. For instance, broccoli contains a chemical called sulforaphane that seems to initiate increased production of cancer-fighting enzymes in the body's cells. Isoflavonoids, found mostly in soy foods, are known as plant **estrogens** or phytoestrogens because they are similar to estrogen and interfere with its actions (estrogen seems to promote breast tumors). Members of the cabbage family (cabbage, broccoli, cauliflower, mustard greens, kale) also called cruciferous vegetables, contain phytochemicals such as indoles and dithiolthiones. They activate enzymes that destroy carcinogens.

- Fruits and vegetables are also low in fat (with the exception of coconuts, avocados, and olives).

Some consumers are concerned about eating more fruits and vegetables that may contain carcinogenic pesticides. The National Academy of Sciences, along with other organizations, feel that the health benefits of eating fresh fruits and vegetables far outweigh any risk associated with pesticide residues. The federal government strictly regulates the kinds and amounts of pesticides used on field crops. The tiny amounts of pesticide residues found on produce are set hundreds of times lower than the amounts that would actually pose any health threat.

Menu Planning to Lower Cancer Risk

1. Offer lower-fat menu items. Also offer more plant-based menu items.

2. Avoid salt-cured, smoked, and nitrite-cured foods. These foods, which are also high in fat, include anchovies, bacon, corned beef, dried chipped beef, herring, pastrami, processed lunch meats such as bologna and hot dogs, sausage such as salami and pepperoni, and smoked meats and cheeses. Conventionally smoked meats and fish contain tars that are thought to be carcinogenic due to the smoking process. Nitrites are known carcinogens.

3. Offer high-fiber foods. For example:

   - Use beans and peas as the basis for entrees, and add them to soups, stews, casseroles, and salads. Nuts and seeds are high in fiber but also contain a significant amount of fat and calories, so use them sparingly.

   - Serve whole-grain breads, rolls, crackers, cereals, and muffins. Bran or wheat germ can be added to some baked goods to increase the fiber content. High-fiber grains such as brown rice and bulgur (cracked wheat) can be used as side dishes instead of white rice.

   - Leave skins on potatoes, fruits, and vegetables as much as possible.

   - Offer salads using lots of fresh fruits and vegetables. Omit shredded cheese, chopped eggs, and bacon bits, which all contribute fat.

4. Include lots of vegetables, especially cruciferous vegetables. Cruciferous vegetables contain substances that are natural anticarcinogens. These vegetables include broccoli, brussels sprouts, cabbage, cauliflower, bok choy, kale, collards, kohlrabi, mustard, rutabagas, spinach, and watercress.

5. Offer foods that are good sources of beta carotene and vitamins C and E. Excellent sources of beta carotene include dark green, yellow, and orange vegetables and fruits such as broccoli, cantaloupe, carrots, spinach, squash, and sweet potatoes. Good sources include apricots, beet greens, brussels sprouts, cabbage, nectarines, peaches, tomatoes, and watermelon. Excellent sources of vitamin C include citrus fruits and juices, any other juices with vitamin C added, strawberries, tomatoes, and broccoli. Good vitamin C sources include berries, brussels sprouts, cabbage, melons, cauliflower, and potatoes. Vitamin E is found in vegetable oils and margarines, whole-grain cereals, wheat germ, soybeans, leafy greens, and spinach.

6. Offer alternatives to alcoholic drinks. Heavy drinkers are more likely to develop cancer in the gastrointestinal tract, such as cancer of the esophagus and stomach.

Capillary Blood vessels composed of only a single layer of endothelium that allows water and other molecules to move across the capillary walls to permit exchanges between the blood and tissue fluid.

Carbonic Acid An **acid** that plays a role with sodium bicarbonate as a **buffer** system in the body.

NUTRIENT FOCUS: CARBOHYDRATE

A group of nutrients containing carbon, hydrogen, and **oxygen** that includes **sugars**, **starch**, and **fibers**. Sugars are known as **simple carbohydrates**. Starch and fibers are known as **complex carbohydrates** because they are long chains of sugar units. Chemically, carbohydrates are a class of compounds made up of polyhydroxy **aldehydes** and **ketones** and their derivatives.

Carbohydrate is the primary source of energy for your body. The **central nervous system** relies almost exclusively on **glucose** and other simple carbohydrates for energy. Carbohydrate is also important to help the body use **fat** efficiently. When fat is burned for energy without any carbohydrate present, the process is incomplete and could result in **ketosis**. Carbohydrates are part of various materials found in the body. See also **sugar**, **starch**, and **fiber**.

Carbohydrate or Glycogen Loading A regimen involving both decreased exercise and increased consumption of **carbohydrates** before an event to increase the amount of **glycogen** stores. The theory behind it is that increased glycogen stores (they normally increase between 50 to 80 percent) will enhance performance by providing more energy during lengthy competition.

Carboxyl Group The –COOH group found in organic **acids**.

Carboxypeptidase A digestive **enzyme** contained in pancreatic juice that is activated by **trypsin**. Carboxypeptidase cleaves the last **amino acid** from the carboxy end of a **polypeptide**.

Carcinoma A malignant tumor that starts with cells that cover an inner or outer body surface, such as the skin or intestinal wall.

Cardiac Output The amount of **blood** pumped by the **heart** in one minute.

Cardiac Rate The pulse rate or number of **heart** beats per minute.

Cardiomegaly An enlarged **heart** due most commonly to **high blood pressure** inside the heart. Cardiomegaly is common and normal in athletes.

Carbon Dioxide A gas produced in the body as a by-product of energy metabolism. Carbon dioxide is transported in the **blood** mostly in the form of bicarbonate (HCO3–), but it can travel as dissolved carbon dioxide or attached to an **amino acid** in **hemoglobin** (then it is called carbaminohemoglobin).

Cardiac Arrest The sudden stopping of the **heart**. In cardiac arrest, the heart stops pumping so **blood** stops flowing and carbon dioxide starts building up. It can quickly damage the heart, lungs, brain, and **kidneys**.

Cardiac Catheterization A procedure in which a catheter, or tube, is inserted into an **artery** or **vein** (usually in an arm or leg) and threaded into the **heart** to detect and measure **blood pressures** and detect patterns of blood flow.

NUTRITION AND DISEASE FOCUS: CARDIOVASCULAR DISEASE (CVD)

A general term for diseases of the **heart** and **blood** vessels as seen in the following.

• Coronary **artery** disease

• **Stroke**

• **High blood pressure**

• Rheumatic heart disease

• Congenital heart defects

About 40 percent of all deaths in 1992 were due to cardiovascular diseases.

Smoking, high blood pressure, and high blood **cholesterol** are three major risk factors for cardiovascular disease. A risk factor is a habit, trait, or condition of an individual that is associated with an increased chance of developing a disease. Preventing or controlling risk factors generally reduces the probability of illness. These three risk factors are modifiable to some extent. Other risk factors are age (CVD increases with age), a family history of premature CVD (**heart attack** in a father before age 55 or before 65 in a mother), cigarette smoking, obesity, and diabetes.

Cholesterol is carried in blood in the form of substances called **lipoproteins**. CHD risk can be assessed by measuring total blood cholesterol, as well as the proportions of the different types of lipoproteins. Total cholesterol refers to the overall level of cholesterol in the blood. **High-density lipoprotein (HDL)** is often referred to as "good" cholesterol, because high levels of HDL are associated with lowered CHD risk. High levels of **low-density lipoprotein (LDL)**—often referred to as "bad" cholesterol—and **very low density lipoprotein (VLDL)** increase CHD risk.

The National Cholesterol Education Program (NCEP) recommends that all adults 20 years of age and older have their total cholesterol and HDL measured at least once every five years. For people without CHD, a total blood cholesterol level of less than 200 mg/dL is considered desirable; from 200 to 239 is borderline-high; and 240 or more is high. An HDL level of less than 35 mg/dL is defined as low and is considered a CHD risk factor (see Table C.3).

Table C.3 If You *Do Not* Have Heart Disease

If your Total and HDL Levels are...		Then...
Total Cholesterol	*HDL Cholesterol*	
less than 200 mg/dL	35 mg/dL or greater	You are doing well and should have your total and HDL-cholesterol levels checked again in about 5 years. In the meantime, take steps to keep your total cholesterol level down: eat foods low in saturated fat and cholesterol, maintain a healthy weight,and be physically active. The last two steps, along with not smoking, will also help keep your HDL level up.
less than 200 mg/DdL or 200-239 mg/dL	less than 35 mg/dL	You will need a lipoprotein profile to find out your LDL-cholesterol level. For this test you need to fast for 9 to 12 hours before the test. Have nothing but water, or coffee or tea with no cream or sugar.
200-239 mg/dL	35 mg/dL or greater	Your doctor will see if you have other risk factors for heart disease and determine whether more tests (including a lipoprotein profile to find out your LDL-cholesterol) need to be done. No matter what your risk is, it is important to eat foods low in saturated fat and cholesterol.
240 mg/dL and above	any level	You will need a lipoprotein profile to find out your LDL-cholesterol level. Again, you need to fast for 9 to 12 hours before the test, having nothing but water, or coffee or tea with no cream or sugar.
If your LDL Level is...		**Then...**
less than 130 mg/dL		You have a desirable LDL-cholesterol level. You will need to have your total and HDL-cholesterol levels tested again need to in 5 years. You should follow an eating plan low in saturated fat and cholesterol, maintain a healthy weight, be physically active, and not smoke.

Table C.3 If You *Do Not* Have Heart Disease (continued)

If your LDL Level is...	Then...
130 mg/dL or above	Your doctor will look at your other heart disease risk factors and decide what you need to do to lower your LDL-cholesterol level. The higher your level and the more other risk factors you have, the more you need to follow a diet low in saturated fat and cholesterol. For example, if your LDL is 160 mg/dL or greater and you have fewer than two other risk factors, your LDL goal is a level below 160 mg/dL. If your LDL is 130 mg/dL or greater and you have two or more other risk factors, your goalis to reduce your LDL level to below 130 mg/dL. It is also important to lose weight if you are overweight, to be physically active, and to not smoke. Discuss your treatment plan with your doctor.

Source: National Institutes of Health: So You Have High Blood Cholesterol. NIH Publication No. 93-2922.

Table C.4 If You *Do Have* Heart Disease

If Your LDL Level is...	Then...
100 mg/dL or less	You do not need to take specific steps to lower your LDL, but you will need to have your level tested again in 1 year. In the meantime, you should closely follow a diet low in saturated fat and cholesterol, maintain a healthy weight, be physically active, and not smoke.
greater than 100 mg/dL	You need to have a complete physical examination done to see if you have a disease or a health condition that is raising your cholesterol levels. You will probably need a diet that is lower in saturated fat and cholesterol, i.e., the Step II diet (see page 49). Since this diet will be more effective, your doctor will likely encourage you to start there, as well as to be physically active, to lose weight if you are overweight, and to not smoke. If your LDL level does not come down, you may need to take medicine.

Source: National Institutes of Health: So You Have High Blood Cholesterol. NIH Publication No. 93-2922.

A lipoprotein analysis that measures LDL as well as HDL is recommended for people with CHD or for those at very high risk of developing CHD. The optimum LDL for patients with CHD is 100 mg/dL or lower. The optimum LDL for high-risk individuals is about 130 mg/dL (see Table C.4).

Dietary therapy is the mainstay of treatment of high blood cholesterol at every age. Unless a young adult (men under age 35, premenopausal women) is at very high risk of CHD with a total cholesterol of more than 300 mg/dL, the NCEP recommends that drug therapy be delayed and dietary modification and lifestyle change be attempted first.

Dietary therapy is prescribed in two steps, called the Step I and Step II Diets. These are designed to help reduce intake of **saturated fat** and cholesterol, and to help achieve a desirable weight by eliminating excess calories. The Step I Diet is usually the starting point of dietary therapy. In the Step I Diet, no more than 8 to 10 percent of calories are in the form of saturated fat; 30 percent or less of calories come from total fat; and less than 300 mg of cholesterol are allowed each day.

If the patient is already following the Step I Diet, and it is not adequate to lower cholesterol to desirable levels, then the Step II Diet should be tried, according to the NCEP report. People with high cholesterol who have CHD or other atherosclerotic disease should begin immediately on this diet, with physician guidance. The Step II Diet calls for reducing daily saturated fat intake to less than 7 percent of calories and cholesterol to less than 200 mg (see Table C.5).

Table C.5 Step I and Step II Diets

	% calories from fat	% calories from saturated fat	Cholesterol
Step I	30% or less	8–10% or less	300 mg or less
Step II	30% or less	7% or less	200 mg or less

Source: National Institutes of Health: Step by Step: Eating to Lower Your High Blood Cholesterol NIH Publication No. 94-2920.

Drug treatment is considered appropriate for adults who have a very high LDL level, especially if they also have other CHD risk factors. The goals of drug therapy are the same as those of dietary therapy: to lower LDL-cholesterol to below 160 mg/dL or to below 130 mg/dL if two other risk factors are present. See also **atherosclerosis, high blood pressure, stroke,** and **cholesterol** (see Table C.6).

Table C.6 Treatment Decisions Based on LDL-Cholesterol

Dietary Therapy	Initiation Level	LDL Goal
Without CHD and with fewer than 2 risk factors	≥160 mg/dL	<160 mg/dL
Without CHD and with 2 or more risk factors	≥130 mg/dL	<130 mg/dL
Without CHD	>100 mg/dL	≤100 mg/dL
Drug Treatment	**Initiation Level**	**LDL Goal**
Without CHD and with fewer than 2 risk factors	≥190 mg/dL*	<160 mg/dL
Without CHD and with 2 or more risk factors	≥160 mg/dL	<130 mg/dL
Without CHD	≥130 mg/dL**	≤100 mg/dL

* In men under 35 years of age and premenopausal women with LDL-cholesterol levels 190-219 mg/dL, drug therapy should be delayed except in high-risk patients such as those with diabetes.

** In CHD patients with LDL-cholesterol levels 100-129 mg/dL, the physician should exercise clinical judgment in deciding whether to initiate drug treatment.

Source: National Institutes of Health. 1993. *Second Report of the Expert Panel on Detection, Evaluation, and Treatment of High Blood Cholesterol in Adults.* NIH Publication No. 93-3096.

Career Sequence of work-related positions occupied throughout a person's life.

Caries See **dental caries**.

Carnitine An **amino acid** made from methionine and lysine that transports long-chain **fatty acids** across the mitochondrial membrane.

Carotenemia A condition in which there is too much carotene in the blood. Carotenemia may be due to excessive intake or abnormal carotene metabolism. In some cases, the skin turns yellow due to excessive carotene pigments.

Carotenoids A class of pigments that contribute red, orange, or yellow color to fruits and vegetables. Carotenoids are divided into two groups: the carotenes (including **beta carotene**, a precursor of **vitamin A**) and the xanthophylls. See also **beta carotene** (see Table C.7).

Table C.7 Some Good Sources of Carotenoids

- Dark-green leafy vegetables (such as spinach, collards, kale, mustard greens, turnip greens), broccoli, carrots, pumpkin and calabasa, red pepper, sweet potatoes, and tomatoes

- Fruits like mango, papaya, cantaloupe

Case Control Studies A type of observational analytic research design that tests a hypothesis or a causal relationship. Case control studies use retrospective means to compare the prevalence of a factor(s), such as sodium intake, in subjects with a disease with subjects who don't have the disease. Case control studies work well with rare diseases and are lower in cost than experimental studies, but bias can be a concern. See also **research.**

Case Study A research design for obtaining descriptive data of what occurred in a single subject or patient. Case studies involve collecting much information on the subject. Case studies are descriptive in nature and therefore can't be used to support or oppose a hypothesis. Also called a *case report.* See also **research.**

Catabolism The metabolic processes in which large, complex molecules are converted to a smaller set of simpler ones, yielding energy.

Catalyst Substances, such as **enzymes**, that speed up chemical reactions without being consumed or changed by the reaction.

Cataracts Thickened lens of the eyes that can lead to blindness.

Catecholamines Hormones produced and secreted by the adrenal medulla in response to stress. The catecholamines includes **epinephrine** and **norepinephrine.**

1. Epinephrine or **adrenaline**—Epinephrine stimulates increased cardiac output, dilates respiratory passageways, increases the respiratory rate, and increases **glycogenolysis** (breakdown of **glycogen** to **glucose**) and **lipolysis** (breakdown of **triglycerides** into **glycerol** and **fatty acids**) so that blood **sugar** and **fatty acid** levels rise.

2. Norepinephrine or **noradrenaline**—Norepinephrine increases **blood pressure** because it constricts blood vessels. It also dilates respiratory passageways, increases the respiratory rate, and increases glycogenolysis and lipolysis, like epinephrine but to a lesser degree.

The catecholamines mimic the actions of the sympathetic nervous system by increasing the heartbeat, respiratory rate, blood pressure, and blood sugar levels during stress.

Cation A positive ion.

Cat Scan (CT Scan) Computed tomography. Tomography means that a series of x-rays are taken around the part of the body that you want to see in depth. Then, a computer processes these x-rays to produce a cross-sectional (transverse) image.

Cecum A pouch connected to the **ileum** of the **small intestine** by the ileocecal valve. The **appendix** is attached to part of the cecum.

Celiac Disease See **gluten sensitive enteropathy.**

Cell Body Part of a **nerve** cell or **neuron.** See also **neuron.**

Cell-Mediated Immunity An **immune response** provided by **T lymphocytes** that use direct action and contact, instead of **antibodies,** to destroy foreign bodies. See also immune system and **T cell lymphocytes.**

Cellulose A type of **fiber** that is the primary component of cell walls of fibrous plants.

Census In a healthcare facility, the number of patients at a point in time (usually midnight). Also called the midnight census.

Center for Disease Control (CDC) A branch of the Department of Health and Human Services that monitors the occurrence of **foodborne illness** as one of its many duties.

Central Nervous System (CNS) The brain and the spinal cord. The central nervous system and the **peripheral nervous system** make up the nervous system of the body. The CNS sends information to and receives information from the peripheral nervous system. The CNS is the main network of coordination and control. See also **peripheral nervous system.**

Cerebral Hemorrhage Rupture of an **artery** in the brain. See **cerebrovasular accident.**

Cerebrospinal Fluid (CSF) Liquid that circulates in the brain and spinal cord.

Cerebrovascular Accident (CVA) A **stroke,** meaning damage to the brain caused by a disorder in the **blood** vessels of the cerebrum. CVA can be due to:

1. A blood clot getting caught in a cerebral artery that has narrowed due to **atherosclerosis** (most frequent)

2. An embolism—a mass such as a blood clot or a bit of tissue—blocks a cerebral artery

3. Hemorrhaging of a cerebral artery (most life-threatening)

See also **stroke**.

Ceruloplasmin A **plasma protein** that carries a copper-containing **enzyme** responsible for oxidizing **iron** from the ferrous to the ferric form so it can be transported.

Cervix Lower part of the uterus that joins with the vagina.

Cesarean Section Removal of the **fetus** by making an abdominal incision into the uterus. Newborns are delivered by cesarean section only when vaginal birth presents dangers to the mother and/or the baby.

Chain of Command The lines along which responsibility and authority are delegated from top to bottom of the organization.

Channels of Communication The organizational lines (corresponding to the chain of command) along which messages are passed from one level to another.

Cheilosis A disorder of the lips and mouth marked by cracks at the corners of the mouth and chapped and swollen lips. Cheilosis is seen in malnourished individuals and individuals lacking **riboflavin**.

Chelating Agents A chemical compound that can bind with a substance to remove it from circulation or from a tissue. For example, some fibers chelate with **iron** in the intestinal tract and carry it out of the body.

Cholangiography X-ray pictures of the **gallbladder** region including the cystic duct and **common bile duct**. These tests use a dye (to provide contrast) that is given orally or with a needle. These tests look for **gallstones**.

Cholecalciferol The chemical name for **vitamin D** in its inactive form, also called D3. Cholecalciferol is hydroxylated in the **liver** to make 25-hydroxy vitamin D3, the major circulating form of the vitamin. The **kidney** adds on another hydroxyl group, making 1, 25-dihydroxy vitamin D3. This is the active form of vitamin D and is called **calcitriol**.

Cholecystetomy Surgical removal of the **gallbladder**.

Cholecystokinin (CCK) A **hormone** secreted by the **small intestine** that stimulates secretion of pancreatic juice **enzymes** and contraction of the **gallbladder**. CCK is secreted by the **duodenum** in response to the presence of **fat** in the **chyme**.

Cholelithiasis **Gallstones**, or small, hard mineral deposits, found in the **gallbladder** and bile ducts. See also **gallstones**.

NUTRIENT FOCUS: CHOLESTEROL

The most abundant sterol (a category of **lipids**). Pure cholesterol is an odorless, white, waxy, powdery substance. You cannot taste it or see it in the foods you eat.

Your body needs cholesterol to function normally. It is present in every cell in your body, including the brain and **nervous system, muscle,** skin, **liver,** intestines, **heart,** and skeleton. Cholesterol is used by the body to make bile acids, which allows us to digest **fats,** and to make cell membranes, many **hormones,** and **vitamin D.** Unfortunately, **high blood cholesterol** is a risk factor for **heart disease** and is found in the walls of clogged arteries.

Table C.8 Cholesterol Content of Foods

Food and Portion	Cholesterol (milligrams)
Liver, braised, 3 ounces	302
Egg, whole, 1	213
Beef, short ribs, braised, 3 ounces	80
Beef, ground, lean, broiled medium, 3 ounces	74
Beef, top round, broiled, 3 ounces	73
Chicken breast, roasted, without skin, 3 ounces	72
Haddock, baked, 3 ounces	63
Flounder of sole, baked, 3 ounces	58
Swordfish, baked, 3 ounces	43
Shrimp, cooked in moist heat, 3 ounces	167
Lobster, cooked in moist heat, 3 ounces	61
Milk, whole, 8 ounces	33
Milk, 2% fat, 8 ounces	18
Milk, 1% fat, 8 ounces	10
Skim milk, 8 ounces	4
Cheddar cheese, 1 ounce	30
American processed cheese, 1 ounce	27
Cottage cheese, low-fat, 1/2 cup	5

Source: National Institutes of Health. 1994. *Step by Step: Eating to Lower Your High Blood Cholesterol*. NIH Publication No. 94-2920.

Which foods contain cholesterol? Cholesterol is found only in foods of animal origin: egg yolks (it's not in the whites), meat, poultry, fish, milk, and milk products. It is not found in foods of plant origin. Egg yolk and organ meats (liver, kidney, sweetbread, brain) contain the most cholesterol—one egg yolk contains 213 milligrams of cholesterol. About four ounces of meat, poultry, or fish (trimmed or untrimmed) contain 100 milligrams of cholesterol (see Table C.8).

In milk products, cholesterol is mostly in the fat, so lower fat products contain less cholesterol. For example, one cup of whole milk contains 33 milligrams of cholesterol, whereas a cup of skim milk contains only four milligrams.

Egg whites and foods that come from plants like fruits, nuts, vegetables, grains, cereals, and seeds have no cholesterol.

We take in about 400 to 500 milligrams of cholesterol daily and the liver also makes a significant amount of cholesterol. Because the body produces cholesterol, it is not considered an essential nutrient. See also **cardiovascular disease.**

NUTRIENT FOCUS: CHLORIDE

A major mineral that functions as an **electrolyte** in the body to maintain **acid-base** balance and water balance. Chloride (with a negative charge) is found mostly in the fluid outside the cells. Chloride is also a part of **hydrochloric acid,** which is found in quite high concentration in the juices of the **stomach.** Hydrochloric acid aids in protein digestion, destroys harmful bacteria, and increases the ability of **calcium** and **iron** to be absorbed. The most important source of chloride in the diet is sodium chloride or **salt.** If sodium intake is adequate, there will be ample chloride as well.

Choline A compound that is not a nutrient.

Chorion During pregnancy, one of the two membranes surrounding the **fetus.** It is the outermost membrane and is part of the placenta.

NUTRIENT FOCUS: CHROMIUM

A trace mineral that works with **insulin** to get **glucose** into the body's cells. A chromium deficiency results in a condition much like diabetes in which the glucose level in the **blood** is abnormally high. Chromium also plays an important role in the body's use of **fats** and **proteins.** Good sources of chromium are whole (unprocessed) foods such as whole grains, lean beef, wheat germ, and brewer's yeast, and some fruits and vegetables such as corn and apples.

Our intake is likely to be less than the **RDA,** but whether this results in identifiable deficiency symptoms has not been established. Although advertised as helping you lose weight and put on **muscle,** research studies have not definitively confirmed this. Although safer than **zinc** or **iron** in supplement form, megadoses are not advised.

Chromosomes Structures in the nucleus of cells that contain **DNA** and **proteins**. The chromosomes contain the genetic master plan.

Chronic Disease A disease that lasts a long time.

Chyme The partially digested food leaving the **stomach** and going into the **duodenum**.

Chylomicron The **lipoprotein** that is responsible for carrying mostly **triglycerides**, and some **cholesterol**, from the intestines through the **lymphatic system** to the bloodstream.

Chymotrypsin A protein-splitting pancreatic **enzyme** that is converted from chymotrypsinogen in the intestine by **trypsin**.

Cirrhosis The final stage of **liver** disease. At this point liver cells harden and die, and the damage is irreversible. Symptoms of cirrhosis include nausea, poor appetite, weight loss, weakness, esophageal varices (varicose veins) that may bleed, **ascites** (accumulation of fluid in the peritoneal cavity), **iron-deficiency anemia**, and **stomach** pain. Nutritional therapy commonly includes extra **protein** (1.5—2.0 g/kg) unless there are signs of **hepatic encephalopathy** in which case protein is restricted, low sodium to reduce fluid retention, soft foods if there are esophageal varices, and a diet high in vitamins and minerals. Cirrhosis most often results from alcoholism.

Citric Acid Cycle A cyclic energy production pathway in the cell mitochondria that oxidizes **acetyl CoA** (from **carbohydrates** and **fats**) to **carbon dioxide** and energy that goes into high-energy phosphate bonds of ATP. Also called the **Krebs cycle**, the **tricarboxylic acid (TCA) cycle**.

Clear Liquid Diet A diet that allows only foods that are clear liquids or become clear liquids at room temperature, such as:

- apple, grape, cranberry, and cranapple juice

- strained orange or grapefruit juice

- fruit punch, lemonade

- carbonated beverages

- clear broth

- flavored gelatin

- fruit ice, popsicle

- tea, coffee

The clear liquid diet may be used before or after surgery, before various diagnostic tests, following periods of vomiting or diarrhea, or in the acute stages of many illnesses. The diet is intended to provide fluids, **electrolytes**, and some energy with minimal stimulation of the digestive tract and minimal fecal material. It is useful in preventing dehydration and relieving thirst but does not provide many nutrients.

Client The person with whom a dietitian is working. In a hospital or nursing facility, the client may be called a **patient**.

Client-Centered Therapy A counseling technique in which counselors take a noncritical, accepting attitude toward the **client**. The goals of client-centered therapy is for clients to feel confident, self-directed, and positive about themselves. Instead of concentrating on cognitive or behavioral aspects, the client-centered therapist looks at the client's emotions. Also called **person-centered therapy** or **humanistic therapy**.

Clinical Dietitian A professional who provides nutrition services, such as nutrition counseling, in a variety of settings but quite often in healthcare environments. The clinical dietitian may practice in hospital units, out-patient clinics, nursing facilities, physicians' offices, or his or her own offices (see Table C.9).

Table C.9 Functions Performed by Clinical Dietitians

I. Client-related activities

    A. Preliminary nutrition screening

    B. Comprehensive nutrition assessment

    C Nutrition care planning

    D. Nutrition care implementation

    E. Nutrition care evaluation and reassessment

    F. Nutrition counseling and education (individual)

    G. Nutrition counseling and education (family)

    H. Nutrition counseling and education (groups)

    I. Nutrition care follow-up

    J. Nutrient intake analysis (limited)

Table C.9 Functions Performed by Clinical Dietitians (continued)

    K. Nutrient intake analysis (comprehensive)

    L. Nutrition history consultation

    M. Health team conference

    N. Recommendation or formulation of enteral nutrition product

    O. Nutrient pattern calculation

    P. Community service or education

    Q. Documentation of nutrition care

    R. Menu preparation for individual patient or client

    S. Nourishment prescriptions

II. Administrative and managerial functions

    A Marketing nutrition services

    B. Preparation and dispensing of nutrition supplements, tube feedings of defined formula diets

    C. Procurement of nutrition supplements or specialized nutrition products

    D. Cycle menu or nourishment development

    E. Nutrition care standards

    F. Quality assurance

    G. Personnel management

    H. Staff and organization meetings

    I. In-service education

    J. Education and training of health professionals

    K. Planning

    L. Budget preparation or accountability

Table C.9 Functions Performed by Clinical Dietitians (continued)

    M. Administrative tasks

    N. Foodservice management responsibilities

    O. Document development and review

III. Professional activities

    A. Literature review

    B. Continuing education

    C. Other professional activities

IV. Nonprofessional activities (clerical tasks)

V. Delay activities

    A. Forced delay

    B. Personal delay

VI. Transit time

Source: Shanklin, C. W., .et al.: Documentation of time expenditures of clinical dietitians: Results of a statewide time study in Texas. Copyright© The American Dietetic Association. Reprinted by permission from *Journal of the American Dietetic Association*, Vol. 88: 39.

Clinical Effectiveness The changes in an individual's health status as a result of an **intervention**, such as **medical nutrition therapy**.

Clinical Trials Medical research using the experimental design. Clinical trials compare the efficacy of two or more medical **interventions** and also are used to establish the safety of an intervention or treatment. Some characteristics of clinical trials include the following.

- Subjects must voluntarily consent to be in the study and be told all the possible risks. A written consent must be signed.

- Subjects are randomly assigned to a control or experimental group. The control group receives the standard treatment. The experimental group receives the intervention being tested.

- A **placebo** may be used if there is no standard treatment.

- Statistical analysis of the results is used to test hypotheses.

Because of the nature of this research, cause and effect relationships can be verified.

Clotting See **blood clotting**.

Coaching A two-part process: observation of employee performance and conversation about job performance between manager and employee. The overall goals of the conversation are to evaluate work performance, then to encourage optimum work performance by either reinforcing good performance or confronting and redirecting poor performance. Coaching therefore provides employees with regular support and feedback about job performance and alerts the manager to exactly what employees need to know (See Table C.10).

Table C.10   General Coaching Guidelines

- Be specific and accurate about job performance.

- Actively listen to the employee. Be supportive and objective. Do not let the conversation drift away to other issues or discussion of other employees. If the conversation starts to drift, make a statement such as "Let's get back to the issue at hand."

- Focus on the employee's behavior, not on the employee. Always affirm the self-respect and self-esteem of the employee.

- The most effective time to reinforce positive performance is while the desired behavior is occurring. If that is not possible, the next best time is immediately afterwards. Confront job performance as soon as possible after observing it. However, if you are at all angry or upset, do not confront the employee. Wait until you are calm.

- Correct in private. Employees are very sensitive about being corrected in front of their peers. Unless the error could have grave consequences, wait until you can at least take the employee aside long enough to tell him or her how to correct it.

- Explain the impact of the employee's job performance on the work group and the total operation.

- Be a coach, not a drill sergeant. Do not stay constantly at a person's side, watching everything he or she does.

Source: Karen Eich Drummond. 1992. *Retaining Your Foodservice Employees.* New York: Van Nostrand Reinhold.

Coagulation The process of **blood clotting**. See also **blood clotting**.

Coagulation or Clotting Time The time needed for venous **blood** to clot in a test tube (usually less than 15 minutes).

NUTRIENT FOCUS: COBALT

A trace mineral that is a part of **vitamin B12** and therefore is needed to form **red blood cells**. The dietary source of cobalt is vitamin B12, which is found in animal foods.

Codon In protein synthesis, the sequence of three **bases** in messenger **RNA** that tells which **amino acid** is needed.

Coenzyme See cofactor.

Coenzyme A (CoA) A coenzyme that contains **pantothenic acid** and is a carrier of acyl groups in energy metabolism. CoA functions in the production of energy from **carbohydrate, fat,** and **protein.** CoA is a part of **acetyl-coA.** See **acetyl-coenzyme A.**

Cofactors Ions or molecules required for the activity of certain **enzymes.** Cofactors that are organic compounds, such as **vitamins,** are called coenzymes.

Cognitive Psychology A contemporary school of psychology that focuses on things you can't see, or mental events. They look at how you use your cognitive processes to process information. Cognitive processes refer to what goes on in your mind, such as perceiving, paying attention, understanding, interpreting, reasoning, problem-solving, storing information, and retrieving information from memory. Cognitive psychology has affected the way teaching, learning, and counseling is viewed. To the cognitivist, instead of the learner passively acquiring knowledge, the learner is actively involved in the learning process through constructing and organizing knowledge. Cognitive counseling techniques look at a **client's** thoughts or beliefs to see if they are contributing to nutrition problems. For example, a client's belief that he or she should never eat after dinner may be restructured to be more realistic.

Cohort Studies A type of observational analytic **research** design that is similar to **clinical trials,** and tests a hypothesis of a causal relationship. Cohort studies collect data on the same research question at different points in time from the same group of persons or cohort. Cohort studies frequently examine the frequency of a disease and possible causal factors within the population. When the study begins, subjects do not have the disease but must be exposed to the possible causal factor. Because cohort studies work forward in time, they are considered prospective studies. Also called *follow-up studies.*

Collagen The most abundant **protein** in the human body. Collagen is a fibrous protein that is a component of skin, **bone,** teeth, ligaments, tendons, and other connective structures. Collagen is a very strong protein.

Collateral Circulation In reference to the **heart**, the widening of smaller **arteries** to supply **blood** to an area where a larger artery is damaged, closed, or narrowed.

Collecting Tubule One of the renal tubules in the **nephron** or functional unit of the **kidney**. Also see **nephron**.

Collective Bargaining Process by which a labor contract between management and a union is negotiated.

College and University Foodservice Foodservices found within colleges and universities that feed students, faculty, and staff.

Colon The **large intestine**. See **large intestine**.

Colostomy The formation of an exit in the abdominal area from the **gastrointestinal tract** by bringing a loop of the **colon** to the surface of the abdomen. The colostomy provides an outlet for feces when the **rectum** can't be used.

Colostrum A yellowish fluid that is the first secretion to come from the breast a day or so after delivery of a baby. It is rich in **proteins**, **antibodies**, and other factors that protect against infectious disease. Colostrum changes to **transitional milk** between the third and sixth days, and then by the tenth day the major changes are finished.

Common Bile Duct A duct that carries **bile** from the cystic duct (which comes from the **gallbladder**) to the **duodenum** of the **small intestine**.

Commission on Dietetic Registration The credentialing agency of The **American Dietetic Association**.

Communication An interaction between sender and receiver. In a successful communication, the sender directs a clear message to someone and the receiver gets the message accurately.

Communication skills include writing, speaking, listening, and interpersonal skills.

Community Based Program A public health program that involves community institutions, organizations, and leaders.

Community Dietitian A **dietitian** who is involved in nutrition and nutrition education in a community setting such a public health agency, day care center, or health and fitness club.

Compact Bone See **cortical bone**.

Complement **Blood proteins** activated by the attachment of **antibodies** to **antigens**. The 11 proteins of complement kill foreign cells.

Complementary Proteins The ability of two **protein** foods to make up for the lack of (or insufficient) **essential amino acids** in each other. See also **vegetarian eating**.

Complete Proteins Food **proteins** that provide all of the **essential amino acids** in the proportions needed.

Complex Carbohydrates **Starch** and **fiber**. Starch and fiber are composed of long chains of **sugar** units. Also called **polysaccharides**. See also **starch** and **fiber**.

Computerized Nutrient Analysis The process by which the nutrient content of a recipe or meal is calculated using the computer. The computer has done a lot to speed up this process and increase its accuracy. Computerized nutrient analysis programs contain the nutrient information of many different resources. By typing in the name of an ingredient, the computer lists similar ingredients so that you can choose exactly which one is appropriate. Then you type in how much of that ingredient you want to be used in the analysis, such as 1 cup. After inputting all the ingredients, you can ask the computer to divide the results by the yield, such as 12 portions. Then the computer will tell you exactly how much of each nutrient (and the percent of the **RDA**) is contained in one portion. Most computer analysis programs also can give you a percentage breakdown of **calories** from **protein, fat, carbohydrate,** and **alcohol**. Of course, these figures can be printed on a printer and/or stored in the computer's memory (see Figure C.2).

Figure C.2 Sample Computerized Nutrient Analysis

Breakfast: 4 Foods

Item	Food Name	Serving	Portion	Amount
441	Pancakes, Home Recipe	3.00	Items	81.00 Gms
3354	Syrup--Pancake with Maple	1.00	Tbsp	20.07 Gms
648	Sausage--Turkey Breakfast	2.00	Ounces	56.80 Gms
362	Orange Juice--From Conc	1.00	Cup	250.00 Gms

Nutrient Values

Kilocalories	454 KC	21% of RDA
Protein	19.50 Gm	39%
Carbohydrate	67.73 Gm	25%
Fat	14.66 Gm	19%
Saturated Fat	1.42 Gm	6%
Cholesterol	109.00 Gm	37%
Fiber--Dietary	1.78 Gm	8%
Vitamin A	37.98 RE	5%
Vitamin C	96.69 Mg	161%
Vitamin D	0.00 Ug	0%
Sodium	934.34 Mg	39%
Potassium	572.22 Mg	29%
Iron	1.35%	10%

Percent of Kcals from: Protein: 16% Carb: 57% Fat: 26%

Diabetic Exchanges: Milk: 0.00 Veg: 0.0 Fruit: 2.0 Bread: 2.0 Meat 1.8 Fat: 1.8

Cones See **retina**.

Confounding Variable Any variable that is not controlled by the study and can therefore affect the outcome of the study.

Congenital Heart Disease Abnormalities of the **heart** that are seen at birth.

Congestive Heart Failure (CHF) The inability of the **heart** to pump an adequate amount of **blood** as a result of **heart disease** or **hypertension**. In CHF, more blood enters the heart from the **veins** than leaves the heart through the **aorta** and **arteries**. Symptoms of CHF include **salt** and water retention and edema (swelling) of the abdomen and legs. Treatment is with drugs to strengthen the heart and increase fluid loss. Diet is usually restricted in **sodium**, fluids, and **fat**.

Congregate Meals Program Meals for older adults that are served in a community setting, such as a senior center, and funded by Title III-C of the Older Americans Act. Participants in this program must be at least 60 years old, although spouses of participants can be any age and receive meals too. Congregate meals usually are served once each weekday, in the middle of the day, at locations such as senior centers, community centers, or churches. The meal site quite often provides other services such as recreation and nutrition education. See also **senior nutrition programs**.

Congressional Record A verbatim recording of activities in the U.S. House of Representatives and Senate. When Congress is in session, the Congressional Record is published each day.

Conjugated Proteins A **protein** that contains one or more nonamino acid units. For example, **hemoglobin** is a conjugated protein: heme- is not an amino acid, globin is the protein constituent.

Constipation Difficulty or delay in passing of feces. Dietary treatment of constipation includes increasing **fiber** and fluids. Exercise also helps.

Consultant Dietitian A **dietitian** who works independently providing services to any of a large variety of **clients**. Consultant dietitians frequently provide dietetic services to nursing homes and other healthcare institutions. They may also advise food companies and restaurants, counsel patients in physician's offices, or provide nutrition services to sports teams.

Contingency Plan An alternate plan for use in case the original plan does not work out.

Continuing Care Retirement Communities (CCRC) Communities that offer retirees their own housing and a variety of services, such as meals, recreational facilities, golf courses, beauty salons, and transportation to nearby shopping. CCRC, also called **lifecare communities,** offer nursing assistance for residents in independent-living apartments, assisted-living housing for those residents who need help performing daily routines, and a skilled nursing facility for the chronically or acutely ill. Foodservices in CCRCs are varied and can be quite elegant, with a focus on serving residents restaurant style in a dining room.

Continuous Quality Improvement (CQI) An organizational philosophy that sets a priority on providing quality services and involves employees in the process. For example, if a hospital implements CQI, it will need to:

1. Identify how quality is to be defined

2. Develop a customer/guest orientation

3. Form teams of employees to study and revise work procedures to meet and exceed customer expectations and focus on making a process better. In CQI, the performance standard is error-free performance. Employee teams use the following procedural steps.

   1. Identify the problem

   2. Analyze the problem

   3. Select a solution and write an action plan

   4. Implement the solution

   5. Evaluate the solution

Contract Foodservice Management The foodservices provided by a professional management company, such as ARAMARK, for a **client.** Foodservice contractors run foodservice operations within many segments such as hospitals, nursing homes, schools, colleges, business and industry, and correctional and recreational facilities. Contract management companies enter into a management contract with their client. Contracts are often one of the following types.

1. Management fee contract—In this arrangement, the client pays a fee which could be a fixed dollar amount, a percentage of gross sales or costs, or a combination of both.

2. Profit and loss contract—With this type of contract, the contractor takes a financial risk to run the operation, and can retain profits or, in the cases of losses, absorbs the loss.

3. Commission-paid contract—This contract is a variation on the profit and loss contract. In addition to the profit and loss aspect of the contract, the contractor pays the client a commission.

Contracting In nutrition counseling, the process in which the **client** forms a written agreement with the counselor to reach a goal or perform a certain behavior. Contracts spell out exactly what the client is to do during a certain time frame, such as lose ten pounds in three months. Contracts sometimes spell out the consequences (rewards) if the goal is reached.

Contractor See **contract foodservice management**.

Control Group A group of subjects in **research** that serves as the comparison for the experimental group(s).

Controlling A managerial activity. Measuring and evaluating results to goals and standards previously agreed upon, such as performance and quality standards, and taking corrective action when necessary to stay on course.

Controls Built-in methods for measuring performance or product against standards.

Coordinating A managerial activity consisting of meshing the work of individuals, work groups, and departments to produce a smoothly running operation.

NUTRIENT FOCUS: COPPER

A trace mineral that works with **iron** to form **hemoglobin**. It also aids in forming **collagen**, a **protein** that gives strength and support to **bones**, teeth, **muscle**, cartilage, and **blood** vessels. Copper is a part of many important **enzymes**, such as those involved in the **nervous system** and energy release.

Copper is found mostly in unprocessed foods. Organ meats, shellfish, legumes, nuts, dried fruits, and whole grain breads and cereals are rich sources.

Copper-deficient diets are linked to heart disease, causing **cholesterol** and **blood pressure** to go up. Copper deficiency is rare, but marginal deficiencies do occur. Single doses of copper only four times the recommended level can cause vomiting and disorders of the nervous system.

Copyright The exclusive ownership of and the right to make use of a literary or artistic work as protected by U.S. copyright laws. A work that is created and fixed in tangible form is automatically protected from the moment of its creation, and is ordinarily given a term enduring the author's life, plus an additional 50 years after the author's death. Only the actual expression of the author can be protected by copyright. The ideas, plans, methods, or systems described or embodied in a work are not protected by copyright. After a work is created, you can place a notice of copyright on the material and apply for copyright registration.

Notice of Copyright: Copyright 1995 by Karen Drummond
                       ©Karen Drummond 1995

See also **trademark**.

Cori Cycle A cycle in which lactic acid produced by the skeletal **muscles** is taken to the **liver** and converted to **glucose** via **gluconeogenesis**, and the glucose is returned to the skeletal muscles. During exercise, some glucose in the muscle is catabolized without **oxygen**, in which case lactic acid is produced. Lactic acid then travels to the liver where, in the presence of oxygen, it is made back into glucose via gluconeogenesis. The glucose then returns to the skeletal muscles. (see Figure C.3.)

Cori's Disease An inherited disorder in which the **enzyme** that debranches **glycogen** is missing, resulting in increased glycogen stores.

Cornea The fibrous transparent tissue over the eyeball.

Figure C.3 Cori Cycle

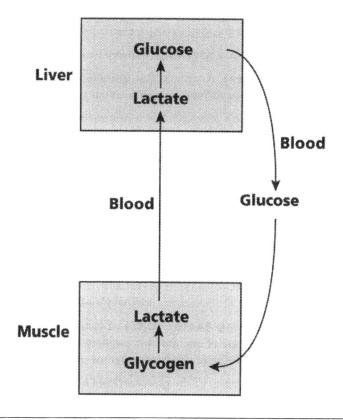

Coronary Arteries A set of **arteries** that branch from the **aorta** to carry **oxygen**-rich **blood** into every part of the **heart muscle**.

Coronary Heart Disease (CHD) A broad term used to describe damage to or malfunction of the **heart** caused by narrowing or blockage of the coronary **arteries**.

More than two-thirds of a coronary artery may be filled with fatty deposits without causing symptoms. Symptoms may manifest themselves as chest pain as in angina or as a **heart attack**. See also **angina pectoris, atherosclerosis, cardiovascular disease,** and **heart attack**.

Coronary Bypass Surgery Major surgery in which portions of leg **veins** or an **artery** in the chest are removed and attached to the **heart** to provide alternate routes for **blood** flow, bypassing blocked arteries.

Corpuscle A **blood cell**.

Corpus Luteum Empty mound of tissue or follicle that forms in the ovary after an egg (ovum) has been released. Even though the egg has been released, the corpus luteum has an important job: to secrete estrogen and progesterone that prepare the body for pregnancy. If the egg is fertilized, the corpus luteum grows bigger and lasts for about three months. If the egg is not fertilized, the corpus luteum shrinks and is shed during menstruation.

Correlation The extent of a relationship between two or more variables.

Correlation Coefficient A statistic that quantifies or measures the relationship between variables without involving causality.

Correlational Research Research that measures the relationships between two or more variables.

Cortex Outer region. For example, the renal cortex is the outer part of the **kidney**.

Cortical Bone A layer of dense **bone** tissue that lies under the **periosteum** of all bones and around the **diaphysis**, or middle region, of a **long bone**. The middle region of long bones contains yellow bone marrow, a specialized **lipid** storage tissue. Also called *compact bone* or *dense bone.*

Corticosteroids Steroid **hormones** made in the adrenal cortex. Corticosteroids include **glucocorticoids** (such as **cortisol**), **mineralocorticoids** (such as **aldosterone**), and sex hormones. See **adrenal glands.**

Corticotropin-Releasing Factor (CRF) A factor in the **hypothalamus** that stimulates the release of the anterior pituitary hormone **adrenocorticotropic hormone (ACTH)**. See also **hypothalamus** and **pituitary gland.**

Cortisol The most important of the **glucocorticoid hormones** produced and secreted by the adrenal cortex. Also called **hydrocortisone**, cortisol suppresses the **immune system** and has an anti-inflammatory effect. Hydrocortisone also stimulates the breakdown of **protein** to **amino acids** in the skeletal **muscle** and increases **gluconeogenesis** in the **liver**.

Cortisone A synthetic **hormone** similar to **cortisol**. See also **cortisol**.

Cost-Benefit Analysis (CBA) A form of economic analysis used to compare the effects and contributions of a program to its costs. CBA is an extension of cost-effectiveness analysis. In CBA, both the costs and the effects are expressed in dollars. See also **economic evaluation.**

Cost-Effectiveness Analysis (CEA) A form of economic analysis used to compare the costs of two different **interventions** when the outcomes are the same. For example, the cost effectiveness of using drugs or diet to lower **blood pressure** a certain amount could be examined. See also **cost-benefit analysis** and **economic evaluation.**

Coumarin An anticoagulant drug.

Counseling See **nutrition counseling.**

Covalent Bond A bond formed when two atoms share a pair of electrons.

Creatine Phosphokinase (CPK) An **enzyme** whose **plasma** concentrations increase within three to six hours after symptoms of a **myocardial infarction** (**heart attack**) and return to normal after three days.

Creatinine A **metabolite** that is produced in the **muscles** and is excreted in the urine. The amount of creatinine excreted daily is fairly constant. Higher than normal levels of creatinine in the urine indicates increased tissue breakdown.

Cretinism **Hypothyroidism** during infancy and childhood. The symptoms are stunted growth, mental retardation, and lethargy. Treatment includes administration of thyroxine.

NUTRITION AND DISEASE FOCUS: CROHN'S DISEASE

A form of inflammatory bowel disease characterized by chronic inflammation of the intestinal tract. In Crohn's disease there are lesions in the mucosal tissue in any part of the **small intestine, large intestine**, and/or **rectum**. The intestinal wall is thickened, inflamed, and rigid, and fistulas are common. Symptoms include persistent diarrhea (often bloody), abdominal pain, and poor appetite. These patients receive medications to reduce the inflammation.

The nutritional care of Crohn's disease often includes a diet high in **protein** (due to protein losses from the mucosal lesions and poor intake) and calories (due to weight loss commonly seen). Fiber is generally limited during times when healing is taking place. Extra vitamins and minerals need to be supplied in foods and/or supplemental form. Enteral and parenteral nutrition may be needed in some cases.

Cross Sectional Design In **research**, a design that examines people of different ages at one point in time.

Cruciferous Vegetables Vegetables in the cabbage family that contain **phytochemicals** (cancer-fighting substances) such as indoles and dithiolthiones. They activate enzymes that destroy carcinogens. Cruciferous vegetables include broccoli, brussels sprouts, cabbage, cauliflower, bok choy, kale, collards, kohlrabi, mustard, rutabagas, spinach, and watercress.

Cyanocobalamin See **vitamin B12**.

Cyanosis Bluish color in the skin due to low levels of oxygen in the **blood**.

Cyclamate An artificial sweetener that dominated the noncaloric sweetener market in the 1960s. It is 30 times sweeter than **sucrose** and is not metabolized by most people. Cyclamate was banned in 1970 after studies showed that large doses of it, given with **saccharin**, were associated with increased risk of **bladder cancer**. Cyclamate continues to be banned in the United States but is approved and used in more than 40 other countries worldwide. Cyclamate is again under consideration for use in specific products, such as tabletop sweeteners and nonalcoholic beverages. It is stable at hot and cold temperatures and has no aftertaste.

Cystic Fibrosis (CF) An inherited disorder of the **exocrine glands** (glands that secrete through **ducts**) that causes the glands to make thick mucus. The glands affected by CF are the **pancreas**, sweat glands, and the mucous membranes of the lungs. Individuals with CF have pancreatic insufficiency and lung infections. There is no cure. Treatment consists of pancreatic enzyme replacement and treatment of the respiratory problems.

Cystitis Inflammation of the **bladder**. The most frequent form of urinary tract infections.

Cystoscopy Visual examination of the urinary **bladder** by means of a cystoscope placed in the **urethra**. This test allows the bladder to be examined for tumors, calculi, or inflammation and for biopsies of growths such as tumors or polyps.

Cytochromes Electron carriers in the **electron transport chain**. See also **electron transport chain**.

Cytoplasm The protoplasm of the cell outside the nucleus in which much cell **metabolism** occurs.

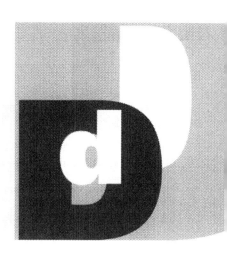

Daily Value On food labels, a guide to the total nutrient amount you need for a day based on a 2,000 **calorie** diet (see Table D.1).

Table D.1 Daily Values Used on Food Labels

Fat	65 grams
Saturated fat	20 grams
Cholesterol	300 milligrams
Total Carbohydrate	300 grams
Fiber	25 grams
Sodium	2,400 milligrams
Protein	50 grams
Vitamin A	5,000 International Units
Vitamin C	60 milligrams
Calcium	1,000 milligrams
Iron	18 milligrams

Data A collection of observations from a survey or experiment.

Deamination The process of removing the amino group from the **amino acid.** Deamination yeilds ammonia. Because ammonia is toxic, the body converts it to urea and then excretes the **urea**. Also called *oxidative deamination*.

Decarboxylase A group of **enzymes** that catalyze the removal of **carboxyl groups** (–COOH) from a compound.

Decarboxylation The removal of a **carboxyl group** (–COOH) from a compound.

Decertification A process in which a **union** is removed from representing a group of employees.

Decision A conscious choice among alternative courses of action directed toward a specific purpose. The steps in decision-making are:

1. Define the problem and set objectives (what do you want to happen?).

2. Analyze the problem: get the facts—the relevant who, what, when, where, how, and why.

3. Develop alternative solutions.

4. Decide on the best solution.

5. Convert the decision into action.

6. Follow up.

NUTRITION AND DISEASE FOCUS: DECUBITUS ULCER

A **skin lesion** caused by unrelieved pressure resulting in damage of underlying tissue. Over one million patients in hospitals and nursing homes, particularly those who are bedridden, suffer from decubitus ulcers. Nutrition plays a vital role in preventing and treating **pressure sores**. Also called **pressure sores** (see Tables D.2 and D.3).

Table D.2 Risk Factors for Decubitus Ulcers (Pressure Sores)

- Impaired transfer or bed mobility

- Bedridden, hemiplegia, quadriplegia

- Urinary or bowel incontinence

- Peripheral vascular disease

- Diabetes mellitus

- Hip fracture

- Weight loss/malnutrition

- Pressure sore history

- Impaired tactile sensory perception

- Medications

Table D.2   Risk Factors for Decubitus Ulcers (continued)

- Restraints

- Severe chronic pulmonary obstructive disease

- Sepsis

- Terminal cancer

- Chronic or end stage renal, liver, and/or heart disease

- Disease or drug-related immunosuppression

- Full body cast

- Steroid, radiation, or chemotherapy

- Renal dialysis

- Head of bed elevated the majority of the day

Table D.3   Staging System to Describe the Extent of Tissue Damage in Pressure Sores

Stage I: A persistent area of skin redness (without a break in the skin) that does not disappear within 30 minutes when pressure is relieved.

Stage II: A partial thickness of skin is lost that presents clinically as an abrasion, blister, or shallow crater.

Stage III: A full thickness of skin is lost, exposing tissues below the skin, presents as a deep crater with or without undermining adjacent tissue.

Stage IV: A full thickness of skin and subcutaneous tissue is lost, exposing muscle and/or bone.

Deglutition   Swallowing food.

Dehydration   Excessive water loss. The first symptom of dehydration is fatigue. When water loss hits five percent, the individual is at risk for heat exhaustion and experiences cramps and reduced strength. At a seven percent water loss, hallucinations may occur, as well as heat stroke, which can be life threatening.

7-Dehydrocholesterol   The precursor of **cholesterol** that is irradiated in the skin by sunlight to produce a form of **vitamin D**.

Dehydrogenase A group of **enzymes** that catalyze the removal of two hydrogens from a compound.

Delegation Giving a portion of one's responsibility and authority to a subordinate.

Dementia A disorder marked by deteriorating mental function, confusion, and lethargy.

Demographic Social statistics of populations such as age, income, education, and births.

Denaturation A process in which a **protein's** shape is distorted, causing it to lose its ability to function. In most cases, the damage cannot be reversed. Denaturation can occur both to proteins in food and to proteins in our bodies.

Denaturation can be caused by high temperatures (as when cooking), ultraviolet radiation, **acids** and **bases**, agitation or whipping, high **salt** concentration, and the salts of mercury, silver, and lead. For example, when you fry an egg, the proteins in the egg white become denatured and turn from clear to white. Denaturation of protein also can occur in the body whenever the **blood** becomes too acidic or too basic.

De Novo To make something new from the beginning of the process.

Dendrite Part of a **nerve** cell or **neuron**. See **neuron**.

Dental Caries Tooth decay. Both **sugar** and **starches** can promote tooth decay. For healthier teeth and gums:

- Eat fewer foods containing sugars and starches between meals. Eat sweets with meals.

- Brush and floss teeth regularly.

- Use a fluoride toothpaste.

- Ask your dentist or doctor about the need for supplemental fluoride, especially for children.

Deoxygenated Blood **Blood** that contains little **oxygen**.

Deoxyribonucleic Acid (DNA) A large molecule found in the cell nucleus that carries the genetic master plan. DNA is a double helix with its strands held together by hydrogen bonding between complementary **bases** and **hydrophobic** interactions.

Deoxyribose A five-carbon **sugar** found in **ribonucleic acid (RNA)**.

Dependent Variable In **research**, the variable that is dependent upon the manipulation of the **independent variable**. The dependent variable is not manipulated by the researcher. Changes that occur in the dependent variable are observed and measured.

Descriptive Research See **research**.

Descriptive Statistics See **statistics**.

Designer Foods See **functional foods**.

Desktop Publishing (DTP) Preparation of a document using a computer to design page layouts, bring in graphic images, and choose type style (also called font) and size.

Diabetic Retinopathy See **retinopathy**.

Diagnosis-Regulated Groups (DRGs) A system of paying Medicare in which the specific diagnosis category allows a certain amount of hospital time and money. DRGs were designed to contain costs.

Dialysis A process in which waste materials such as **urea** are separated from the bloodstream when the **kidneys** can no longer do this. There are two types of dialysis: hemodialysis and **peritoneal dialysis**. In hemodialysis, the individual's **blood** is filtered using an artificial kidney machine. In peritoneal dialysis, fluid is introduced into the abdominal cavity by a catheter or tube permanently placed in the **abdomen**. The fluid causes wastes in the capillaries to pass out of the blood and into the fluid. Fluid with wastes is then removed by the catheter. Peritoneal dialysis may be performed intermittently (called *intermittent peritoneal dialysis—IPD*) with a mechanical device or continuously by the patient without a mechanical device (called *continuous ambulatory peritoneal dialysis—CAPD*).

Diabetes Insipidus A condition in which not enough **antidiuretic hormone** is secreted. Symptoms include **polyuria** and **polydipsia**. Treatment is with synthetic **ADH**.

NUTRITION AND DISEASE FOCUS: DIABETES MELLITUS

A disease in which there is insufficient or ineffective **insulin**, a **hormone** that helps regulate your **blood sugar** level. When the blood sugar is above normal, such as after eating a meal, insulin is released by the **pancreas**. The insulin causes **glucose** to enter the body's cells to be used for energy. If there is no insulin or the insulin is not working, sugar can't enter the cells; high blood sugar levels (called *hyperglycemia*) result and sugar spills into the urine.

About 13 million Americans are diabetic—that's about six percent of the entire population. The life expectancy for a diabetic is only two-thirds that of the nondiabetic, and diabetes is the fourth leading cause of death. Risk factors for the most common type of diabetes include advanced age, family history, obesity, high waist-to-hip ratio, and a high fat/low carbohydrate diet.

People with diabetes are more than ordinarily vulnerable to many kinds of infections and to deterioration of the **kidneys, heart, blood** vessels, **nerves,** and vision. The National Institute of Health estimates that more than 250,000 Americans a year die from the complications of this illness, largely because it doubles their chances of having **heart attacks** and **strokes.** In addition, diabetes is the nation's leading cause of kidney failure and adult blindness. Because of the damage it can do to the blood vessels and nerves of the lower limbs, only accidents necessitate more amputations of the toes, feet, and legs.

There are two types of diabetes.

1. Type I (insulin-dependent diabetes mellitus)—This form of diabetes is seen mostly in children and adolescents. These patients make no insulin at all and therefore require frequent injections of insulin to maintain a normal level of glucose in the blood. Fewer than 10 percent of Americans who have diabetes have Type I.

2. Type II (noninsulin-dependent diabetes mellitus)—This form of diabetes is a separate disease from Type I. Patients usually are older and obesity is very common; in fact 80 percent of patients weigh 20 percent or more than they should. In Type II, the person's beta cells do make insulin and may, in fact, make too much. Here the problem is that the patient's tissues aren't sensitive enough to the hormone and so use it inefficiently. Some of these patients require insulin but many do not. Treatment is with diet, weight reduction when appropriate, exercise, and if necessary, oral hypoglycemic agents (medications taken by mouth that can stimulate the release of insulin and improve the body's sensitivity to insulin). Most diabetics fall into this category.

Although both types of diabetes are popularly called "sugar diabetes," they are not caused by eating too many sweets. High sugar levels in the blood and urine are a result of these illnesses; their exact causes are unknown. What is clear is that Type II runs in families far more often than Type I does, and that—unlike Type I which cannot be prevented—it can frequently be avoided by staying in shape.

Symptoms of Type I diabetes typically appear abruptly and include excessive, frequent urination, insatiable hunger, and unquenchable thirst. Unexplained weight loss is also common, as are blurred vision (or other vision changes), nausea and vomiting, weakness, drowsiness, and extreme fatigue.

The most immediately life-threatening aspect of Type I diabetes is the formation of poisonous acids called **ketone bodies.** They occur as an end-product of burning **fat** for energy because glucose does not get in the cells to be burned for energy. Like glucose, ketone bodies accumulate in the blood and spill into the urine.

Symptoms of Type II diabetes may include any or all those of Type I, but they are often overlooked because they tend to come on gradually and be less pronounced. Other symptoms are tingling or numbness in the lower legs, feet, or hands; skin or genital itching; and gum, **skin,** or **bladder** infections that recur and are slow to clear up. Again, many people fail to connect them with possible diabetes.

Measuring glucose levels in samples of the patient's blood is key to the diagnosis of both types of diabetes. This is first done early in the morning on an empty stomach. For more information, the blood test is repeated, usually on another day, before the patient drinks a liquid containing a known amount of glucose and at intervals afterwards.

Treatment for either type seeks to do what the human body normally does naturally: maintain a proper balance between glucose and insulin. The guiding principle is that food makes the blood glucose level rise whereas insulin and exercise make it fall. The trick is to juggle the three factors to avoid both hyperglycemia, meaning a blood glucose level that is too high, and **hypoglycemia**, meaning one that is too low. Either problem causes problems for the patient.

The cornerstone of treatment is diet, exercise, and medication.

Diabetic Diets Diets used to treat diabetes. The exact nature of the diabetic diet has changed over the years from starvation diets to more liberal diets. The current diabetic diet is based on the following principles.

- No one diet is suitable for everyone with diabetes. The diet needs to be individualized based on each person's type of diabetes, food preferences, culture, age, lifestyle, medication, other health concerns, education, nutrition status, medical treatment goals, and other factors.

- The goals for meal planning are to maintain the best **glucose** control possible, keep **blood** levels of **fat** and **cholesterol** in normal ranges, maintain or get body weight within a desirable range, and meet all nutrient needs.

- **Sugar** does not have to be avoided because **sucrose** and other sugars do not impair blood sugar control any more than starchy foods do. Sugars can be incorporated into the diabetic diet as part of the total **carbohydrate** allowance. The total amount of carbohydrate consumed, rather than the source of carbohydrate, should be the priority. Because sugars appear in foods that usually contain a lot of **calories** and fat, sweets can be eaten occasionally.

- Instead of setting rigid percentages of **protein**, fat, and carbohydrates, the new guidelines recommend that protein make up 10 to 20 percent of the calories consumed. **Saturated fat** and **polyunsaturated fat** should be maintained at less than 10 percent each. The remaining 60 to 70 percent of calories will come from carbohydrates and **monounsaturated fats**. The distribution of the calories depends on the individual's nutritional assessment and treatment goals.

The **Exchange Lists for Meal Planning** have been developed by the American Diabetes and **American Dietetic Association** for use primarily by diabetics who need to regulate what and how much they eat. There are seven exchange lists of like foods. Each food on a list has approximately the same amount of calories, carbohydrate, fat, and protein as another in the portions listed, so that any food on a list can be exchanged, or traded, for any other food on the same list. The seven exchange lists are starch, fruit, milk, other carbohydrates, vegetables, meat and meat substitutes, and fat. Diabetics can exchange starch, fruit, or milk choices within their meal plans because they all have about the same amount of carbohydrate per serving. A patient works with the dietitian to set up an appropriate meal plan that sets up how many exchanges of each food group can be eaten at each meal and snack.

Each exchange list has a typical member with specific portion size that can be remembered:

Starch–1 slice bread, 80 calories

Meat–1 ounce lean meat, 55 calories

Vegetable–1/2 cup cooked vegetable, 25 calories

Fruit–1 small apple, 60 calories

Milk–1 cup skim milk, 90 calories

Fat–1 teaspoon margarine, 45 calories

The meat exchange is broken down into very lean, lean, medium-fat and high-fat meat, and meat alternates. Very lean and lean meats are encouraged. The milk exchange contains skim, low-fat, and whole milk exchanges. Fats are divided into three groups, based on the main type of fat they contain: monounsaturated, polyunsaturated, and saturated. There is also a listing of free foods that contain negligible calories.

Diaphram The muscle that separates the thoracic from the abdominal cavity.

Diaphysis Shift or middle region of a **long bone**.

Diarrhea Loose, watery bowel movements or stool.

Diastole A phase of the heartbeat in which the **heart muscle** relaxes. During diastole, the ventricles relax and **blood** flows into the right and left atria from the venae cavae and the pulmonary **veins**. The tricuspid and **mitral valves** are open during diastole to allow the blood to pass from the atria into the ventricles. See also **systole**.

Diastolic Pressure The bottom number in the **blood pressure** fraction that represents the pressure in the **arteries** when the **heart** is resting between beats. See also **systolic pressure** and **hypertension**.

Dicoumarol A drug that is an antagonist of **vitamin K** which is essential for **blood clotting**.

Didactic Program or Experience Learning in a classroom situation such as the typical college lecture, discussion, or laboratory.

Dietary Fiber See **fiber**.

PRACTICAL NUTRITION FOCUS: DIETARY GUIDELINES FOR AMERICANS

1. **Eat a variety of foods.**

   To obtain the nutrients and other substances needed for good health, vary the foods you eat. Foods contain combinations of nutrients and other healthful substances. No single food can supply all nutrients in the amounts you need. To make sure you get all of the nutrients and other substances needed for health, choose the recommended number of daily servings from each of the five major food groups displayed in the Food Guide Pyramid (see Table D.4).

Table D.4 Choose Foods from Each of Five Food Groups

The Food Guide Pyramid illustrates the importance of balance among food groups in a daily eating pattern. Most of the daily servings of food should be selected from the food groups closest to the base of the Pyramid, such as grains, vegetables, and fruits.

- Choose most of your foods from the grain products group (6–11 servings), the vegetable group (3–5 servings), and the fruit group (2–4 servings).

- Eat moderate amounts of foods from the milk group (2–3 servings) and the meat and beans group (2–3 servings).

- Choose sparingly foods that provide few nutrients and are high in fat and sugars.

Table D.4 Choose Foods From Each of Five Food Groups (continued)

Note: A range of servings is given for each food group. The smaller number is for people who consume about 1,600 calories a day, such as many sedentary women. The larger number is for those who consume about 2,800 calories a day, such as active men.

Source: U. S. Department of Agriculture and U. S. Department of Health and Human Services. 1995. *Nutrition and Your Health: Dietary Guidelines for Americans,* Home and Garden Bulletin No. 232.

Foods vary in their amounts of calories and nutrients. Some foods such as grain products, vegetables, and fruits have many nutrients and other healthful substances but are relatively low in calories. Fat and alcohol are high in calories. Foods high in both sugars and fat contain many calories but often are low in **vitamins, minerals,** or **fiber** (see Table D.5).

Table D.5 What Counts as a Serving *

Grain Products Group (bread, cereal, rice, and pasta)

- 1 slice of bread

- 1 ounce of ready-to-eat cereal

- 1/2 cup of cooked cereal, rice, or pasta

Vegetable Group

- 1 cup of raw leafy vegetables

- 1/2 cup of other vegetables—cooked or chopped raw

- 3/4 cup of vegetable juice

Fruit Group

- 1 medium apple, banana, orange

- 1/2 cup of chopped, cooked, or canned fruit

- 3/4 cup of fruit juice

Milk Group (milk, yogurt, and cheese)

- 1 cup of milk or yogurt

Table D.5 What Counts As a Serving * (continued)

* 1-1/2 ounces of natural cheese

* 2 ounces of processed cheese

Meat and Beans Group (meat, poultry, fish, dry beans, eggs, and nuts)

* 2-3 ounces of cooked lean meat, poultry, or fish

* 1/2 cup of cooked dry beans or 1 egg counts as 1 ounce of lean meat. Two tablespoons of peanut butter or 1/3 cup of nuts count as 1 ounce of meat.

* Some foods fit into more than one group. Dry beans, peas, and lentils can be counted as servings in either the meat and beans group or vegetable group. These "cross over" foods can be counted as servings from either one or the other group, but not both. Serving sizes indicated here are those used in the Food Guide Pyramid and based on both suggested and usually consumed portions necessary to achieve adequate nutrient intake. They differ from serving sizes on the Nutrition Facts Label, which reflect portions usually consumed.

Source: U.S. Department of Agriculture and U. S. Department of Health and Human Services. 1995. *Nutrition and Your Health: Dietary Guidelines for Americans,* Home and Garden Bulletin No. 232.

Growing children, teenage girls, and women have higher needs for some nutrients such as *calcium* and *iron* (see Tables D.6 and D.7).

Table D.6 Some Good Sources of Calcium

* Most foods in the milk group*

  * milk and dishes made with milk, such as puddings and soups made with milk

  * cheeses such as Mozzarella, Cheddar, Swiss, and Parmesan

  * yogurt

* Canned fish with soft bones such as sardines, anchovies, and salmon**

* Dark-green leafy vegetables, such as kale, mustard greens, turnip greens, and pak-choi

Table D.6 Some Good Sources of Calcium (continued)

• Tofu, if processed with calcium sulfate; read the labels

• Tortillas made from lime-processed corn; read the labels

*Some foods in this group are high in fat, cholesterol, or both. Choose lower fat, lower cholesterol foods most often. Read the labels.

Source: U.S. Department of Agriculture and U. S. Department of Health and Human Services. 1995. *Nutrition and Your Health: Dietary Guidelines for Americans*, Home and Garden Bulletin No. 232.

Where do vitamin, mineral, and fiber supplements fit in? Supplements of vitamins, minerals, or fiber also may help to meet special nutritional needs. However, supplements do not supply all of the nutrients and other substances present in foods that are important to health. Supplements of some nutrients taken regularly in large amounts are harmful. Daily vitamin and mineral supplements at or below the **Recommended Dietary Allowances** are considered safe, but are usually not needed by people who eat the variety of foods in the Food Guide Pyramid.

Table D.7 Some Good Sources of Iron

• Meats—beef, pork, lamb, liver, and other organ meats*

• Poultry—chicken, duck, and turkey, especially dark meat; liver*

• Fish—shellfish, like clams, mussels, and oysters; sardines; anchovies; and other fish*

• Leafy greens of the cabbage family, such as broccoli, kale, turnip greens, collards

• Legumes, such as lima beans and green peas; dry beans and peas, such as pinto beans, black-eyed peas, and canned baked beans

• Yeast-leavened whole-wheat bread and rolls

• Iron-enriched white bread, pasta, rice, and cereals; read the labels

* Some foods in this group are high in fat, cholesterol, or both. Choose lean, lower fat, lower cholesterol foods most often. Read the labels.

Source: U.S. Department of Agriculture and U. S. Department of Health and Human Services. 1995. *Nutrition and Your Health: Dietary Guidelines for Americans*, Home and Garden Bulletin No. 232.

Sometimes supplements are needed to meet specific nutrient requirements. For example, older women and others with little exposure to sunlight may need a **vitamin D** supplement.

Enjoy eating a variety of foods. Get the many nutrients your body needs by choosing among the varied foods you enjoy from these groups: grain products, vegetables, fruits, milk, and milk products, **protein**-rich plant foods (beans, nuts), and protein-rich animal foods (lean meat, poultry, fish, and eggs). Remember to choose lean and low-fat foods and beverages most often. Many foods you eat contain servings from more than one food group. For example, soups and stews may contain meat, beans, noodles, and vegetables.

2. **Balance the food you eat with physical activity—maintain or improve your weight.**

   Many Americans gain weight in adulthood, increasing their risk for high blood pressure, heart disease, stroke, diabetes, certain types of cancer, arthritis, breathing problems, and other illness. Therefore, most adults should not gain weight. If you are overweight and have one of these problems, you should try to lose weight, or at the very least, not gain weight (see Table D.8).

Table D.8   Healthy Adult Weights

Height*	Healthy Weight in pounds **
4'10"	91–119
4'11"	94–124
5'0"	97–128
5'1"	101–132
5'2"	104–137
5'3"	107–141
5'4"	111–146
5'5"	114–150
5'6"	118–155
5'7"	121–160
5'8"	125–164
5'9"	129–169
5'10"	132–174
5'11"	136–179
6'0"	140–184

Table D.8 Healthy Adult Weights (continued)

6'1"	144–189
6'2"	148–195
6'3"	152–200
6'4"	156–205
6'5"	160–211
6'6"	164–216

*Without shoes

**Without clothes. The higher weights apply to people with more muscle and bone, such as many men.

Source: Report of the Dietary Guidelines Advisory Committee on the Dietary Guidelines for Americans, 1995, pages 23–24.

Healthy diets and exercise can help people maintain a healthy weight, and may also help them lose weight. It is important to recognize that overweight is a chronic condition that can only be controlled with long-term changes. To reduce caloric intake:

- Eat a variety of foods that are low in **calories** and high in nutrients—read the Nutrition Facts label.
- Eat less fat and fewer high-fat foods.
- Eat smaller portions and limit second helpings of foods high in fat and calories.
- Eat more vegetables and fruits without fats and **sugars** added in preparation or at the table.
- Eat pasta, rice, breads, and cereals without fats and sugars added in preparation or at the table.
- Eat less sugars and fewer sweets (like candy, cookies, cakes, soda).
- Drink less or no **alcohol**.

If you are not physically active, spend less time in sedentary activities such as watching television, and be more active throughout the day. As people lose weight, the body becomes more efficient at using energy and the rate of weight loss may decrease. Increased physical activity will help you to continue losing weight and to avoid gaining it back (see Table D.9).

Table D.9 To Increase Calorie Expenditure by Physical Activity

Remember to accumulate 30 minutes or more of moderate physical activity on most—preferably all—days of the week.

Examples of moderate physical activities for healthy U.S. adults

- walking briskly (3–4 miles per hour)

- conditioning or general calisthenics

- home care, general cleaning

- racket sports such as table tennis

- mowing lawn, power mower

- golf—pulling cart or carrying clubs

- home repair, painting

- fishing, standing/casting

- jogging

- swimming (moderate effort)

- cycling, moderate speed (10 miles per hour)

- gardening

- canoeing leisurely (2.0–3.9 miles per hour)

- dancing

Source: U.S. Department of Agriculture and U. S. Department of Health and Human Services. 1995. *Nutrition and Your Health: Dietary Guidelines for Americans*, Home and Garden Bulletin No. 232.

3. **Choose a diet with plenty of grain products, vegetables, and fruits.**
   Grain products, vegetables, and fruits are key parts of a varied diet. They are emphasized in this guideline because they provide vitamins, minerals, **complex carbohydrates (starch and dietary fiber)**, and other substances that are important for good health. They are also generally low in fat, depending on how they are prepared and what is added to them at the table. Most

Americans of all ages eat fewer than the recommended number of servings of grain products, vegetables, and fruits, even though consumption of these foods is associated with a substantially lower risk for many chronic diseases, including certain types of cancer.

Most of the calories in your diet should come from grain products, vegetables, and fruits. These include grain products high in complex carbohydrates—breads, cereals, pasta, rice—found at the base of the Food Guide Pyramid, as well as vegetables such as potatoes and corn. Dry beans (like pinto, navy, kidney, and black beans) are included in the meat and beans group of the Pyramid, but they can count as servings of vegetables instead of meat alternatives (see Table D.10).

Table D.10   For a Diet with Plenty of Grain Products, Vegetables, and Fruits, Eat Daily

6-11 servings* of grain products (breads, cereals, pasta, and rice)

- Eat products made from a variety of whole grains, such as wheat, rice, oats, corn, and barley.

- Eat several servings of whole-grain breads and cereals daily.

- Prepare and serve grain products with little or no fats and sugars.

3-5 servings* of various vegetables and vegetable juices

- Choose dark-green leafy and deep-yellow vegetables often.

- Eat dry beans, peas, and lentils often.

- Eat starchy vegetables, such as potatoes and corn.

- Prepare and serve vegetables with little or no fats.

2-4 servings* of various fruits and fruit juices

- Choose citrus fruits or juices, melons, or berries regularly.

- Eat fruits as desserts or snacks.

- Drink fruit juices.

- Prepare and serve fruits with little or no added sugars.

Table D.10   For a Diet with Plenty of Grain Products, Vegetables, and
Fruits, Eat Daily (continued)

Source: U. S. Department of Agriculture and U. S. Department of Health and
Human Services. 1995. *Nutrition and Your Health: Dietary Guidelines for Americans*, Home and Garden Bulletin No. 232.

Plant foods provide fiber. Fiber is found only in plant foods like whole-grain breads and cereals, beans and peas, and other vegetables and fruits. Because there are different types of fiber in foods, choose a variety of foods daily. Eating a variety of fiber-containing plant foods is important for proper bowel function, can reduce symptoms of chronic constipation, diverticular disease, and hemorrhoids, and may lower the risk for heart disease and some cancers. However, some of the health benefits associated with a high-fiber diet may come from other components present in these foods, not just from fiber itself.

Plant foods provide a variety of vitamins and minerals essential for health, such as **vitamin C, vitamin B6, carotenoids,** and **folate**.

The **antioxidant** nutrients found in plant foods (e.g., vitamin C, carotenoids, **vitamin E,** and certain minerals) are presently of great interest to scientists and the public because of their potentially beneficial role in reducing the risk for cancer and certain other chronic diseases (see Table D.11).

Table D.11   Some Good Sources of Carotenoids and Folate

Carotenoids	Folate
• Dark-green leafy vegetables (such as spinach, collards, kale, mustard greens, turnip greens, broccoli, carrots, pumpkin, calabasa, red pepper, sweet potatoes, and tomatoes	• Dry beans (like red beans, navy beans, and soybeans)
	• Lentils
	• Chickpeas, cowpeas, and peanuts
• Fruits like mango, papaya, cantaloupe	• Many vegetables, especially leafy greens (spinach, cabbage, brussels sprouts, romaine, looseleaf lettuce), peas, okra, sweet corn, beets and broccoli
	• Fruits such as oranges, orange juice, blackberries, boysenberries, kiwifruit, oranges, plantains, strawberries, and pineapple juice

4. Choose a diet low in fat, saturated fat, and cholesterol.

Some dietary fat is needed for good health. Fats supply energy and **essential fatty acids** and promote absorption of the fat-soluble vitamins A, D, E, and K. Most people are aware that high levels of saturated fat and cholesterol in the diet are linked to increased blood cholesterol levels and a greater risk for heart disease. More Americans are now eating less fat, saturated fat, and cholesterol-rich foods than in the recent past, and fewer people are dying from the most common form of heart disease. Still, many people continue to eat high-fat diets, the number of overweight people has increased, and the risk of heart disease and certain cancers (also linked to fat intake) remains high. This guideline emphasizes the continued importance of choosing a diet with less total fat, saturated fat, and cholesterol (see Table D.12).

Table D.12   For a Diet Low in Fat, Saturated Fat, and Cholesterol

Fats and Oils

- Use fats and oils sparingly in cooking and at the table.

- Use small amounts of salad dressings and spreads such as butter, margarine, and mayonnaise.

- Consider using low-fat or fat-free dressings for salads

- Choose vegetable oils and soft margarines most often because they are lower in saturated fat than solid shortenings and animal fats, even though their caloric content is the same.

- Check the Nutrition Facts Label to see how much fat and saturated fat are in a serving; choose foods lower in fat and saturated fat.

Grain Products, Vegetables, and Fruits

- Choose low-fat sauces with pasta, rice, and potatoes.

- Use as little fat as possible to cook vegetables and grain products.

- Season with herbs, spices, lemon juice, and fat-free or low-fat salad dressings.

Meat, Poultry, Fish, Eggs, Beans, and Nuts

- Choose two to three servings of lean fish, poultry, meats, or other protein-rich foods, such as beans, daily. Use meats labeled "lean" or "extra lean." Trim fat from meat; take skin off poultry. (Three ounces of cooked lean beef or chicken without skin—a piece the size of a deck of cards—provides about 6 grams of fat; a piece of chicken with skin or untrimmed meat of that size may have as much as twice this amount of fat.) Most beans and bean products are almost fat-free and are a good source of protein and fiber.

Table D.12 For a Diet Low in Fat, Saturated Fat, and Cholesterol (Continued)

- Limit intake of high-fat processed meats such as sausages, salami, and other cold cuts; choose lower fat varieties by reading the Nutrition Facts Label.

- Limit the intake of organ meats (three ounces of cooked chicken liver have about 540 mg of cholesterol); use egg yolks in moderation (one egg yolk has about 215 mg of cholesterol). Egg whites contain no cholesterol and can be used freely.

Milk and Milk Products

- Choose skim or low-fat milk, fat-free or low-fat yogurt, and low-fat cheese.

- Have two to three low-fat servings daily. Add extra calcium to your diet without added fat by choosing fat-free yogurt and low-fat milk more often. [One cup of skim milk has almost no fat, 1 cup of 1 percent milk has 2.5 grams of fat, 1 cup of 2 percent milk has 5 grams (one teaspoon) of fat, and 1 cup of whole milk has 8 grams of fat.] If you do not consume foods from this group, eat other calcium-rich foods (Table D.6).

Source: U.S. Department of Agriculture and U. S. Department of Health and Human Services. 1995. *Nutrition and Your Health: Dietary Guidelines for Americans*, Home and Garden Bulletin No. 232.

Choose a diet that provides no more than 30 percent of total calories from fat. The upper limit on the grams of fat in your diet will depend on the calories you need (see Table D.13).

Table D.13 Maximum Total Fat Intake at Different Calorie Levels

Calories	1,600	2,200	2,800
Total fat (grams)	53	73	93

Mono- and polyunsaturated fat sources should replace saturated fats within this 30 percent limit. Partially hydrogenated vegetable oils, such as those used in many **margarines** and shortenings, contain a particular form of unsaturated fat known as **trans-fatty acids** that may raise blood cholesterol levels, although not as much as saturated fat.

Advice in the previous sections does not apply to infants and toddlers below the age of 2 years. After that age, children should gradually adopt a diet that, by about 5 years of age, contains no more than 30 percent of calories from fat.

5. **Choose a diet moderate in sugars. Sugars come in many forms.**
    Sugars are carbohydrates. Dietary carbohydrates also include the complex carbohydrates starch and fiber. During digestion all carbohydrates except fiber break down into sugars. Sugars and starches occur naturally in many foods that also supply other nutrients. Examples of these foods include milk, fruits, some vegetables, breads, cereals, and grains. Americans eat sugars in many forms, and most people like their taste. Some sugars are used as natural preservatives, thickeners, and baking aids in foods; they are often added to foods during processing and preparation or when they are eaten. The body cannot tell the difference between naturally occurring and added sugars because they are identical chemically (see Table D.14).

Table D.14 On a Food Label, Sugars Include

- brown sugar

- corn sweetener

- corn syrup

- fructose

- fruit juice concentrate

- glucose (dextrose)

- high-fructose corn syrup

- honey

- invert sugar

- lactose

- maltose

- molasses

- raw sugar

- [table] sugar (sucrose)

- syrup

A food is likely to be high in sugars if one of the above terms appears first or second in the ingredients list, or if several of them are listed.

Source: U.S. Department of Agriculture and U. S. Department of Health and Human Services. 1995. *Nutrition and Your Health: Dietary Guidelines for Americans,* Home and Garden Bulletin No. 232.

Scientific evidence indicates that diets high in sugars do not cause hyperactivity or diabetes.

If you wish to maintain your weight when you eat less fat, replace the lost calories from fat with equal calories from fruits, vegetables, and grain products, found in the lower half of the Food Guide Pyramid. Some foods that contain a lot of sugars supply calories but few or no nutrients. These foods are located at the top of the Pyramid. For very active people with high calorie needs, sugars can be an additional source of energy.

Sugar substitutes such as **sorbitol, saccharin,** and **aspartame** are ingredients in many foods. Most sugar substitutes do not provide significant calories and therefore may be useful in the diets of people concerned about calorie intake. Foods containing sugar substitutes, however, may not always be lower in calories than similar products that contain sugars.

Both sugar and starches can promote tooth decay. For healthier teeth and gums:

- Eat fewer foods containing sugars and starches between meals.

- Brush and floss teeth regularly.

- Use a fluoride toothpaste.

- Ask your dentist or doctor about the need for supplemental fluoride, especially for children.

6. **Choose a diet moderate in salt and sodium.**
   Sodium and salt are found mainly in processed and prepared foods. Sodium and sodium chloride—known commonly as salt—occur naturally in foods, usually in small amounts. Salt and other sodium-containing ingredients are often used in food processing. Some people add salt and salty sauces, such as soy sauce, to their food at the table, but most dietary sodium or salt comes from foods to which salt has already been added during processing or preparation. Although many people add salt to enhance the taste of foods, their preference may weaken with eating less salt.

   Sodium is associated with **high blood pressure**. In the body, sodium plays an essential role in regulation of fluids and blood pressure. Many studies in diverse populations have shown that a high sodium intake is associated with higher blood pressure. Most evidence suggests that many people at risk for high blood pressure reduce their chances of developing this condition by consuming less salt or sodium. Some questions remain, partly because other factors may interact with sodium to affect blood pressure (see Table D.15).

Table D.15   To Consume Less Salt and Sodium

- Read the Nutrition Facts Label to determine the amount of sodium in the foods you purchase. The sodium content of processed foods—such as cereals, breads, soups, and salad dressings—often varies widely.

- Choose foods lower in sodium and ask your grocer or supermarket to offer more low-sodium foods. Request less salt in your meals when eating out or traveling.

- If you salt foods in cooking or at the table, add small amounts. Learn to use spices and herbs, rather than salt, to enhance the flavor of food.

- When planning meals, consider that fresh and most plain frozen vegetables are low in sodium.

- When selecting canned foods, select those prepared with reduced or no sodium. Remember that fresh fish, poultry, and meat are lower in sodium than most canned and processed ones.

- Choose foods lower in sodium content. Many frozen dinners, packaged mixes, canned soups, and salad dressings contain a considerable amount of sodium. Remember that condiments such as soy and many other sauces, pickles, and olives are high in sodium. Ketchup and mustard, when eaten in large amounts, can also contribute significant amounts of sodium to the diet. Choose lower-sodium varieties.

- Choose fresh fruits and vegetables as a lower-sodium alternative to salted snack foods.

Source: U.S. Department of Agriculture and U. S. Department of Health and Human Services. 1995. *Nutrition and Your Health: Dietary Guidelines for Americans*, Home and Garden Bulletin No. 232.

Following other guidelines in the **Dietary Guidelines for Americans** may also help prevent high blood pressure. An important example is the guideline on weight and physical activity. The role of body weight in blood pressure control is well documented. Blood pressure increases with weight and decreases when weight is reduced. The guideline to consume a diet with plenty of fruits and vegetables is relevant because fruits and vegetables are naturally lower in sodium and fat and may help with weight reduction and control. Consuming more fruits and vegetables also increases potassium intake, which may help to reduce blood pressure. Increased physical activity helps lower blood pressure and control weight (see Table D.16).

Table D.16 Some Good Sources of Potassium

- Vegetables and fruits in general, especially
  - potatoes and sweet potatoes
  - spinach, swiss chard, broccoli, winter squashes, and parsnips
  - dates, bananas, cantaloupes, mangoes, plantains, dried apricots, raisins, prunes, orange juice, and grapefruit juice
  - dry beans, peas, lentils
- Milk and yogurt are good sources of potassium and have less sodium than cheese; cheese has much less potassium and usually has added salt

Source: U.S. Department of Agriculture and U. S. Department of Health and Human Services. 1995. *Nutrition and Your Health: Dietary Guidelines for Americans*, Home and Garden Bulletin No. 232.

Most Americans consume more salt than is needed. The Nutrition Facts Label lists a **Daily Value** of 2,400 mg per day for sodium. One level teaspoon of salt provides about 2,300 milligrams of sodium.

Fresh fruits and vegetables have very little sodium. The food groups in the Food Guide Pyramid include some foods that are high in sodium and other foods that have very little sodium, or can be prepared in ways that add flavor without adding salt. Read the Nutrition Facts Label to compare and help identify foods lower in sodium within each group. Use herbs and spices to flavor food. Try to choose forms of foods that you frequently consume that are lower in sodium and salt.

7. **If you drink alcoholic beverages, do so in moderation.**
Alcoholic beverages supply calories but few or no nutrients. The alcohol in these beverages has effects that are harmful when consumed in excess. These effects of alcohol may alter judgment and can lead to dependency and a great many other serious health problems. Alcoholic beverages have been used to enhance the enjoyment of meals by many societies throughout human history. If adults choose to drink alcoholic beverages, they should consume them only in moderation. Moderate drinking is defined as no more than one drink per day for women and no more than two drinks per day for men. Count as one drink:

- 12 ounces of regular beer (150 calories)
- 5 ounces of wine (100 calories)
- 1.5 ounces of 80-proof distilled spirits (100 calories)

(Adapted from *Nutrition and Your Health: Dietary Guidelines for Americans*, Fourth Edition, 1995, U.S. Department of Agriculture and U. S. Department of Health and Human Services.)

Dietetic Internship A structured educational program that provides dietetic students the opportunity to develop entry level dietetic performance skills through supervised practice in healthcare facilities and other settings. Dietetic internships are designed to meet the **American Dietetic Association's** Performance Requirements. Internships normally take place after completion of the A.D.A. **Didactic Program.**

Dietetics The profession of the science and art of human nutritional care.

Dietetic Practice The performance of activities in **dietetics.**

Dietetic Technician A professional who works as a member of a foodservice or health team often under the supervision of a dietitian in a healthcare setting. By completing an **American Dietetic Association**-approved Dietetic Technician Program, earning an associate degree, and passing a credentialing exam, dietetic technicians can become registered. Registered dietetic technicians are permitted to use the initials DTR to signify professional competence.

Diet History A unique assessment tool of the **client's** food intake patterns. A diet history has two features.

1. It describes actual food intake.

2. It gives information about why the patient makes certain food choices.

The most frequently used diet history is a 24-hour diet recall in which the patient is asked to recall everything taken in during the previous day. A client's diet history is a valuable screening tool for long- and short-term nutritional deficiencies. (*Screening* is the term used to describe the use of preliminary nutrition assessment techniques, such as diet history, to identify people who are at nutritional risk.) It is a preliminary step to planning and implementing the nutritional program for the client. The task of gathering diet history information should be part of the first contact with the client (see Figure D.1).

Three-day food records and **food frequency questionnaires** are also used to obtain more diet history information. A weekly food frequency questionnaire is a useful tool. When used in combination with a 24-hour diet recall, the food frequency questionnaire can verify the accuracy, or inaccuracy, of the diet recall. It has two parts: a list of foods and an indication of how frequently they are eaten each day or each week.

Diet Therapy The use of food and drink to treat a disease, correct a nutritional deficiency, maintain normal nutrition, change body weight, allow rest to the body or an **organ**, or generally act as a supplement to medical or surgical care.

Figure D.1   24-Hour Diet Recall

Time	Food (Describe how cooked, brand name, etc.)	Portion Size

Comments: _____

Special Likes: _____

Special Dislikes: _____

Food Group Omitted?(Specify): _____

Calories Appropriate	☐ Yes	☐ No
Fat Level Appropriate	☐ Yes	☐ No
Sodium Level Appropriate	☐ Yes	☐ No
Sugar Level Appropriate	☐ Yes	☐ No

Patient Name: _____ Date: _____

Differentiation   A change in the structure and function of a cell as it matures.

Diffusion   The net movement of molecules or ions from regions of greater to regions of lesser concentration.

Digestion   The breakdown of food into its components in the mouth, **stomach**, and **small intestine** with the help of **digestive enzymes**. Complex

proteins are digested or broken down into their building blocks called **amino acids**; complicated **sugars** are reduced to simple sugars such as **glucose**; and **fat** molecules are broken down into **fatty acids** and **glycerol**.

Digestive Enzymes **Enzymes** that break down food into its components to be absorbed (see Table D.17).

Table D.17 Major Digestive Enzymes

Site*	Enzyme Name	Action
Mouth	Salivary amylase	Breaks down starch into dextrins.
Stomach	Pepsin	Breaks down proteins to make them shorter in length.
Small intestine	Pancreatic amylase	Breaks down starch to maltose.
	Sucrase	Breaks down sucrose to glucose and fructose.
	Lactase	Breaks down lactose to glucose and galactose.
	Maltase	Breaks down maltose to glucose.
	Pancreatic lipase	Breaks down triglycerides to fatty acids and glycerol.

Table D.17 Major Digestive Enzymes (continued)

	Intestinal lipase	Breaks down triglycerides to fatty acids and glycerol.
	Aminopeptidase	Breaks peptide bonds of protein from amino- terminal end.
	Dipeptidase	Breaks peptide bonds of dipeptides to free amino acids.
	Trypsin	Breaks peptide bonds inside protein.
	Chymotrypsin	Breaks peptide bonds inside protein.
	Carboxypeptidase	Breaks peptide bonds of protein from carboxyl- terminal end.

* This is the site where the enzymes are made and act with one exception. The pancreas makes pancreatic amylase, pancreatic lipase, trypsin, chymotrypsin, and carboxypeptidase.

Diglyceride Glycerol attached to two **fatty acids.**

Dipeptide A **peptide** containing two **amino acids.**

Dipeptidases See **digestive enzymes.**

Directing A managerial activity consisting of assigning tasks, giving instructions, training, and guiding and controlling performance.

Disaccharide Two single **sugars** linked together. The most common are **sucrose, lactose,** and **maltose.**

Discharge Planning In hospitals and some other institutions, the plans made for the patient when leaving the institution so that appropriate medical and nutritional care continues.

Discipline (1) A condition or state of orderly conduct and adherence to rules, regulations, and procedures; (2) action to enforce orderly conduct and adherence to rules, regulations, and procedures.

Distal Convoluted Tubule One of the renal tubules in the **nephron** or funtional unit of the **kidney.** Also see **nephron.**

Diuresis Increased formation and excretion of urine.

Diuretics A category of drugs frequently used to treat **hypertension.** Diuretics stimulate urination and some also deplete **potassium.**

Diversity The physical and cultural dimensions that separate and distinguish individuals and groups: age, gender, physical abilities and qualities, ethnicity, race, and sexual preference. Culture includes many aspects of our lives—the language we speak, our values, the way we dress, the music we like, the way we interact, and the food we eat.

The population of the United States is diverse, and its racial and ethnic diversity is growing rapidly. In fact, according to the 1990 census, almost one in four Americans has African, Asian, Hispanic, or American Indian ancestry. That figure is projected to rise to almost one in three by the year 2020 and almost one in two by the year 2050. The growth of culturally distinct groups in the United States has two main origins: a higher birth rate for many ethnic groups and an increase in immigration, including the entry of refugees as well as undocumented persons. See also counseling (see Table D.18).

Table D.18 Guidelines for Cross-Cultural Counseling

Preparing for Counseling

- Understand your own cultural values and biases.
- Acquire basic knowledge of cultural values, health beliefs, and nutrition practices for client groups you routinely serve.

Table D.18 Guidelines for Cross-Cultural Counseling (continued)

- Be respectful of, interested in, and understanding of other cultures without being judgmental.

Enhancing Communication

- Determine the level of fluency in English and arrange for an interpreter, if needed.

- Ask how the client prefers to be addressed.

- Learn greetings, proper pronunciation of names, and attitudes towards personal space and eye contact.

- Allow the client to choose seating for comfortable personal space and eye contact.

- Avoid body language that may be offensive or misunderstood.

- Speak directly to the client, whether an interpreter is present or not.

- Choose a speech rate and style that promotes understanding and demonstrates respect for the client.

- Avoid slang, technical jargon, and complex sentences.

- Use open-ended questions or questions phrased in several ways to obtain information.

- Determine the client's reading ability before using written materials in the process.

- Write numbers down for the client—for example, with recipe amounts. People easily confuse numbers spoken in a new language.

- Don't think that people who are struggling with English are stupid. Applaud them for trying to make things easier for you. They are trying to learn your language instead of asking you to learn theirs.

- Be friendly, accepting, and approachable. Everyone relates to a smile.

Promoting Positive Change

- Build on cultural practices, reinforcing those which are positive, and promoting change only in those that are harmful.

- Check for client understanding and acceptance of recommendations.

Diverticulitis Inflammation of the diverticula in the intestines. Diverticulitis occurs in patients who have **diverticulosis**. Dietary treatment often restricts **fiber** so that it doesn't add to the inflammation. See also **diverticulosis**.

Diverticulosis A disease of the intestine in which the intestinal walls become weakened and bulge out into pockets called diverticula. These pockets can become inflamed (which is called **diverticulitis**). A low-**fiber** diet may be the cause for this condition so increased fiber is often recommended to decrease the pressure in the intestine that causes the pockets to form.

Docosahexanoic Acid (DHA) A **polyunsaturated omega-3 fatty acid** found in seafood, especially fatty fish. DHA is a precursor of the **eicosanoids**, **hormone**-like substances. See also **eicosanoids**.

Dopamine A **neurotransmitter** that is deficient in persons with **Parkinson's disease**. See **Parkinson's disease**.

Double Bond A covalent bond in which two atoms share two pairs of electrons.

Down's Syndrome A birth defect due to chromosomal abnormality that is marked by mental retardation and physical defects. Children with Down's syndrome often are short with low-set ears and a mongoloid slant to the eyes. Also called **mongolism**.

Drug-Nutrient Interaction The effects foods and drugs have on each other which can determine whether medications do their job and whether your body gets the nutrients it needs. The extent of interaction between foods and drugs depends on the drug dosage and on the individual's age, size, and specific medical condition. In general, though, the presence of food in the **stomach** and intestines can influence a drug's effectiveness by slowing down or speeding up the time it takes the medicine to go through the **gastrointestinal tract** to the site in the body where it is needed.

Food also contains natural and added chemicals that can react with certain drugs in ways that make the drugs virtually useless. Some reactions can be downright dangerous, triggering a medical crisis or, in rare instances, even death. It is because of these interactions that your doctor tells you to take certain medications on an empty stomach, some just before meals, and some with meals.

A major way food affects drugs is by enhancing or impeding **absorption** of the drug into the bloodstream. There are a few cases in which foods speed up absorption. For example, **blood** levels of griseofulvin, a substance that combats fungus infections such as ringworm, rise markedly if the patient eats fatty foods before taking the drug.

More commonly, though, food and beverages interfere with absorption. A classic interaction is the one between tetracycline compounds and dairy products. The **calcium** in milk, cheese, and yogurt impairs absorption of tetracycline. On the other hand, taking some **iron** supplements with citrus fruits or juices that contain **ascorbic acid** enhances absorption of the iron.

Just as some foods can affect the way drugs behave in the body, some drugs can affect the way the body uses food. Drugs may act in various ways to impair proper **nutrition**: by hastening excretion of certain nutrients, by hindering absorption of nutrients, or by interfering with the body's ability to convert nutrients into usable forms. Nutrient depletion of the body occurs gradually, but for those taking drugs over long periods of time, these interactions can lead to deficiencies of certain **vitamins** and **minerals** especially in children, the elderly, those with poor diets, and the chronically ill.

Some drugs inhibit nutrient absorption by their effect on the wall of the intestine. Among these are colchicine, a drug prescribed for gout, and mineral oil, an ingredient used in some over-the-counter laxatives. Mineral oil can interfere with absorption of **vitamin D**, **vitamin K**, and **carotene**.

A number of drugs affect specific vitamins and minerals. The antihypertension drug hydralazine and the antituberculosis drug INH can deplete the body's supply of **vitamin B6** by inhibiting production of the **enzyme** necessary to convert the vitamin into a form the body can use or by combining with the vitamin to form a compound that is excreted.

Duodenum The first section of the **small intestine**. About one foot long, the duodenum receives the digested food from the **stomach** as well as **bile** from the **liver** and **gallbladder**, and pancreatic juice from the **pancreas**. In the wall of the duodenum (and throughout the entire small intestine) are tiny, fingerlike projections (villi). The muscular walls mix the **chyme** with the digestive juices and bring the nutrients into contact with the villi and the projections on the villi, called microvilli or the **brush border**. The microvilli contain **digestive enzymes** (called brush border enzymes) that are not secreted into the intestine but instead remain attached to the cell membrane.

Most nutrients pass through the villi of the duodenum into either the **blood** or **lymph** vessels where they are transported to the liver and to the cells of the body. The duodenum connects with the second section of the small intestine (**jejunum**).

Dysgeusia Abnormal taste.

Dysphagia Difficulty in swallowing.

Dyspnea Difficulty breathing.

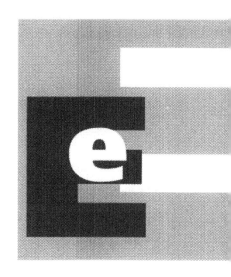

Eating Disorders Each year millions of people in the United States develop serious and sometimes life-threatening eating disorders. The vast majority—more than 90 percent—of those afflicted with eating disorders are adolescent and young adult women. One reason that women in this age group are particularly vulnerable to eating disorders is their tendency to go on strict diets to achieve an "ideal" figure. Researchers have found that such stringent dieting can play a key role in triggering eating disorders. The actual cause of eating disorders is not entirely understood, but many risk factors have been identified. Risk factors may include a high degree of perfectionism, low self-esteem, genetics, or family preoccupation with dieting and weight.

Eating disorder patients deal with two sets of issues: those surrounding their eating behaviors and those surrounding their **interactions** with others and themselves. Eating disorders are considered a mental disorder and both psychotherapy and medical nutrition therapy are cornerstones of treatment.

Table E.1 Common Symptoms of Eating Disorders

Symptoms	Anorexia Nervosa*	Bulimia Nervosa*	Binge Eating Disorder
Excessive weight loss in relatively short period of time	•		
Continuation of dieting although bone-thin	•		
Dissatisfaction with appearance; belief that body is fat, even though severely underweight	•		
Loss of monthly menstrual periods	•	•	
Unusual interest in food and development of strange eating rituals	•	•	

Table E.1 Common Symptoms of Eating Disorders (continued)

Symptoms	Anorexia Nervosa*	Bulimia Nervosa*	Binge Eating Disorder
Eating in secret	•	•	•
Obsession with exercise	•	•	
Serious depression	•	•	•
Binging—consumption of large amounts of food		•	•
Vomiting or use of drugs to stimulate vomiting, bowel movements, and urination		•	
Binging but no noticeable weight gain		•	
Disappearance into bathroom for long periods of time to induce vomiting		•	
Abuse of drugs or alcohol		•	•

*Some individuals suffer from anorexia and bulimia and have symptoms of both disorders.

Source: National Institute of Mental Health. 1993. *Eating Disorders* NIH Publication No. 93–3477.

Approximately one percent of adolescent girls develop **anorexia nervosa**, a dangerous condition in which they can literally starve themselves to dealth. Another two to three percent of young women develop **bulimia nervosa**, a destructive pattern of excessive overeating followed by vomiting or other "purging" behaviors to control their weight. The most recently recognized eating disorder, **binge eating disorder**, could turn out to be the most common. With this disorder, binges are not followed by purges so these individuals often become overweight. Eating disorders also occur in men and older women, but much less frequently (see Table E.1).

The consequences of eating disorders can be severe, with 1 in 10 cases leading to death from starvation, **cardiac arrest**, or suicide over the course of 10 years. The outlook is better for bulimia than for anorexia. Anorexia patients tend to relapse more. Many patients with anorexia or bulimia also suffer from other psychiatric illnesses such as clinical depression, anxiety, obsessive-compulsive disorder, or substance abuse. Fortunately, increasing awareness of the dangers of eating disorders—sparked by medical studies and extensive media coverage of the illness—has led many people to seek help. Nevertheless, some people with eating disorders refuse to admit that they have a problem and do not get treatment. Family members and friends can help recognize the problem and encourage the person to seek treatment. The earlier treatment is started, the better the chance of a full recovery (see Table E.2).

Table E.2 Do You Have an Eating Disorder?

A positive answer to one or more of these questions may indicate an eating disorder.

1. Do you eat large amounts of food within an hour or two while feeling out of control and by yourself?

2. Do you frequently eat a lot of food when you are not hungry and usually when you are alone?

3. Do you feel very guilty after overeating?

4. Do you make yourself vomit or use laxatives or diurectics to purge yourself?

5. Do you carefully make sure you only eat a small amount of calories each day, such as 500 calories or less, and exercise a lot?

6. Do you avoid going out to maintain your eating and exercise schedule?

7. Do you feel food controls your life?

Eclampsia See **pregnancy-induced hypertension.**

Economic Evaluation Methods used to determine the economic impact of programs. (See Table E.3.)

Edema Swelling due to an abnormal accumulation of fluid in the intercellular spaces.

Edentulous Without natural teeth.

Efferent Neurons **Neurons** that conduct impulses out of the central nervous to **muscles, glands,** and **organs.** Also called **motor neurons.** See also **neuron.**

Eicosanoids The **hormone**-like substances made from the **essential fatty acids, linoleic acid** and **linolenic acid.** The eicosanoids include three **lipid** families: **prostaglandins,** thromboxanes, and leukotrienes. The eicosanoids affect many important physiological functions such as **blood pressure, blood clotting,** and the **immune response.** See also **prostaglandins.**

Table E.3 Definitions, Objectives, and Calculations of Types of Economic Evaluations

Variable	Cost-effectiveness analysis	Cost-benefit analysis	Cost-utility analysis	Cost-of-illness studies
Definition	Measures the costs and outcomes of programs or services provided. Costs may include expenditures only or expenditures minus savings. Consequences are measured in terms of a concrete desired health outcome.	Inputs and outcomes of program are expressed in dollar terms; the benefits of the program minus the costs of the program are determined to be the net benefit or cost.	Similar to cost-effectiveness analysis, but measures the consequences of program alternatives in terms of preferences or quality (e.g., quality-adjusted life years, quality of life).	Computes lifetime costs and financial consequences of an illness in current dollar value. Direct costs (medical care) plus indirect costs (dollar value of lost productivity) over a lifetime equal the cost of an illness.
Objective	To compare two or more alternative means of achieving a desired outcome in terms of efficiency of dollar cost per unit of outcome.	To assess whether the investment in a program yields a positive return.	To compare two or more alternatives in terms of a uniform quality or preference measure.	To determine economic impact to society of an illness.

Table E.3 Definitions, Objectives, and Calculations of Types of Economic Evaluations (continued)

Variable	Cost-effectiveness analysis	Cost-benefit analysis	Cost-utility analysis	Cost-of-illness studies
Calculation	Costs are in dollar terms and outcomes are in natural units. Cost-effectiveness ratio = $\dfrac{(\$) \text{ cost}}{\text{unit of outcome}}$ compared to another alternative $\dfrac{(\$) \text{ cost}}{\text{unit of outcome}}$	$\$$ net benefits = $\$$ benefits of a program − $\$$ costs of a program. Benefit-cost ratio = $\dfrac{(\$) \text{ benefits}}{(\$) \text{ costs}}$	Same ratio as cost-effectiveness, but the denominator outcome reflects quality of life or patient preferences	Cost-of-illness = direct costs + indirect costs

Source: Franz, Marion J.; Splett, Patricia L.; Monk, Arlene; Barry, Barbara; McClain, Kathryn; Weaver, Tanya; Upham, Paul; Bergenstal, Richard; and Mazze, Roger S.: Cost-effectiveness of medical nutrition therapy provided by dietitians for persons with noninsulin-dependent diabetes mellitus. Copyright The American Dietetic Association. Reprinted by permission from *Journal of The American Dietetic Association,* Vol. 95: 1019.

Eicosapentaenoic Acid (EPA) An **omega-3 polyunsaturated fatty acid** found in seafood, especially fatty fish, that is found in the brain, eyes, and other tissues. EPA is a precursor of the **eicosanoids**, hormone-like substances. See also **eicosanoids**.

Elastin A type of fibrous **protein** that stretches like rubber bands. Elastin is found in the lungs, the walls of large **blood** vessels, and elastic ligaments.

Electrocardiogram (ECG, EKG) A picture made by an electrocardiograph. An electrocardiograph is a device that records the electric activity of the **heart**, and thereby helps in diagnosis of cardiac abnormalities.

Electroencephalography (EEG) The process of recording brainwave activity. EEG is used to diagnose seizure disorders, tumors, clots, and other diseases and injury to the brain.

Electrolyte A chemical element or compound that ionizes in solution and can carry an electric current. The most common electrolytes in the **blood** are **sodium, potassium**, and **chloride**. Potassium, with a positive charge, is found mainly within the cells. Sodium (with a positive charge) and chloride (with a negative charge) are found mostly in the fluid outside the cells. The electrolytes maintain two critical balancing acts in the body: **water balance** and **acid-base balance**. See also **water balance** and **acid-base balance**.

Electron Transport Chain A series of oxidative-reduction reactions that transport electrons via the **coenzymes NADH** and **FADH2**. NADH and FADH2 are reoxidized. In the electron transport chain, a series of electron carriers transport electrons from the reduced coenzymes to **oxygen**, with energy going into **ATP**. The electron transport chain takes place in the mitochondria. Also called the *respiratory chain*.

Electrophoresis A biochemical technique of separating substances by their movement in an electric field.

Electronic Mail (E Mail) Mail that is typed into a computer and transmitted over phone lines connecting the computers. E mail is commonly available in organizations to allow quick distribution of mail to many people.

Elemental Formula A formula made of nutrients that require no digesting and are readily absorbed. Elemental formulas are used in nutrition support. Also called *chemically defined diets*.

Emboli (Singular: embolus) A traveling **blood** clot or other substance that blocks a blood vessel.

Embryo The name of the fertilized egg from conception to the eighth week. After the eighth week, it is called a **fetus**.

Emetic Causing vomiting. An emetic medicine causes vomiting, which may be useful in certain poisoning situations.

Empathy Understanding and identifying with the feelings, thoughts, and concerns of someone else. In **counseling**, empathy helps to build rapport and establish a safe arena in which to encourage change.

Employee Assistance Program (EAP) **Counseling** programs available to employees to provide a confidential and professional counseling and referral service.

Employment-at-Will A common-law that states employers have the right to hire, fire, demote, or promote who they want, unless there is a contract or law that states otherwise.

Empty Calories Foods that provide few nutrients for the number of **calories** they have.

Emulsification The process of breaking up **fat** globules into small droplets so **enzymes** can get in and break them down further.

Emulsifier A substance that can break up **fat** globules into small droplets. Emulsifiers can mix with both fat and water.

Endarterectomy Surgical removal of the innermost lining (**tunica intima**) of an **artery** thickened by fatty deposits and thromboses.

Encephalopathy Any degenerative disease of the brain.

Endemic A disease or infection common to a population or geographical area but only in a small number of cases.

Endergonic Reactions Chemical reactions that require energy.

Endocardium The inner lining of the **heart** chambers.

Endocarditis Inflammation of the **endocardium** caused by bacteria. Also called bacterial endocarditis. Endocarditis is treated with antibiotics. See also **mitral valve prolapse**.

Endocrine System A system of **glands** found in many locations in the body that secrete **hormones** or chemical messengers directly into the **blood**. Examples of endocrine glands include the **pancreas (islets of Langerhans), adrenal glands, pituitary gland, thyroid gland, ovaries** in females, and the testes in males. Hormones travel in the blood to target tissues where they bind to receptor **proteins** on the target tissue's cells. When the hormone combines with its receptor protein, a sequence of changes takes place in the target cells.

Endoenzymes **Enzymes** located in the cell.

Endogenous Coming from inside the organism.

Endometriosis A growth of endometrial tissue outside of the uterus. In endometriosis, endometrial tissue is found in places such as the **ovaries** and **small intestine.**

Endometrium The inner lining of the uterus.

Endoplasmic Reticulum In the cytoplasm of the cell, a network of canals.

Endorphin A **peptide** in the brain that acts like morphine.

Energy Balance The balance between energy intake (**calories** taken in) and energy output (calories burned in normal metabolic activities plus exercise).

Energy-Yielding Nutrients The nutrients that can be burned as fuel to provide energy for the body. They include **carbohydrate, fat,** and **protein.**

Enriched Foods Foods to which nutrients have been added that were originally in the food but were removed during processing. For example, when whole wheat is milled to produce white flour, nutrients are lost. White flour must be enriched by law with three **vitamins** and **iron** to make up for some of these lost nutrients.

Enteral Feeding Feeding that uses the **gastrointestinal tract,** either by mouth or through a feeding tube. See also **tube feeding.**

Enteral Formulas Formulas, usually liquids, that contain essential nutrients in a caloric concentration appreciably in excess of normal requirements (see Table E.4).

Enteritis Inflammation of the intestine.

Enterohepatic Circulation The path of **bile salts** from the **liver** to the **gallbladder** and the intestines where much of them are reabsorbed from the **ileum** and sent back to the liver.

Entitlement Program A federal program that provides funds to all qualified applicants.

Enuresis Inability to control the need to urinate, especially while sleeping.

Environmental Protection Agency (EPA) A federal agency that regulates pesticide use and clean water.

Enzyme Specialized **proteins** that can speed up chemical changes in other substances without being changed or consumed themselves. Enzymes have an active site where the catalytic reaction takes place between the enzyme and the substrate. In most cases, the active site and the substrate fit together like a key in a lock. See also **digestive enzymes.**

Eosinophils A type of **leukocyte** (**white blood cell**) that functions in the allergic response to detoxify foreign substances. Eosinophils also secrete **enzymes** that break down **blood** clots. See also **leukocyte.**

Table E.4 Enteral Tube Feeding Formulas

Type	Description	Indication for use	Advantages	Disadvantages
Standard	Isotonic, low residue. Nutritionally complete. Supplies 1.0-2.0 kcal/mL. Supplies 40 g/L protein.	Maintenance to mild stress.	Inexpensive, well tolerated.	Lacks fiber.
Fiber-containing	Low osmolarity. Nutritionally complete. Supplies 1.0-2.0 kcal/mL. Supplies approximately 44 gL protein. Whole food or soy polysaccharides provide fiber source.	Maintenance to mild stress bowel dysfunction.	Provides a well-tolerated fiber source.	May cause gas, bloating, or constipation if adequate water is not supplied.
High-nitrogen	Low osmolarity. Nutritionally complete. Supplies 1.0-1.2 kcal/mL. Supplies 44-55 g/L protein.	Residents with elevated protein needs. High. stress situations.	Well tolerated. Increased protein content without increasing caloric level.	Higher protein level may require more water. May not be suitable for patients with renal insufficiency. Usually lacks fiber.

Table E.4 Enteral Tube Feeding Formulas (continued)

Type	Description	Indication for use	Advantages	Disadvantages
High-calorie/ high-nitrogen	Nutritionally complete. Concentrated high fat content. Supplies 1.5–2.0 kcal/mL. Supplies 70–84 g/L protein.	High-stress situations for residents who have both elevated caloric and protein needs.	Concentrated formula that can be useful in residents who need to be fluid restricted.	Higher osmolarity and fat content may cause intolerance.
Elemental or chemically defined	Low residue, low fat. Predigested (may contain peptides and/or amino acids). Nutritionally °complete. Supplies 1.0 kcal/mL. Supplies 40 g/L protein.	Malabsorption syndromes, fat intolerances, or high-stress situations.	Easily digested. Well tolerated (may contain significant amounts of glutamine).	Lacks fiber. May have higher osmolarity. Expensive. Only moderate level of protein.
Disease-specific	Vary in nutritional composition, depending on disease-specific recommendations.	Specific diseases (diabetes, renal failure, respiratory failure).	May help meet nutrition requirements in residents with specific problems.	May be expensive. Questionable efficiency.

Source: Consultant Dietitians in Health Care Facilities: *Nutrition Care in Nursing Facilities.* Copyright The American Dietetic Association. Reprinted with permission, page 132.

Epidemiology The study of the distribution and determinants of disease. Epidemiological **research** can be descriptive or analytical.

Epidermis See **integumentary system**.

Epiglottis The flap that covers the **larynx** and the opening to the trachea so that food does not enter during swallowing.

Epinephrine A **hormone** produced and secreted by the adrenal medulla. Epinephrine is classified as a **catecholamine** along with **norepinephrine**. Epinephrine stimulates increased **cardiac output**, dilates respiratory passageways, increases the respiratory rate, and increases **glycogenolysis** (breakdown of **glycogen** to **glucose**) and **lipolysis** (breakdown of **triglycerides** into **glycerol** and **fatty acids**) so that blood **sugar** and fatty acid levels rise. The catecholamines work together to mimic the actions of the sympathetic nervous system by increasing the heartbeat, respiratory rate, **blood pressure**, and blood sugar levels during stress. Also called **adrenaline**.

Epiphysis End of a **long bone**.

Epiphyseal Line or Plate In the end of a **long bone**, an area of cartilage tissue that is constantly being replaced by new bony tissue as the **bone** grows.

Equal Employment Opportunity (EEO) The legal requirement that all people must be treated equally in all aspects of employment regardless of race, creed, color, national origin, age, sex, and disability unrelated to the job (see Table E.5).

Table E.5 Equal Employment Opportunity (EEO) Laws

Federal Laws and Executive Orders	Type of Employment Discrimination Prohibited	Employers Covered
Equal Pay Act of 1963	Sex differences in pay, fringe benefits, and pension for substantially equal work	Private
Title VII, 1964 Civil Rights Act	Discrimination in all human resource activities based on race, color, sex, religion, or national origin; established Equal Employment Opportunity Commission to administer the law	Private; federal, state, and local governments; unions; employment agencies
Age Discrimination in Employment Act of 1967 (as amended in 1986)	Age discrimination against those 40 years of age or older	Private; unions; employment agencies

Table E.5 Equal Employment Opportunity (EEO) Laws (continued)

Federal Laws and Executive Orders	Type of Employment Discrimination Prohibited	Employers Covered
Executive Order 11478 (1969)	Discrimination based on race, color, religion, sex, national origin, political affiliation, marital status, or physical handicap	Federal government
Equal Employment Opportunity Act of 1972	Amended Title VII; gave Equal Employment Opportunity Commission (EEOC) more power to enforce and extended coverage	Educational institutions; other employers
Vocational Rehabilitation Act of 1973, Executive Order 11914 (1974)	Discrimination based on physical or mental handicap	Federal government and federal contractors
Vietnam Era Veterans Readjustment Act of 1974	Discrimination against disabled veterans and Vietnam veterans	Same as above
Pregnancy Discrimination Act of 1978	Discrimination in hiring, promoting, or terminating because of pregnancy; pregnancy to be treated as a medical disability	Same as Title VII
Immigration Reform and Control Act (1986)	Requires employer to verify identity and eligibility of new hires using Form I-9	Must be done on all new hires
Americans with Disabilities Act of 1990	Discrimination of disabled individuals in hiring and employment	Businesses with 15 or more employees
Fair Employment Practice Acts of States and Local Governments	Discrimination of various types	Varies

Ergogenic Aids Substances, commonly foods and supplements, that supposedly enhance an athlete's performance.

Ergosterol A **steroid** in plants that can be activated by irradiation to ergocalciferol or vitamin D2.

Erythrocytes **Red blood cells** or RBCs. RBCs are flattened, biconcave discs that transport **oxygen** around the body. Each RBC contains about 280 million **hemoglobin** molecules which actually carry the oxygen molecules. RBCs have no nuclei or mitochondria so they have a life span of about 120 days before being destroyed by phagocytic cells (called **macrophages**) in the **liver, spleen,** and bone marrow. See also **hemoglobin** and **macrophages** (see Table E.6).

Table E.6 Laboratory Tests on Erythrocytes

Red Blood Cell Count	The number of red blood cells in a cubic millimeter of blood.
Hemoglobin (Hgb)	The amount of hemoglobin (in grams) per 100 ml of blood.
Hematocrit	Percentage of red blood cells in 100 ml of blood. A percentage of 42 percent means that there are 42 ml of red blood cells in 100 ml of blood.
Mean Cell Hemoglobin (MCH)	The hemoglobin content of each individual red blood cell. MCH is expressed as micromicrograms or picograms of hemoglobin per red blood cell.
Mean Cell Hemoglobin Concentration (MCHC)	A laboratory test that measures the concentration of hemoglobin in grams per 100 ml of red blood cells. MCHC is the average concentration of hemoglobin per red blood cell.
Mean Cell Volume (MCV)	A laboratory test that describes the red blood cells in terms of individual cell size. Cell size is expressed as microcubic millimeters per red cell.

Erythrocyte Sedimentation Rate (ESR) A **blood** test that measures the rate at which **red blood cells** settle out of unclotted blood in a test tube. The distance the **erythrocytes** fall in the tube is measured. ESR is high in cases of inflammation, swelling, and tumors.

Erythropoiesis The production of **erythrocytes** (**red blood cells**).

Erythropoietin A **hormone** secreted by the **kidney** that stimulates **red blood cell** production.

Essential or Indispensable Amino Acids Amino acids that either cannot be made in the body or cannot be made in the quantities needed by the body. These amino acids must therefore be obtained in foods for the body to function properly.

Essential Fatty Acids Fatty acids that the body can't make itself so they are necessary in the diet: **linoleic acid** and **linolenic acid**.

Essential Nutrients The nutrients that either cannot be made in the body or cannot be made in the quantities needed by the body. Essential nutrients need to be taken in with food.

Esophageal Varices Enlarged, twisted **veins** in the **esophagus** that can occur in **liver** disease, such as **cirrhosis**.

Esophagus The part of the **gastrointestinal tract** that connects the **pharynx** to the **stomach**. The esophagus is about a 10-inch muscular tube, at the bottom of which is the lower esohageal **sphincter**. Food is propelled down the esophagus by rhythmic contractions of **muscles** in the wall of the esophagus called **peristalsis**.

Essential Hypertension See **primary hypertension**.

Ester A compound made by the reaction between an **acid** and an **alcohol**.

Estimated Minimum Requirements Nutrient requirements for **sodium**, **chloride**, and **potassium** set by the National Academy of Sciences' Food and Nutrition Board. They are based on what is needed for growth and for replacement of normal daily losses.

Estimated Safe and Adequate Daily Dietary Intake Nutrient intake recommendations by the National Academy of Sciences' Food and Nutrition Board in cases when there is not enough scientific evidence to develop an **RDA**.

Estradiol A form of **estrogen** made by the female **ovaries**.

Estrogen A **hormone** produced by the **ovaries** that is responsible for female secondary sex characteristics; preparation of the uterine wall for fertilization, implantation, and nutrition of the early **embryo**; and stimulation of bone growth.

Ethanol See **alcohol**.

Ethics The rules of conduct recognized by a group (see Table E.7).

Table E.7 Code of Ethics for the Profession of Dietetics

Preamble

The American Dietetic Association and its credentialing agency, the Commission on Dietetic Registration, believe it is in the best interests of the profession and the public it serves that a Code of Ethics provide guidance to dietetic practitioners in their professional practice and conduct. Dietetic practitioners have voluntarily developed a Code of Ethics to reflect the ethical principles guiding the dietetic profession and to outline commitments and obligations of the dietetic practitioner to self, client, society, and the profession.

The purpose of the Commission on Dietetic Registration is to assist in protecting the nutritional health, safety, and welfare of the public by establishing and enforcing qualifications for dietetic registration and for issuing voluntary credentials to individuals who have attained those qualifications. The Commission has adopted this Code to apply to individuals who hold these credentials.

The Ethics Code applies in its entirety to members of The American Dietetic Association who are Registered Dietitians (RDs) or Dietetic Technicians Registered (DTRs). Except for sections solely dealing with the credential, the Code applies to all American Dietetic Association members who are not RDs or DTRs. Except for aspects solely dealing with membership, the Code applies to all RDs and DTRs who are not ADA members. All of the aforementioned are referred to in the Code as "dietetic" practitioners."

Principles

1. The dietetic practitioner provides professional services with objectivity and with respect for the unique needs and values of individuals.

2. The dietetic practitioner avoids discrimination against other individuals on the basis of race, creed, religion, sex, age, and national origin.

3. The dietetic practitioner fulfills professional commitments in good faith.

4. The dietetic practitioner conducts himself/herself with honesty, integrity, and fairness.

5. The dietetic practitioner remains free of conflict of interest while fulfilling the objectives and maintaining the integrity of the dietetic profession.

6. The dietetic practitioner maintains confidentiality of information.

7. The dietetic practitioner practices dietetics based on scientific principles and current information.

Table E.7 Code of Ethics for the Profession of Dietetics (continued)

8. The dietetic practitioner assumes responsibility and accountability for personal competence in practice.

9. The dietetic practitioner recognizes and exercises professional judgment within the limits of his/her qualifications and seeks counsel or makes referrals as appropriate.

10. The dietetic practitioner provides sufficient information to enable clients to make their own informed decisions.

11. The dietetic practitioner who wishes to inform the public and colleagues of his/her services does so by using factual information. The dietetic practitioner does not advertise in a false or misleading manner.

12. The dietetic practitioner promotes or endorses products in a manner that is neither false nor misleading.

13. The dietetic practitioner permits use of his/her name for the purpose of certifying that dietetic services have been rendered only if he/she has provided or supervised the provision of those services.

14. The dietetic practitioner accurately presents professional qualifications and credentials.

    a. The dietetic practitioner uses "RD" or "registered dietitian" and "DTR" or "dietetic technician registered" only when registration is current and authorized by the Commission on Dietetic Registration.

    b. The dietetic practitioner provides accurate information and complies with all requirements of the Commission on Dietetic Registration program in which he/she is seeking initial or continued credentials from the Commission on Dietetic Registration.

    c. The dietetic practitioner is subject to disciplinary action for aiding another person in violating any Commission on Dietetic Registration requirements or aiding another person in representing himself/herself as an RD or DTR when he/she is not.

15. The dietetic practitioner presents substantiated information and interprets controversial information without personal bias, recognizing that legitimate differences of opinion exist.

Table E.7 Code of Ethics for the Profession of Dietetics (continued)

16. The dietetic practitioner makes all reasonable effort to avoid bias in any kind of professional evaluation. The dietetic practitioner provides objective evaluation of candidates for professional association memberships, awards, scholarships, or job advancements.

17. The dietetic practitioner voluntarily withdraws from professional practice under the following circumstances:

   a. The dietetic practitioner has engaged in any substance abuse that could affect his/her practice;

   b. The dietetic practitioner has been adjudged by a court to be mentally incompetent;

   c. The dietetic practitioner has an emotional or mental disability that affects his/her practice in a manner that could harm the client.

18. The dietetic practitioner complies with all applicable laws and regulations concerning the profession. The dietetic practitioner is subject to disciplinary action under the following circumstances:

   a. The dietetic practitioner has been convicted of a crime under the laws of the United States which is a felony or a misdemeanor, an essential element of which is dishonesty and which is related to the practice of the profession.

   b. The dietetic practitioner has been disciplined by a state and at least one of the grounds for the discipline is the same or substantially equivalent to these principles.

   c. The dietetic practitioner has committed an act of misfeasance or malfeasance which is directly related to the practice of the profession as determined by a court of competent jurisdiction, a licensing board, or an agency of a governmental body.

19. The dietetic practitioner accepts the obligation to protect society and the profession by upholding the Code of Ethics for the Profession of Dietetics and by reporting alleged violations of the Code through the defined review process of The American Dietetic Association and its credentialing agency, the Commission on Dietetic Registration.

Source: American Dietetic Association: Code of Ethics for the Profession of Dietetics. Copyright The American Dietetic Association. Reprinted by permission from *Journal of The American Dietetic Association*, Vol. 88: 1292–1293.

Ethnic Foods Foods associated with a particular ethnic/cultural group.

Evaluation The process of determining if a program met its objectives or goals.

Exchange Lists A menu planning guide that groups foods by their **calorie, carbohydrate, fat,** and **protein** content. Each food on a list has approximately the same amount of calories, carbohydrate, fat, and protein as another in the portions listed so that any food on a list can be exchanged for any other food on the same list.

The *Exchange Lists for Meal Planning* have been developed by the American Diabetes and **American Dietetic Association** for use primarily by diabetics who need to regulate what and how much they eat. They are also often used in weight control because they are relatively easy to learn and master, and they afford a good deal of control over calorie intake. There are seven exchange lists of like foods. Each food on a list has approximately the same amount of calories, carbohydrate, fat, and protein as another in the portions listed, so that any food on a list can be exchanged, or traded, for any other food on the same list. The six exchange lists are **starch,** fruit, milk, other carbohydrates, vegetables, meat and meat substitutes, and fat. Diabetics can exchange starch, fruit, or milk choices within their meal plans because they all have about the same amount of carbohydrate per serving.

Each exchange list has a typical member with specific portion size that can be remembered:

Starch—1 slice bread, 80 calories

Meat—1 ounce lean meat, 55 calories

Vegetable—1/2 cup cooked vegetable, 25 calories

Fruit—1 small apple, 60 calories

Milk—1 cup skim milk, 90 calories

Fat—1 teaspoon margarine, 45 calories

The meat exchange is broken down into very lean, lean, medium-fat, and high-fat meat and meat alternates. Very lean and lean meats are encouraged. The milk exchange contains skim, low-fat, and whole milk exchanges. Fats are divided into three groups, based on the main type of fat they contain: **monounsaturated, polyunsaturated,** and **saturated.** There is also a listing of free foods that contain negligible calories.

Exercise Bodily exertion especially for training or conditioning.

Exercise is a prerequisite to good health. Frequent exercise helps prevent **heart disease,** some forms of **cancer,** and **obesity.**

Table E.8 Calories Spent per Hour in Physical Activity

Activity	Calories Burned*
Bicycling, 6 mph	240 calories
Bicycling, 12 mph	410 calories
Cross-country skiing	700 calories
Jogging, 5-1/2 mph	740 calories
Jogging, 7 mph	920 calories
Jumping rope	750 calories
Running in place	650 calories
Running, 10 mph	1280 calories
Swimming, 25 yards/minute	275 calories
Swimming, 50 yards/minute	500 calories
Tennis, singles	400 calories
Walking, 2 mph	240 calories
Walking, 3 mph	320 calories
Walking, 4-1/2 mph	440 calories

* The calories burned in a particular activity vary in proportion to one's body weight. For example, a 100-pound person burns 1/3 fewer calories, so you would multiply the number of calories by 0.7. For a 200-pound person, multiply by 1.3.

Source: National Heart, Lung, and Blood Institute and the American Heart Association. 1993. *Exercise and your heart: A guide to physical activity.*

Menu Planning for Athletes

1. Offer a variety of foods from all food groups.

2. Good sources of **complex carbohydrates** to emphasize on menus include pasta, rice, other grain products such as breads and cereals, legumes, and fruits and vegetables.

3. Don't offer too much protein and fat in the thought that athletes need the calories in them. They do, but much of those extra calories should be coming from complex carbohydrates. The days of steak-and-egg dinners are over for athletes. The protein and fat present in these meals did nothing to improve performance.

4. Offer a variety of fluids, not just soft drinks and other sugared drinks. Good beverage choices include fruit juices, iced tea, and iced coffee (hopefully freshly brewed decaffeinated), and plain and flavored mineral and seltzer water, spritzers (fruit juice and mineral water), and milkshakes made with yogurt or ice milk and fruit. Soft drinks and juice drinks, which are both loaded with sugar, should be offered in moderation.

5. Make sure iodized **salt** is on the table.

6. Be sure to include sources of **iron** at each meal. Good iron sources include **liver**, red meats, legumes, and iron-fortified breakfast cereal. Moderate iron sources include raisins, dried fruit, bananas, nuts, whole-grain and fortified grain products. Be sure to include good **vitamin C** sources at each meal as vitamin C helps iron to be absorbed into the body. Vitamin C sources include citrus fruits and juices, cantaloupe, strawberries, broccoli, potatoes, and brussels sprouts.

7. After competition and workouts, again emphasize complex carbohydrates to ensure that **glycogen** will be restored. The sooner an athlete fuels up after exercising, the larger the amount of glycogen that will be stored in the muscle. Food is also important to restore the **minerals** lost in sweating. See also **precompetition meal**.

Exergonic Reactions Chemical reactions that release energy.

Exit Interview A meeting with employees leaving the organization to identify why they are leaving and their impressions about the organization.

Exocrine Glands Glands that secrete their chemical substances to an epithelial surface either directly or through ducts. Sweat, **mammary**, mucous, and **salivary glands** are all exocrine glands.

Exoenzymes Enzymes excreted by cells.

Expanded Food and Nutrition Education Program (EFNEP) See **Extension Service.**

Experimental Research See **clinical trials.**

Extension Service A food and nutrition education program for the public administered by the **United States Department of Agriculture.** The Extension Service employs specialists based at land grant colleges who give **research-**based information to agents located in each county. There is a home economics component of this program that addresses food and nutrition topics.

Extension Service also administers the **Expanded Food and Nutrition Education Program (EFNEP).** EFNEP offers education to low-income families to help them select and prepare a nutritious diet. Trained paraprofessionals often deliver this training.

External Respiration The exchange of gases (**oxygen** and **carbon dioxide**) between the air and **blood** that occurs in the lungs.

Extracellular Fluid (ECF) The water compartment consisting of the water outside of the body's cells.

Extraneous Variable In a **research** study, any variable (other than the **independent variable**) that might affect the **dependent variable**. Extraneous variables may also be **confounding variables** if not controlled.

Exudate Fluid, cells, and other substances that have come through small pores or breaks in cell membranes or **blood** vessels, usually due to inflammation. Examples include pus and perspiration.

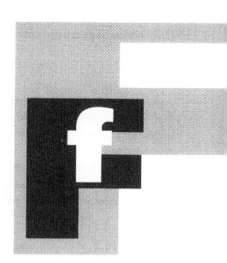

Facilitated Diffusion Diffusion or transport across the cell membrane that is speeded up by **proteins**. As in **simple diffusion**, movement is always from a region of higher to lower concentration.

Failure to Thrive (FTT) In pediatrics, a condition in which an infant or child has weight gain and increase in height two standard deviations below the mean for a period of time.

Fasting Hypoglycemia A type of **hypoglycemia** in which symptoms occur after not eating for eight or more hours, so it usually occurs during the night or before breakfast.

NUTRIENT FOCUS: FAT

The most common form of fat is the **triglyceride**, which is three **fatty acids** attached to a **glycerol** molecule. Triglycerides that are solid at room temperature are usually of animal origin, such as butter. If the triglycerides are liquid at room temperature, they are called oils. Fats are part of the group called **lipids**, which also includes **phospholipids** (such as **lecithin**) and sterols (such as **cholesterol**).

In foods, fats enhance taste, flavor, aroma, crispness, juiciness, tenderness, and texture. Fats also have satiety value. Fats also have many functions in the body. Many fat cells are located just under the **skin** where fat provides insulation for the body, a cushion around critical **organs**, and optimum body temperature in the cold. Fat stores are a very compact way to store lots of energy (9 **calories** per gram). Fat also is present in all cell membranes and transports the **fat-soluble vitamins** through the body.

Triglycerides are made up of a mixture of **saturated** and **unsaturated fatty acids**. Saturated fats (triglycerides with mostly saturated fatty acids) raise your blood cholesterol level more than anything else you eat. It is found in greatest amounts in foods from animals, such as fatty cuts of meat, poultry with the skin, whole-milk dairy products, lard, and in some vegetable oils like coconut, palm kernel, and palm oils. Unsaturated fats may be either **polyunsaturated** or **monounsaturated**. Polyunsaturated fats are found in vegetable oils such as safflower, sunflower, soybean, corn, cottonseed, and sesame oils, as well as fish oils. Monounsaturated fats include olive, canola, and peanut oils. Polyunsaturated fats and monounsaturated fats both lower the levels of LDL (the bad cholesterol) in the body, but only polyunsaturated fat also lowers HDL (the good cholesterol). Monounsaturated fats, such as olive oil, don't affect the level of HDLs (see Table F.1).

Table F.1 Recommended Fat and Saturated Fat Intake

If Your Total Daily Calories Are	Total Fat* (grams)	Saturated Fat* (grams)
1,200	40	13
1,500	50	17
1,800	60	20
2,000	67	22
2,200	73	24
2,400	80	27
2,600	86	29
2,800	93	31
3,000	100	33

* Total fat is 30 percent of total calories. Saturated fat is 10 percent of total calories.

The following tips will help guide you in making food choices that are lower in fat, saturated fat, and/or cholesterol.

Meat

1. You can still eat red meat as long as you choose lean cuts. Choosing lean red meat gives you all the benefits of the meat's **protein** and **iron**. Lean beef cuts include top round and eye of the round. Lean veal cuts include shoulder, sirloin, ground veal, and veal cutlets. Lean pork cuts include tenderloin, sirloin, and top loin.

2. Limit high-fat processed meats like bacon, bologna, salami, hot dogs, and sausage. They are high in saturated fat and total fat. Look for low-fat processed meats.

3. Limit organ meats, like liver, sweetbreads, and kidneys. Organ meats are high in cholesterol even though they are fairly low in fat.

Poultry

1. You can buy chicken and turkey pieces with the skin already removed, or buy the pieces with the skin on and remove it yourself before eating. Remember, the white meat always contains less saturated fat than the dark meat. Removing the skin, particularly from the white meat pieces, can help you get rid of almost all of the saturated fat. Removing the skin from the dark meat thighs and drumsticks also helps, but not as much.

2. Limit goose and duck. They are high in saturated fat, even with the skin removed.

3. Try fresh ground turkey or chicken that is made only from breast meat. Types that don't say "white meat" or "breast" on the label may include the skin and dark meat, so they are higher in fat. Substitute ground turkey or chicken for ground beef.

4. Remember that some (but not all) chicken and turkey hot dogs are lower in saturated fat and total fat than pork and beef hot dogs. There are also "lean" beef hot dogs that are low in fat and saturated fat.

Fish and Shellfish

1. Most fish is lower in fat, saturated fat, and cholesterol than meat and poultry.

2. Shellfish varies in cholesterol content. Some, like shrimp, are fairly high in cholesterol. Others, like scallops, mussels, and clams, are low. Shellfish have little saturated fat and total fat.

Dairy Foods

1. Buy skim and 1 percent milk rather than whole or 2 percent milk. They have just as much or more calcium and other nutrients as whole milk—with much less saturated fat, cholesterol, and calories.

2. Because they are made with whole milk or cream, most cheeses are high in saturated fat and cholesterol. Ounce for ounce, meat, poultry, and regular cheeses have about the same amount of cholesterol, but regular cheeses have much more saturated fat. Fortunately, many cheese makers are starting to offer low-fat versions of cheese favorites like cheddar, swiss, and mozzarella. They use skim milk and vegetable oils to replace some of the cream and other fat. The result is more reduced-fat and fat-free cheeses to choose from.

When looking for hard cheeses, go for versions that are "fat-free," "reduced-fat," "low-fat," "light," or "part- skim." When looking for soft cheeses, choose low-fat (1 percent) or nonfat cottage cheese, farmer cheese, or part skim or light ricotta.

Ideally, try to pick a cheese with 3 grams of fat or less in an ounce.

3. Because ice cream is made from whole milk and cream, it is fairly high in saturated fat and cholesterol. Instead, try to buy other frozen desserts that are low in saturated fat such as ice milk, low-fat frozen yogurt, low-fat frozen dairy desserts, fruit ices, sorbet, and popsicles.

4. Buy low-fat or nonfat yogurt. Use it as toppings or in recipes.

5. Try low-fat or nonfat sour cream or creamy cheese blends. Many taste as rich as the real thing, but have less fat and calories.

Eggs

1. Limit how many egg yolks you eat, preferably to four a week, including the egg yolks in baked goods and processed foods.

2. Substitute two egg whites for each whole egg in recipes. For cakes or cookies, this substitution is acceptable for one or two eggs in most recipes and for three or four in some others. For scrambled eggs and omelets, you can use one whole egg and two egg whites or a commercial egg substitute that contains virtually no cholesterol.

Fat and Oils

1. Choose liquid vegetable oils that are high in unsaturated fats—like canola, corn, olive, peanut, safflower, sesame, soybean, and sunflower oils.

2. Buy margarine made with unsaturated liquid vegetable oils as the first ingredient. Choose tub or liquid margarine or vegetable oil spreads. The softer the margarine, the more unsaturated it is.

3. Limit butter, lard, and solid shortenings. They are high in saturated fat.

4. Buy light or nonfat mayonnaise and salad dressings instead of the regular kinds that are high in fat.

Fruits and Vegetables

1. Buy fruits and vegetables to eat as snacks, desserts, salads, side dishes, and in main dishes. Season with herbs, spices, lemon juice, fat-free or low-fat mayonnaise. Limit the use of regular mayonnaise or other fatty sauces.

Breads, Cereals, Pasta, Rice and Other Grains, and Dry Peas and Beans

1. Choose whole-grain breads and rolls often.

2. Buy dry cereals; most are low in fat. Limit the high-fat granola, muesli, and oat bran types that are made with coconut or coconut oil. Granola and muesli often have nuts as well, which increases total fat and calories.

3. Buy pasta, rice, and dry peas and beans to use as entrees, or in casseroles or soups. Hold the high fat sauces.

4. Limit baked goods that are made with lots of saturated fat like croissants, muffins, biscuits, butter rolls, doughnuts, and brioche.

Sweets and Snacks

1. For a delicious cake with no fat, try angel food cake and top it with fruit puree or fresh fruit slices.

2. Try fat-free or low-fat cakes, cupcakes, brownies, and pastries.

3. Try fat-free or low-fat cookies like animal crackers, fig and other fruit bars, ginger snaps, graham crackers, and vanilla or lemon wafers.

4. Avoid baked goods, cookies, and crackers with the fats listed.

5. Bake your own sweets and snacks at home using a recipe that contains a moderate amount of fat, preferably high in polyunsaturated fat.

6. Gelatin desserts contain no fat. Make puddings with 1 percent or skim milk.

7. Instead of chips, pick pretzels or air-popped popcorn.

In addition to these tips, choose cooking methods such as broiling, roasting, poaching, stir-frying, or baking rather than frying. When roasting, place the meat on a rack so that the fat can drip away. For basting, substitute wine or tomato or lemon juice for fat. Limit the amount of fat used in cooking and, if need be, use vegetable oil or margarine rather than butter, shortening, or lard. Use nonstick cooking equipment. When sauteing, substitute vegetable juice, wine, or defatted stock for the fat or use vegetable oil cooking spray. Vegetables can be steamed or microwaved for best appearance, flavor, texture, and nutrient retention.

Fat Cell Theory A theory of **obesity**. Obese people usually have a larger than normal number of fat cells and/or enlarged fat cells. Fat cells can be added but never subtracted, so when an obese person loses weight, the cells must reduce in size, not number. The fat cell theory states that weight loss will be met with internal resistance when cells are to be reduced below their normal size.

Fat-Soluble Vitamins A group of **vitamins** that include **vitamins A, D, E, and K**. They generally occur in foods containing **fats** and they are stored in the body either in the **liver** or in **adipose** (fatty) **tissue** until they are needed. Fat-soluble vitamins are absorbed and transported around the body like other fats. If anything interferes with normal fat digestion and absorption, these vitamins may not be absorbed. See also **vitamin A, vitamin D, vitamin E**, and **vitamin K**.

Fat Substitutes Ingredients that mimic the functions of fat in foods, and either contain fewer **calories** than fat or no calories. Reduced-fat foods almost always use more than one fat substitute to replace the fat. There are three categories of fat substitutes: **carbohydrate**-based, **lipid**-based, and **protein**-based.

Carbohydrate-Based Fat Substitutes

In many food products with lowered fat content, various types and forms of carbohydrates are used to produce the texture that fat normally supplies. In fact, carbohydrates such as **starches** and gums were commonly used in foods as thickening agents to supply texture long before their use in development of lower-fat and fat-free food product choices. Today, carbohydrates continue to play key roles as thickeners, bulking agents, moisturizers and stabilizers in foods including lower-fat and fat-free frozen desserts, baked goods, cheeses, salad dressings, sauces and gravies, sour cream, yogurt, and puddings.

For instance, modified food starches, maltodextrins and dextrins, which are made from starches, absorb water to form gels that mimic the texture and mouth feel of fat. Polydextrose, a bland starch polymer, acts as a bulking agent to replace some of the volume lost when fat and/or **sugar** are removed from a food. It also helps keep the food moist. It has been used as a partial fat substitute in baked goods, cake frostings, puddings, and frozen desserts. Gums provide a creamy mouth feel and help stabilize emulsions such as in salad dressings. Cellulose gel is a purified form of cellulose ground to microparticles that supply mouth feel and flow properties for products such as frozen desserts, sauces, and salad dressings. Algins such as sodium alginate and calcium alginate can also be used as part of a fat reduction process.

As compared with traditional fats that contain 9 calories per gram, carbohdyrate-based ingredients provide from 0 to 4 calories per gram, depending on the type of ingredient and the concentration in which it is used. For example, dry forms of maltodextrins provide 4 calories per gram. But when hydrated with water, as required for some products, their caloric contribution drops to 1 to 2 calories per gram of the finished product. Other carbohydrates, such as cellulose and xanthan gums, are not digested except by bacteria in the lower intestine, and contribute negligible calories.

Carbohydrate-based fat reduction ingredients do have their limitations. They cannot replace oils and shortenings used to fry foods. Most are not suitable for cooking or frying. Another problem with starches is taste: they do not always mimic the mouth feel of fat at different levels of concentration. The next category of fat substitutes overcomes these problems, but also introduces new concerns.

Lipid-Based Fat Substitutes

Some lipid-based ingredients are actually fats tailored to contribute fewer calories and less available fat to foods. Others are structurally modified to provide no calories or fat.

As with other fat-reduction techniques, fat-based ingredients are very versatile and can be used in a variety of foods including chocolate, **margarine**, spreads, sour cream, and cheese. In addition, some may be used to fry foods. Because these ingredients are made from fats, they have the same physical properties as fats, including taste, texture, and mouth feel.

The caloric values of fat-based ingredients vary. **Olestra** is not absorbed so it contributes no calories. Other fat-based ingredients, such as caprenin, are not completely absorbed. Caprenin contains about five calories per gram.

Olestra was developed for use in hot foods (such as in shortenings and frying) as well as cold (such as in salad dressings). Olestra keeps its fat-like qualities when heated. It is similar in structure to fat (it has eight **fatty acids** attached to a core of sugar) so it has the mouth feel of regular fat. It also carries flavors well.

Because it is a new molecular structure that can't be digested in the digestive tract (it is simply excreted), olestra had to be approved as a new food additive, which means that studies were required to prove its safety. Studies on olestra have shown two concerns. First, research has shown that olestra can cause gastrointestinal problems such as cramping, bloating, and diarrhea. The more olestra eaten, the more severe the problems. Second, as olestra moves through the **gastrointestinal tract**, it takes some **fat-soluble vitamins** (A, D, E, and K) as well as beta carotene along with it to be excreted. Research has started to show that beta carotene, which belongs to a group called the **carotenoids**, seems to protect the body against diseases such as **cancer**. Beta carotene is found in carrots and other foods and is converted into vitamin A in the body.

One study showed that eating one ounce of potato chips made with olestra each day for four weeks caused a 60 percent reduction in carotenoids in the blood. Fat-soluble vitamins A, D, and E also were reduced (see Table F.2).

Table F.2 A Guide to Fat Substitutes

1. Carbohydrate-Based
   (Starches and gums stabilize water in a gel-like structure. They are hydrophilic and add texture and structure.)

Name	Description	Other Functions	Cal/Gm.
Dextrins	Bland, nonsweet. Made from hydrolyzed starches.	Some thickening ability. Stabilizer	1–4 calories (depends on concentration) Fully digestible.
Uses: Salad dressings.			
Maltodextrin	Nonsweet. Made from hydrolyzed cornstarch.	Bulking agent. Fully	4 calories. digestible.
Uses: Baked products, margarines, salad dressings, mayonnaise.			
Modified Food Starches (A starch that has been altered by physical or chemical means.)	Made from corn, rice, potato, tapioca.	Stabilizers. Thickeners. Texturizers.	4 calories. Fully digestible.
Uses: Baked goods, mayonnaise, sour cream, puddings, pie fillings, gravies, sauces, gum drops.			
Polydextrose	Randomly cross-linked polymer of glucose. Made from dextrose and small amounts of sorbitol and citric acid.	Bulking agent.	1 calorie. Partially absorbable.
Uses: Frozen desserts, puddings, cake frostings, candy, baked goods and mixes.			
Gums	Made from seeds, seaweed extracts, and plants	Thickening agents Stabilizers. Increase fiber. Replaces starch and/or fat.	1–3 calories. Limited digestion and absorption.

Table F.2 A Guide to Fat Substitutes (continued)

Some Gums:
Xanthum gum (1 cal/gm)—synthetic, thickener in salad dressings.
Guar gum (1-3 cal/gm)—in dressings, soups, baked goods, ice cream.
Alginates—in salad dressings.
Carageenan (1 cal/gm)—in salad dressings, ice cream, milk products, and
                reduced-fat ground beef.
Cellulose gum—bulking agent in low-cal foods.

2. Lipid-Based

Name	Description	Other Functions	Cal/Gm.
Olestra	Fatty acid esters of sucrose. 6–8 fatty acids on a sucrose core. Good carrier of flavors.	--	0 Not absorbed
Uses: Snack foods such as chips and crackers.			
Caprenin	Esterification of glycerol with 3 fatty acids. Like cocoa butter.	--	5 calories. 1 of fatty acids only partially absorbed.
Uses: Candy.			

3. Protein-Based

Name	Description	Other Functions	Cal/Gm.
Simplesse	Microparticulated protein of milk and egg white proteins. Retains water within its structure	--	1–2 calories.
Uses: Frozen desserts, cheese foods (will denature if heated too much)			

Protein-Based Fat Substitutes

Some of these ingredients are made through a process called microparticula-tion. For example, **simplesse** is made from egg white and milk protein blended and heated using microparticulation. The protein is shaped into microscopic round particles that roll easily over one another. The aim of the process is to create the feel of a creamy liquid with the texture of fat. Simplesse cannot be used to fry foods but can be used in some cooking and baking. It contains one to two calories per gram (see Table F.2).

Fatty Acid   Organic acids made of carbon atoms joined like links in a straight chain that occur mainly in **triglycerides**. The number of carbons is interestingly always an even number. Fatty acids differ from one another in two respects: the length of the carbon chain and the degree of saturation. The length of the chain may be categorized as short chain (6 carbons or less), medium chain (8 to 12 carbons), and long chain (14 to 20 carbons). Most **lipids** in food contain long-chain fatty acids. The length of the chain influences the **fat's** ability to dissolve in water. Generally, triglycerides do not dissolve in water, but the short- and medium-chain fatty acids have some solubility in water (see Figure F.1).

Figure F.1   Types of Fatty Acids

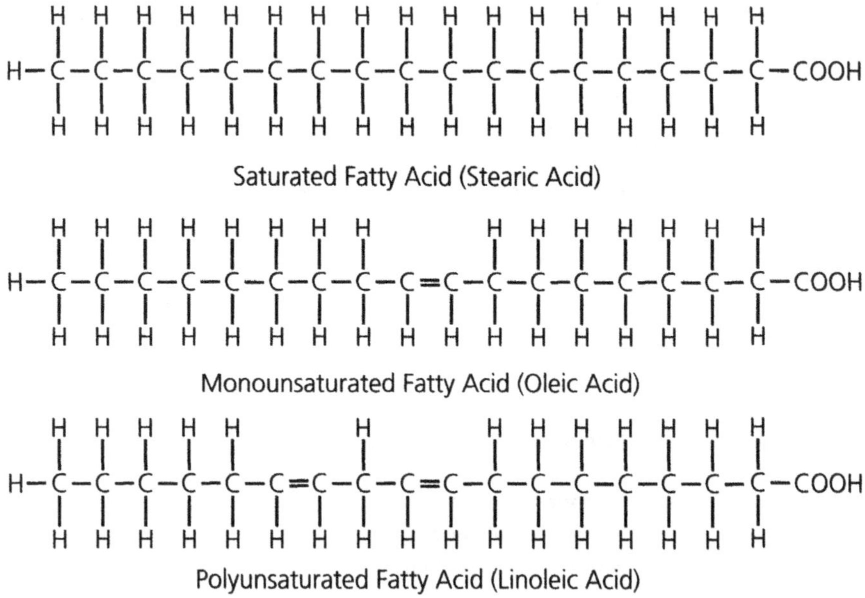

Saturated Fatty Acid (Stearic Acid)

Monounsaturated Fatty Acid (Oleic Acid)

Polyunsaturated Fatty Acid (Linoleic Acid)

Fatty acids are referred to as saturated or unsaturated. To understand this concept, think of each carbon atom in the fatty acid chain as having hydrogen atoms attached just like charms on a bracelet. Each carbon atom can have a maximum of four bonds so it can attached to four other atoms. Typically a carbon atom has one bond each to the two carbon atoms on its sides and one bond each to two hydrogens. If each carbon atom in the chain is filled to capacity with hydrogens, it is considered a saturated fatty acid. That's how **saturated**

fatty acid got its name: it is saturated with hydrogen atoms. When a hydrogen is missing from two neighboring carbons, a double bond forms between the carbon atoms, and this type of fatty acid is considered unsaturated.

Each "C" in a fatty acid represents a carbon atom, each "H" represents a hydrogen atom, and each "O" represents an oxygen atom. The top fatty acid in the illustration is saturated, meaning that it is filled to capacity with hydrogens. By comparison, the middle and lower fatty acids are unsaturated. This is evident because there are empty spaces without hydrogens in the picture. Wherever hydrogens are missing, the carbons are joined by two lines, meaning a double bond. The spot where the double bond is located is called the point of unsaturation.

Unsaturated fatty acids are either monounsaturated or polyunsaturated. A fatty acid that contains only one (*mono* means one) double bond in the chain is called monounsaturated; if the chain has two or more double bonds, the fatty acid is called polyunsaturated. The **monounsaturated fatty acid** is missing one pair of hydrogen atoms in the middle of the molecule. The **polyunsaturated fatty acid** is missing two pairs of hydrogen atoms.

Fatty Acid Synthetase A group of enzymes that regulate the synthesis of new **fatty acids**.

Ferritin The storage form of **iron**.

Fertilization The union of the sperm and ovum (egg) to form a zygote from which the embryo develops.

Fetal Alcohol Syndrome (FAS) A set of symptoms occurring in newborn babies due to **alcohol** use of the mother during pregnancy. FAS children may show signs of mental retardation, growth retardation, brain damage, and facial deformities. Newborns with FAS are generally small in size and irritable after birth because of alcohol withdrawal. The most serious concern with FAS infants is their impaired physical and mental development. They have problems gaining weight and frequently are mentally retarded.

You don't have to be a chronic alcoholic to have problems with FAS. Moderate drinkers may have babies with more subtle features of FAS. These women also have a higher rate of miscarriages and low-birth-weight babies. The American Academy of Pediatrics recommends that women stop drinking alcohol as soon as they plan to become pregnant because harm can be done during the first six to eight weeks when a woman doesn't yet know for sure if she is pregnant.

Fetus The infant in the mother's uterus from eight weeks after conception until birth.

NUTRIENT FOCUS: FIBER

The indigestible **carbohydrates** including soluble and insoluble fibers. Soluble fibers have more water-holding capacity than the insoluble fibers which only hold a limited amount of water. Pectin, gums, and mucilages are soluble fibers. Soluble fibers tend to decrease blood cholesterol levels and delay stomach emptying. Cellulose and lignin are insoluble fibers. Hemicellulose is both a soluble and insoluble fiber. Insoluble fiber seems to decrease the chance of constipation or colon cancer.

Following are tips to increase your fiber consumption.

General

1. The majority of breads and baked goods available are made with white flour, a poor source of fiber. For more fiber, choose whole-wheat bread (made with 100 percent whole-wheat flour) or another whole grain listed first on the ingredient label. Other whole-grain ingredients include cracked wheat, oatmeal, whole cornmeal, and whole rye.

2. Eat fruits, in their whole form preferably, at any meal or for snacks, at least two times each day.

Breakfast

3. Choose whole-grain and bran cereals for good fiber sources and make sure the cereal contains at least four grams of dietary fiber per serving.

4. Whole fruits have more fiber than fruit juice so include whole fruits with your breakfast.

5. Bran muffins are a tasty high-fiber breakfast food.

Lunch and Dinner

6. For fiber, select soups rich in split peas, beans, lentils, and vegetables. Use barley to thicken vegetable soups.

7. Use whole-wheat or other whole-grain pasta instead of refined pasta products. For example, make macaroni salad with whole-wheat macaroni for added fiber and flavor or serve whole-wheat spaghetti with homemade tomato sauce with vegetables.

8. Top casseroles with wheat germ.

9. Try recipes using grains such as bulgur and couscous.

10. Use cooked or canned dry beans and peas in main dishes, side dishes, and salads. For example:

   Combine black beans and rice with chili powder or other peppery seasoning for a Caribbean-style dish. Try a mixture of any of these with a vinegar and oil dressing for a three- or four-bean salad: green beans, wax beans, kidney beans, lima beans, great northern beans, or chickpeas. Add kidney beans or chickpeas to a lettuce or spinach salad.

11. Use brown rice instead of white rice.

12. Leave the skin on potatoes.

13. Have a bean salad or mixed green salad with plenty of vegetables such as carrots, broccoli, and cauliflower. Include kidney or garbanzo beans as well.

Snacks

14. Most commercial cookies contain little fiber, unless made with whole grains, such as oats, or dried fruits, such as raisins, dates, and figs.

15. For fiber in crackers, choose whole-grain crackers, such as whole-wheat crackers, or crackers made with bran.

16. Fresh fruits and popcorn are two high-fiber snacks.

Desserts and Baking

17. Bake or broil fruits for dessert.

18. Use fresh, frozen, canned, or dried fruits when baking muffins, pancakes, quick breads or other baked products. Dried apricots, raisins, bananas, blueberries, or apples add extra fiber and variety in flavor.

19. White flour, and baking mixes using white flour, contain little fiber. For more fiber, choose whole-grain flours, such as whole wheat, and mixes using whole-grain flour.

20. When baking, use plenty of fresh, frozen, canned, and dried fruits to increase fiber.

21. For puddings, try rice (use brown rice), tapioca, and bread (use whole-wheat bread).

Fibrinogen A **blood plasma protein** made by the **liver** that is involved in **blood clotting**. See also **blood clotting**.

Fibroids **Benign** (noncancerous) tumors of the uterus. They are often found in women between 30 and 50 years old.

Fibrillation A **heart** condition in which the electrical impulses that regulate heart contractions become random, rapid, and continuously changing. During fibrillation, the timing of the electrical impulses of the heart and the time when the heart rests becomes totally uncoordinated. It can occur because of damage to the myocardium. Fibrillation sometimes can be stopped by an electrical device called a defibrillator. The defibrillator applies a strong electric shock to the chest to cause all the heart cells to rest, then hopefully begin normal electrical impulses.

Fibrous Proteins Fiber-like **proteins**, such as **collagen** and **elastin**, that are generally insoluble in water. Collagen is a fibrous protein that is a component of **skin, bone**, teeth, ligaments, tendons, and other connective structures. Elastin fibers can be stretched like rubber bands.

Filtration The process by which some substances pass through a filter, and some don't.

First Trimester The first 13 weeks of pregnancy.

Fistula An abnormal passage from an internal **organ** to a body surface or to another internal organ.

PRACTICAL NUTRITION FOCUS: FIVE A DAY

A program developed by the National Cancer Institute to encourage Americans to eat five or more servings of fruits and vegetables every day (the **Food Guide Pyramid** recommends at least three servings of vegetables and two servings of fruits). Surveys continually show that most Americans eat less than five servings a day. The program is a venture of the National Cancer Institute along with the Produce for Better Health Foundation, a nonprofit foundation representing the fruit and vegetable industry.

Many fruits and vegetables are rich sources of **vitamins** and other nutrients and most contain **dietary fiber**. They have no **cholesterol** and almost all are naturally low in **calories, fat,** and **sodium**. Leading health authorities recommend that you eat five servings of fruits and vegetables every day along with a variety of foods. One serving is 1/2 cup of fruit, 3/4 cup juice, 1/2 cup cooked vegetable, 1 cup leafy vegetable (such as leaf lettuce), or 1/4 cup dried fruit. It is recommended that you eat at least one **vitamin A**-rich selection (such as apricots, cantaloupe, papaya, broccoli, carrots, spinach, sweet potatoes, or tomatoes) and one **vitamin C**-rich selection (such as citrus fruits, cantaloupe, honeydew, strawberries, watermelon, broccoli, or tomatoes) every day.

Fruits and vegetables lower your risk of **cancer**. It is estimated that 35 percent of all cancer deaths may be related to what we eat—a diet high in fat and low in fiber. Fruits and vegetables help reduce your risk of cancer because they are low in fat and are rich sources of vitamin A, vitamin C, and fiber. A low-fat diet that is low in **saturated fat** and cholesterol and includes plenty of high-fiber foods also decreases the risk of **heart disease**.

Flatulence Excessive gas in the **gastrointestinal tract** that is often expelled through the **anus**.

Flat Bones **Bones** covering soft body parts such as the shoulder bone and ribs.

Flatus Gas expelled through the **anus**.

Flavin Adenine Dinucleotide (FAD/FADH2) A **nucleotide** that is involved in removal and storage of electrons for oxidation-reduction reactions. FAD can accept two hydrogen ions and two electrons to be reduced to FADH2. When FADH2 is oxidized (the reverse reaction) to FAD, it transfers two hydrogen atoms to the oxidizing agent and heat is released. FAD is derived from the B vitamin **riboflavin**.

Flavin Mononucleotide (FMN) A **riboflavin**-containing **coenzyme** involved in deaminating some **amino acids**.

Fluorosis Discoloration of the teeth in children because of high ingestion of fluoride during tooth development.

Focus Groups A method used to obtain information from consumers on what their needs and wants are, and how certain ideas and products appeal to them.

NUTRIENT FOCUS: FOLATE

A water-soluble **vitamin** that is a component of the **enzymes** required to form **DNA**, the genetic material that appears within every body cell. Folate is therefore needed to make all new cells. Much folate is used to produce adequate numbers of **red blood cells, white blood cells**, and digestive tract cells.

Excellent sources of folate include green leafy vegetables (the word folate comes from the word foliage, meaning leafy) such as spinach and romaine, organ meats such as liver and kidney, legumes, and orange juice. Good sources include beef, whole-grain breads and cereals, and fortified ready-to-eat cereals. Much folate is lost during food preparation and cooking, so fresh and lightly cooked foods are more likely to contain more folate.

A deficiency of folate can cause **megaloblastic anemia,** a condition in which the red blood cells are larger in size than normal and function poorly. Other symptoms may include digestive tract problems such as **diarrhea,** and mental depression. Groups particularly at risk for folate deficiency are pregnant women, low-birthweight infants, and the elderly.

A deficiency of folate may have especially serious consequences during the first few weeks of pregnancy when it can cause serious birth defects. For this reason, most grain products will be fortified with folate by 1998. Also called **folic acid** or **folacin.** See also **neural tube defects.**

Follicle-Stimulating Hormone (FSH) A **hormone** produced by the **pituitary gland** after the onset of menstruation that stimulates the development of the ovum (egg cell) and ovulation. The high levels of **estrogen** and **progesterone** during pregnancy shut down the production of FSH so ovulation cannot occur. In males, FSH stimulates sperm production in the testes.

Food Additives Any substance added to food. If a substance is added to a food for a specific purpose in that food, it is referred to as a direct additive. Indirect food additives are those that become part of the food in trace amounts due to its packaging, storage, or other handling. Food additives play a vital role in today's bountiful and nutritious food supply. Additives perform a variety of useful functions in foods (see Table F.3).

Table F.3 Common Uses of Additives

Additive Function/Examples*	Foods Where Likely Used
Impart/Maintain Desired Consistency	
Alginates, lecithin, mono- & diglycerides, methyl cellulose, carrageenan, glycerine, pectin, guar gum, sodium aluminosilicate	Baked goods, cake mixes, salad dressings, ice cream, process cheese, coconut, table salt, chocolate
Improve/Maintain Nutritive Value	
Vitamins A and D, thiamin, niacin, riboflavin, pyridoxine, folic acid, ascorbic acid, calcium carbonate, zinc oxide, iron	Flour, bread, biscuits, breakfast cereals, pasta, margarine, milk, iodized salt, gelatin desserts
Maintain Palatability and Wholesomeness	
Propionic acid and its salts, ascorbic acid, butylated hydroxyanisole (BHA), butylated hydroxytoluene (BHT), benzoates, sodium nitrite, citric acid	Bread, cheese, crackers, frozen and dried fruit, margarine, lard, potato chips, cake mixes, meat

Table F.3 Common Uses of Additives (continued)

Additive Function/Examples*	Foods Where Likely Used
Produce Light Texture; Control Acidity/Alkalinity Yeast, sodium bicarbonate, citric acid, fumaric acid, phosphoric acid, lactic acid, tartrates	Cakes, cookies, quick breads, crackers, butter, soft drinks
Enhance Flavor or Impart Desired Color Cloves, ginger, fructose, aspartame, saccharin, FD&C Red No. 40, monosodium glutamate, caramel, annatto, limonene, turmeric	Spice cake, gingerbread, soft drinks, yogurt, soup, confections, baked goods, cheeses, jams, gum

Source: Food and Drug Administration.

Food Allergens Those parts of food causing allergic reactions. See also **food allergy.**

NUTRITION AND DISEASE FOCUS: FOOD ALLERGY

An abnormal response of the **immune system** to an otherwise harmless food. True food allergies affect a relatively small percentage of people. Experts estimate that only two percent of adults, and from four to eight percent of children, are truly allergic to certain foods.

Food allergy symptoms are very specific. When a food allergen (the part of the food that causes the allergic reaction) passes from the mouth into the **stomach,** the body recognizes it as a foreign substance, producing **antibodies** to halt the invasion. In allergic individuals, as the body fights off the invasion, symptoms begin to appear throughout the body. The most common sites are the mouth (swelling of the lips or tongue, itching lips), digestive tract (**stomach** cramps, vomiting, **diarrhea**), the **skin** (hives, rashes, or eczema), and the airways (wheezing or breathing problems). Allergic reactions to foods usually begin within minutes to a few hours after eating.

Food allergies are much more common in infants and young children, who often later outgrow them. Cow's milk, peanuts, eggs, wheat, and soy are the most common food allergies in children. In many cases, children outgrow these allergies later on in childhood. In general, the more severe the first allergic reaction was, the longer it takes to outgrow. Adults are usually most affected by nuts, fish, shellfish, and peanuts.

Most cases of allergic reactions to foods are mild, but some are violent and life-threatening. The greatest danger in food allergy comes from anaphylaxis, a rare allergic reaction involving a number of parts of the body simultaneously. Anaphylaxis is also known as anaphylactic shock. Like less serious allergic reactions, anaphylaxis usually occurs after a person is exposed to an allergen to which he or she was sensitized by previous exposure. That is, it does not usually occur the first time a person eats a particular food. Anaphylaxis can produce severe symptoms in as little as 5 to 15 minutes. Signs of such a reaction include: difficulty breathing, swelling of the mouth and throat, drop in **blood pressure**, and loss of consciousness. The sooner anaphylaxis is treated, the greater the person's chance of surviving.

Although any food can trigger anaphylaxis, peanuts, nuts, shellfish, milk, eggs, and fish are the most common culprits. Peanuts are the leading cause of death from food allergies. See also **food intolerance**. (See Table F.4.)

Table F.4 Foods to Omit for Specific Allergies

Food Allergen	Foods to Omit	Check Food Labels for These
Milk	All fluid milk including buttermilk, evaporated or condensed milk, nonfat dry milk, all cheeses, all yogurts, ice cream and ice milk, butter, many margarines, most nondairy creamers and whipped toppings, hot cocoa mixes, creamed soups, many breads, crackers and cereals, pancakes, waffles, many baked goods such as cakes and cookies (check the label), fudge, instant potatoes, custards, puddings, some hot dogs and luncheon meats.	Instant nonfat dry milk, nonfat milk, milk solids, whey, curds, casein, caseinate, milk, lactose-free milk, lactalbumin, lactoglobulin, sour cream, butter, cheese, cheese food, milk chocolate, buttermilk.
Eggs	All forms of eggs, most egg substitutes, eggnog, any baked good made with eggs such as muffins and cookies or glazed with eggs such as sweet rolls, ice cream, sherbet,	Eggs, albumin, globulin, livetin, ovalbumin, ovomucin, ovomucoid, ovoglobulin egg albumin, ovovitellin, vitellin.

Table F.4 Foods to Omit for Specific Allergies (continued)

Food Allergen	Foods to Omit	Check Food Labels for These
	custards, meringues, cream pies, puddings, French toast, pancakes, waffles, some candies, some salad dressings and sandwich spreads such as mayonnaise, any sauce made with egg such as hollandaise, souffles, any meat or potato made with egg, all pastas unless egg-free, soups made with eggs or noodles, soups made with stocks that were cleared with eggs, marshmallows.	
Gluten	All foods containing wheat, oats, barley or rye as flour or in any other form, salad dressings, gravies, malted beverages, postum, soy sauce, instant puddings, distilled vinegar, beer, ale, some wines, gin, whiskey, vodka.	Flour (unless from sources noted below), modified food starch, monosodium glutamate, hydrolyzed vegetable protein, cereals, malt or cereal extracts, food starch, vegetable starch, vegetable gum, wheat germ, wheat bran, bran, semolina, malt flavoring, distilled vinegar, emulsifiers, stabilizers.

(Corn, rice, soy, arrowroot, tapioca, and potato do not contain gluten so they can be used.)

Food and Drug Administration A branch of the Department of Health and Human Services' Public Health Service that ensures the safety and wholesomeness of all foods (except meat, poultry, and egg) that travel across state lines, inspects food plants and imported foods, and sets standards for food composition and food labels.

Food Assistance Programs See **United States Department of Agriculture.**

Table F.5 Major Foodborne Diseases of Bacterial Origin

	Salmonellosis Infection	Shigellosis Infection	Listeriosis Infection	Staphyloccal Intoxication	Clostridium Perfringens Toxin Mediated Infection	Bacillus Cereus Intoxication	Botulism Intoxication
Bacteria	Salmonella (facultative)	Shigella (facultative)	Listeria monocytogenes (reduced oxygen)	Staphylococcus aureus (facultative)	Clostridium perfringens (anaerobic)	Bacillus Cereus (facultative)	Clostridium botulinum (anaerobic)
Incubation Period	6–72 hours	1–7 days	1 day to 3 weeks	1–6 hours	8–22 hours	1/2–5 hours; 8–16 hours	12–36 hours + 72
Duration of Illness	2–3 days	Indefinite, depends on treatment	Indefinite, depends on treatment, but has high fatality in the immuno-compromised	24–48 hours	24 hours	6–24 hours; 12 hours	Several days to a year
Symptoms	Abdominal, pain, headache, nausea, vomiting, fever, diarrhea	Diarrhea, fever, chills, lassitude, dehydration	Nausea, vomiting, headache, fever, chills, backache, meningitis	Nausea, vomiting, diarrhea, dehydration	Abdominal pain, diarrhea	Nausea and vomiting; diarrhea, abdominal cramps	Vertigo, visual disturbances, inability to swallow, respiratory paralysis

Table F.5 Major Foodborne Diseases of Bacterial Origin (continued)

	Salmonellosis Infection	Shigellosis Infection	Listeriosis Infection	Staphyloccal Intoxication	Clostridium Perfringens Toxin Mediated Infection	Bacillus Cereus Intoxication	Botulism Intoxication
Reservoir	Domestic and wild animals; also humans; especially as carriers	Human feces, flies	Humans, domestic and wild animals, fowl, soil water, mud	Humans (skin, nose, throat, infected sores); also, animals	Humans (intestinal tract), animals, and soil	Soil and dust	Soil, water
Foods Implicated	Poultry and poultry salads, meat and meat products, milk, shell eggs, egg custards and sauces, and other protein foods	Potato, tuna, shrimp, turkey and macaroni salads, lettuce, moist and mixed foods	Unpasteurized milk and cheese, vegetables, poultry and meats, seafood, and prepared, chilled, ready-to-eat foods	Warmed-over foods, ham and other meats, dairy products, custards, potato salad, cream-filled pastries, and other protein foods	Meat that has been boiled, steamed, braised, stewed or roasted at low temperature for a long time, or cooled slowly before serving	Rice and rice dishes, custards, seasonings, dry food mixes, spices, puddings, cereal products, sauces, vegetable dishes, meat loaf	Improperly processed canned goods of low-acid food, garlic-in-oil products, grilled onions, stews, meat/poultry loaves

Table F.5 Major Foodborne Diseases of Bacterial Origin (continued)

	Salmonellosis Infection	Shigellosis Infection	Listeriosis Infection	Staphyloccal Intoxication	Clostridium Perfringens Toxin Mediated Infection	Bacillus Cereus Intoxication	Botulism Intoxication
Spore Former	No	No	No	No	Yes	Yes	Yes
Prevention	Avoid cross-contamination, refrigerate foods, cool cooked meats and meat products properly, avoid fecal contamination from foodhandlers by practicing good personal hygiene	Avoid cross-contamination, avoid fecal contamination from food-handlers by practicing good personal hygiene, use sanitary food and water sources, control flies	Use only pasteurized milk and dairy products, cook foods to proper temperatures, avoid cross-contamination	Avoid contamination from bare hands, exclude sick foodhandlers from food preparation and serving, practice good personal hygiene, practice sanitary habits, proper heating and refrigeration of food	Use careful time and temperature control in cooling and reheating cooked meat dishes and products	Use careful time and temperature control and quick chilling methods to cool foods, hold hot foods above 140° F (60° C), keep sous-vide packages refrigerated, reheat leftovers to 165° F (74° C)	Do not use home-canned products, use careful time and temperature control for sous-vide items, and all large, bulky foods, keep sous-vide packages refrigerated, purchase garlic-in-oil in small quantities for immediate use, cook onions only on request

Source: Reprinted with permission from *Applied Foodservice Sanitation*, Fourth Edition. Copyright © 1992 by the Educational Foundation of the National Restaurant Association.

Table F.6 Emerging Pathogens that Cause Foodbourne Illness

	Campylobacteriosis Infection	E. Coli 0157: H7 Infection/Intoxication	Norwalk Virus Illness
Pathogen	*Campylobacter jejuni*	*Escherichia coli*	Norwalk and Norwalk-like viral agent
Incubation period	3–5 days	12–72 hours	24–48 hours
Duration of illness	1–4 days	1–3 days	24–48 hours
Symptoms	Diarrhea, fever, nausea, abdominal pain, headache	Bloody diarrhea; severe abdominal pain, nausea, vomiting, diarrhea, and occassionally fever	Nausea, vomiting, diarrhea, abdominal pain, headache, and low-grade fever
Reservoir	Domestic and wild animals	Humans (intestinal tract); animals, particularly cattle	Humans (intestinal tract)
Foods implicated	Raw vegetables, unpasteurized milk and dairy products, poultry, pork, beef, and lamb	Raw and undercooked beef and other red meats, imported cheeses, unpasteurized milk, raw finfish, cream pies, mashed potatoes, and other prepared foods	Raw vegetables, prepared salads, raw shellfish, and water contaminated from human feces
Spore former	No	No	No
Prevention	Avoid cross-contamination, cook foods thoroughly	Cook beef and red meats thoroughly, avoid cross-contamination, use safe food and water supplies, avoid fecal contamination from foodhandlers by practicing good personal hygiene	Use safe food and water supplies, avoid fecal contamination from foodhandlers by practicing good personal hygiene, thoroughly cook foods

Source: Reprinted with permission from *Applied Foodservice Sanitation*, Fourth Edition. Copyright © 1992 by the Educational Foundation of the National Restaurant Association.

Foodborne Illness A preventable disease carried to people through food. Symptoms include vomiting, **stomach** cramps, and **diarrhea**, and vary depending on the type. Foodborne illness is often due to bacteria and viruses. Foodborne infections are diseases that result from eating food containing living harmful microorganisms. A *foodborne intoxication* occurs when toxins (poisons) from bacteria or molds are present in the ingested food and cause illness. A foodborne toxin-mediated infection is a disease due to eating a food with a large amount of disease-causing microorganims that produce toxins in the host's intestine that make him sick (see Tables F.5 and F.6).

Food Diary A written record of what an individual eats and drinks during the day, normally noting when, where, and how one felt. The food diary is useful in weight control to show situations where one overeats and then use **behavior modification** techniques.

Food Disappearance Data Per capita consumption of foods compiled by the Economic Research Service of the **U.S. Department of Agriculture**. Consumption is calculated by determining the total available food at the beginning of the period and then subtracting the amount of food exported, used by the military, put to nonfood use, and ending inventory of food. Food disappearance data overestimates per capita usage.

Food Jag A food behavior found particularly in young children in which they eat mostly one food, such as peanut butter, for a period of time. Food jags usually don't last long enough to cause any harm.

Food Frequency Questionnaire (FFQ) A questionnaire form used to get eating habit information from **clients** (see Figure F.2).

Figure F.2 Food Frequency Questionnaire

| | | Average Intake | | |
Food Group	Never	Times Per Day	Times Per Week	Times Per Month
Milk: Whole				
Skim				
Low-fat				
Cheese: Regular				
Low-fat				
Meat, fish, poultry:				
Lean				
With fat				
Luncheon meat:				
Low-fat				
Regular				

Figure F.2   Food Frequency Questionnaire (continued)

		Average Intake		
Food Group	**Never**	**Times Per Day**	**Times Per Week**	**Times Per Month**
Eggs				
Fruit: Citrus				
Others				
Vegetables:				
Deep green or leafy				
Dark yellow				
Potato				
Dried peas or beans				
Cereals				
Bread:				
Whole grain				
Other				
Rice, pasta				
Margarine, oil				
Cake, cookies, etc.:				
Commercial				
Homemade				
Candy:				
Chocolate				
Nuts and peanut butter				
Ice cream:				
Low-fat				
Yogurt				
Regular				
Jam or jelly				
Salt: Cooking				
Added				
Soups: Cream				
Broth base				
Alcohol: Wine				
Beer				
Other				
Coffee or tea/decaf:				
coffee or tea				
Soft drinks:				
Regular				
Sugar-free				
Convenience foods				

PRACTICAL NUTRITION FOCUS: FOOD GUIDE PYRAMID

The most recent food guidance system developed by the **U.S. Department of Agriculture (USDA)**. The Pyramid is based on USDA's research on what foods Americans eat, what nutrients are in these foods, and how to apply variety, moderation, and balance to your daily meals and snack choices. The Pyramid focuses on **fat** because most Americans' diets are too high in fat. Following the Pyramid will help you keep your intake of total fat and **saturated fat** low.

The Pyramid includes foods from the five food groups shown in the three lower sections.

1. Breads, cereals, rice, and pasta

2. Fruits

3. Vegetables

4. Meat, poultry, fish, dry beans, eggs, and nuts

5. Milk, cheese, and yogurt

At the base of the Pyramid are breads, cereals, rice, and pasta—all foods from grains. You need the most servings of these foods each day. Foods from the grain products group, along with vegetables and fruits on the next level, are the basis of healthful diets. Vegetables and fruits are placed on the same level because they both include foods that come from plants. On the next level are two groups of foods that come mostly from animals: milk, yogurt, and cheese; and meats, poultry, fish, dry beans, eggs, and nuts (see Figure F.3).

The Pyramid shows a range of servings for each major food group. The number of servings that are right for you depends on how many **calories** you need, which in turn depends on your age, sex, size, and how active you are. Almost everyone should have at least the lowest number of servings in the ranges. Unfortunately the Pyramid's serving sizes do not always correspond to the serving sizes on the new food labels. This is because the serving sizes on food labels are meant to reflect what people normally eat, whereas the serving sizes for the Pyramid are what is recommended (see Table F.7).

Figure F.3 Food Pyramid

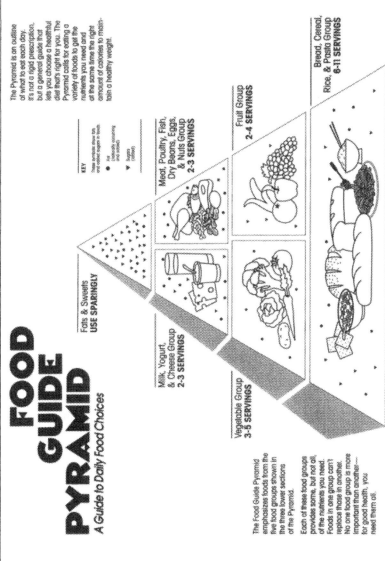

Table F.7 What Counts as a Serving?*

Grain Products Group (bread, cereal, rice, and pasta)

- 1 slice of bread

- 1 ounce of ready-to-eat cereal

- 1/2 cup of cooked cereal, rice, or pasta

Vegetable Group

- 1 cup of raw leafy vegetables

- 1/2 cup of other vegetables—cooked or chopped raw

- 3/4 cup of vegetable juice

Fruit Group

- 1 medium apple, banana, orange

- 1/2 cup of chopped, cooked, or canned fruit

- 3/4 cup of fruit juice

Milk Group (milk, yogurt, and cheese)

- 1 cup of milk or yogurt

- 1-1/2 ounces of natural cheese

- 2 ounces of processed cheese

Meat and Beans Group (meat, poultry, fish, dry beans, eggs, and nuts)

- 2-3 ounces of cooked lean meat, poultry, or fish

- 1/2 cup of cooked dry beans or 1 egg counts as 1 ounce of lean meat. Two tablespoons of peanut butter or 1/3 cup of nuts count as 1 ounce of meat.

* Some foods fit into more than one group. Dry beans, peas, and lentils can be counted as servings in either the meat and beans group or vegetable group. These "cross over" foods can be counted as servings from either one or the other group, but not both. Serving sizes indicated here are those used in the Food Guide Pyramid and based on both suggested and usually consumed

Table F.7 What Counts as a Serving?* (continued)

portions necessary to achieve adequate nutrient intake. They differ from serving sizes on the Nutrition Facts Label, which reflect portions usually consumed.

Source: U.S. Department of Agriculture. 1994. *The Food Guide Pyramid.*

The following calorie level suggestions are based on recommendations of the National Academy of Sciences and on calorie intakes reported by people in national food consumption surveys (see Table F.8).

- 1,600 calories is about right for many sedentary women and some older adults.

- 2,200 calories is about right for most children, teenage girls, active women, and many sedentary men. Women who are pregnant or breastfeeding may need somewhat more.

- 2,800 calories is about right for teenage boys, many active men, and some very active women.

Table F.8 Caloric Distribution

Calories	2,000	2,500	2,800	3,500	4,000
Total fat (g)	65	80	95	120	135
Saturated fat (g)	20	25	30	40	45
Cholesterol (mg)	300	300	300	300	300
Total carbohydrate (g)	300	375	425	525	600
Dietary Fiber (g)	25	30	30	40	45
Protein (g)	50	65	70	90	100
For each of these nutrients, your % Daily Value can add up to...	100%	125%	140%	175%	200%

Source: U.S. Food and Drug Administration and International Food Information Council Foundation. 1994. *The New Food Label: There's Something In It For Everyone.*

The small tip of the Pyramid shows fats, oils, and sweets, such as salad dressings, cream, butter, margarine, sugar, soft drinks, candies, and sweet desserts, but these do not make a food group (there are no pictures at the tip of the Pyramid). These foods supply calories and little else nutritionally. Most people should use them sparingly. Some fat symbols (dots) or added sugar symbols (triangles) are shown in the other food groups. That's to remind you that some foods in these groups can also be high in fat and added **sugars**. Many foods in the milk group and in the meat and beans group (which includes eggs and nuts, as well as meat, poultry, and fish) are also high in fat, as are some processed foods in the grain group. Choosing lower fat options among these foods allows you to eat the recommended servings from these groups and increase the amount and variety of grain products, fruits, and vegetables in your diet without going over your calorie needs. When choosing foods for a healthful diet, consider the fat and added sugars in your choices from all the food groups, not just fats and sweets from the Pyramid tip.

You can achieve a healthful, nutritious eating pattern with many combinations of foods from the five major food groups. Choosing a variety of foods within and across food groups improves dietary patterns because foods within the same group have different combinations of nutrients and other beneficial substances. It also makes meals more interesting. Meals can have rice, pasta, potatoes, or bread at the center of the plate, accompanied by other vegetables and fruit, and lean and low-fat foods from the other groups.

Food Intolerance Symptoms of gas, bloating, constipation, dizziness, or difficulty sleeping, after eating certain foods. Food intolerance may produce symptoms similar to **food allergies,** such as abdominal cramping. Although people with true food allergies must avoid offending foods altogether, people with food intolerance can often eat small amounts of the offending food without experiencing symptoms, and don't have any immunological reaction to the food. See also **food allergy.**

Food Labeling The information shown on food labels. Since 1938 the federal government has required basic information on food labels. The **Food and Drug Administration (FDA)** regulates labels on all packaged foods except for meat, poultry, and egg products, which is regulated by the **U.S. Department of Agriculture (USDA).** The amount of information on food labels varies, but all food labels must contain at least the following information also: (see Figure F.4).

- The name of the food

- The net contents or net weight–this is the quantity of the food itself without the packaging (in English and metric units)

- The name and place of business of the manufacturer, packer, or distributor

- A list of ingredients

Nutrition information is also required for most foods.

For most foods, all of the ingredients must be listed on the label and must be identified by their common or usual names to help consumers identify ingre-

Figure F.4 Food Label

Nutrition Facts

Serving Size 1 cup (228g)
Servings Per Container 2

Amount Per Serving

Calories 250 Calories from Fat 110

	% **Daily Value***
Total Fat 12g	**18**%
Saturated Fat 3g	**15**%
Cholesterol 30mg	**10**%
Sodium 470mg	**20**%
Total Carbohydrate 31g	**10**%
Dietary Fiber 0g	**0**%
Sugars 5g	
Protein 5g	

Vitamin A 4%	•	Vitamin C 2%
Calcium 20%	•	Iron 4%

* Percent Daily Values are based on a 2,000 calorie diet. Your daily values may be higher or lower depending on your calorie needs:

	Calories:	2,000	2,500
Total Fat	Less than	65g	80g
Sat Fat	Less than	20g	25g
Cholesterol	Less than	300mg	300mg
Sodium	Less than	2,400mg	2,400mg
Total Carbohydrate		300g	375g
Dietary Fiber		25g	30g

Calories per gram:
Fat 9 • Carbohydrate 4 • Protein 4

INGREDIENTS: WATER, ENRICHED MACARONI (ENRICHED FLOUR [NIACIN, FERROUS SULFATE (IRON), THIAMINE MONONITRATE AND RIBOFLAVIN], EGG WHITE), FLOUR, CHEDDAR CHEESE (MILK, CHEESE CULTURE, SALT, ENZYME), SPICES, MARGARINE (PARTIALLY HYDROGEN-ATED SOYBEAN OIL, WATER, SOY LECITHIN, MONO- AND DIGLYCERIDES, BETA CAROTENE FOR COLOR,VITAMIN A PALMITATE), AND MALTODEXTRIN.

dients that they are allergic to or want to avoid for other reasons. The ingredient that is present in the largest amount, by weight, must be listed first. Other ingredients follow in descending order according to weight.

See also **nutrition labeling.**

Food Poisoning See **foodborne illness.**

Food Preservation Any treatment of food and its immediate surroundings that serves to minimize undesirable changes in the food, such as those caused by microbes or chemical changes. Some methods of food preservation follow.

1. Use of preservatives, such as **citric acid.**

2. Use of heat (thermal processing) as when foods are canned or milk is pasteurized.

3. Use of cold temperatures (refrigeration or freezing).

4. Removing water (**dehydration**).

5. Exposing food to high-energy radiation (**irradiation**).

Food Products Foods that contain parts of whole foods and often have ingredients such as **sugars,** sugar or **fat substitutes,** and nutrients added to them. For instance, cookies are made with white flour from grains and eggs. Then sugar, shortening, and nutrients are added. The supermarket shelves are jammed with food products such as most breakfast cereals, cookies, crackers, sauces, soups, baking mixes, frozen entrees, pasta, snack foods, and condiments.

Foodservice Contractor See **contract foodservice management.**

Forecasting A technique that uses appropriate and available data to predict what is likely to occur in the future. It amounts to intelligent, educated guesswork about future events.

Fore Milk The breast milk that is present in the ducts and sinuses between the cells where it is made and the nipple. Fore milk contains less **protein** and fat than **hind milk.** Hind milk is the milk stored in the milk-producing cells. When an infant breastfeeds, the fore milk is readily available. Once suckling causes **oxytocin** to be produced, the milk-producing cells contract and release the hind milk.

Fortification Foods that have had nutrients added to them that were never present in the original food. For example, orange juice with **calcium** is a fortified food because calcium was added to a product that never had calcium before.

Fresh Foods Raw foods that have not been frozen, processed (such as canned or frozen), or heated. Fresh foods also cannot contain any preservatives. Examples of fresh foods in the supermarket include fresh fruits and vegetables, and fresh meats, poultry, and fish.

Fructose A **monosaccharide** (simple sugar) found in fruits and honey. Fructose is the sweetest natural sugar (see Figure F.5).

Full Liquid Diet A diet of clear and opaque foods, such as milk, that are either liquid at room temperature or become liquid at room temperature (such as ice cream). It differs from the **clear liquid diet** mostly by the addition of milk products and hot cereals. The full liquid diet is indicated in post-operative situations when the patient has not fully recovered the ability to consume and tolerate solid food. In this case the full liquid diet acts as a transition between a clear liquid and **soft** or regular **diet**. It may also be used for patients with chewing problems or with esophageal or **stomach** disorders that interfere with the handling of solid foods.

Figure F.5 Fructose

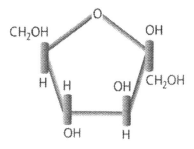

Functional Disability A disability that interferes with the normal activities of daily life such as getting dressing, cooking, or going to the store.

Functional Foods Foods that are supplemented with ingredients thought to help prevent disease or improve health. In some cases, they are developed through **biotechnology**. Some of the health-promoting ingredients being touted are a variety of **vitamins** and **phytochemicals**, substances found in fruits and vegetables that may be helpful in preventing **cancer**.

Fundus The upper dome-shaped region of the **stomach**. See also **stomach**.

Furanose **Monosaccharides** with five-membered rings such as **fructose**.

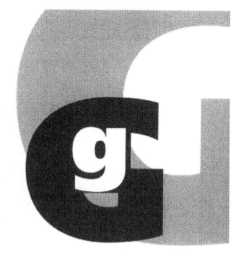

Gag Reflex A normal reflex stimulated by touching the back of the throat. The gag reflex pulls the tongue back and contracts the throat **muscles**. When eating, if something gets stuck in the back of the throat, the gag reflex often results in vomiting of the food so that the food doesn't obstruct the windpipe.

Galactose A **monosaccharide** (**simple sugar**) found linked to **glucose** to form **lactose** or milk **sugar** (see Figure G.1).

Figure G.1 Galactose

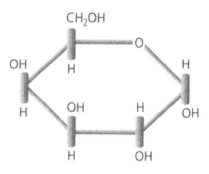

Galactosemia A rare genetic disease seen in newborns. Babies with galactosemia lack the **enzyme** required to convert **galactose** (found in milk **sugar— lactose**) to **glucose**, so they must use a soy-based formula and avoid foods containing milk and milk products.

Gallbladder An **organ** under the **liver** that stores and concentrates **bile** until food is in the **stomach** and **duodenum**. Then the gallbladder contracts and bile travels down the cystic duct to the **common bile duct** to the duodenum. See also **bile**. (See Figure G.2.)

Figure G.2 Gallbladder

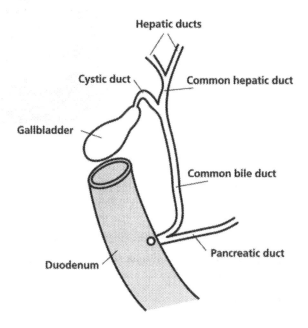

Gallstones Small, hard **mineral** deposits that can obstruct the cystic or **common bile ducts** and cause pain. Gallstones are mostly made of **cholesterol**.

Gamete Sex cell—either sperm (male gamete) or ovum (female gamete).

Ganglion (Ganglia—Plural) 1) A group of many **nerve** cell bodies outside the brain and spinal cord. 2) A mass arising from a tendon in the wrist.

Gastrectomy Surgical removal of all or part of the **stomach**.

Gastric Bypass A surgical procedure for severely obese individuals. In the gastric bypass, a section of the **small intestine** is connected to the **stomach** to decrease the amount of nutrients that are digested and absorbed.

Gastric Lipase A **fat**-splitting **enzyme** produced in the **stomach**.

Gastrin A **hormone** secreted by the **stomach** that stimulates the stomach to make **hydrochloric acid** and **pepsinogen**, the inactive form of the **protein**-splitting **enzyme pepsin**.

Gastritis Inflammation of the **stomach**.

Gastroenteritis Inflammation of the **stomach** and intestines.

Gastroenterologist A physician who diagnoses and treats **alimentary tract** disorders.

Gastroesophageal Reflux See **heartburn**.

Gastrointestinal Endoscopy A medical procedure in which a flexible fiberoptic tube is placed through the mouth or **anus** to see parts of the **gastrointestinal tract**.

Gastrointestinal Tract A hollow tube running down the middle of your body in which digestion of food and absorption of nutrients takes place. At the top of the tube is your mouth, which is connected in turn to your **pharynx**, **esophagus, stomach, small intestine, large intestine, rectum**, and **anus**, where solid wastes leave the body. See also **pharynx, esophagus, stomach, small intestine, large intestine, rectum**, and **anus**. (See Figure G.3.)

Figure G.3 Human Digestive Tract

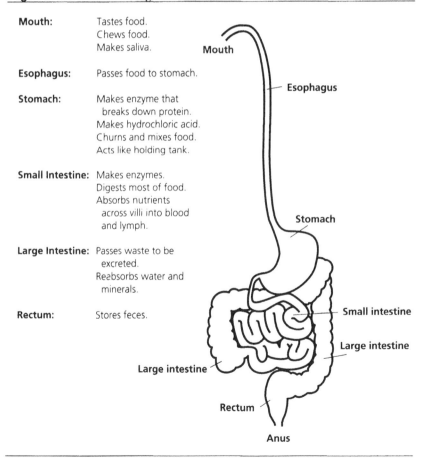

Mouth:	Tastes food. Chews food. Makes saliva.
Esophagus:	Passes food to stomach.
Stomach:	Makes enzyme that breaks down protein. Makes hydrochloric acid. Churns and mixes food. Acts like holding tank.
Small Intestine:	Makes enzymes. Digests most of food. Absorbs nutrients across villi into blood and lymph.
Large Intestine:	Passes waste to be excreted. Reabsorbs water and minerals.
Rectum:	Stores feces.

Mouth

Esophagus

Stomach

Small intestine

Large intestine

Large intestine

Rectum

Anus

Gastrojejunostomy A surgically-created opening between the **stomach** and the **jejunum**.

Gastroplasty Surgery that makes the **stomach** pouch smaller such as by stapling. Gastroplasty has been used to enable obese individuals to eat less.

Gatekeeper In **nutrition**, the individual who controls to an extent what someone else can eat. For example, a mother of a young child quite often is a gatekeeper until the child is older.

Gene The information in **DNA** that contains the code for one **polypeptide**. Generally speaking, gene refers to the genetic code found in DNA. Genes are found in the cell's **chromosomes**.

Generally Regarded as Safe (GRAS) **Food additives** that were determined to be safe in part because of their long use. The GRAS list was established by the **Food and Drug Administration**.

Generalize In **research**, the extent to which the results of a study are applicable to other similar situations.

Genetic Engineering A process that allows plant breeders to modify the genetic makeup of a plant species precisely and predictably, creating improved varieties faster and easier than can be done using more traditional plant-breeding techniques. New methods allow scientists to identify a **gene** that produces a particular trait and transfer a copy of it to another plant used for human food or animal feed.

Geriatrics The branch of medicine that looks at older people and their medical problems.

Gerontology The study of aging.

Gestation The period from when a baby is conceived to when it is born.

Gestational Diabetes A diabetic state that occurs during pregnancy and disappears when pregnancy is over.

Glass Ceiling Discriminatory practices that keep women and other protected classes from advancing to top managerial jobs.

Globulins One of the **blood plasma proteins**. About one-third of the plasma proteins are **globulins**. Globulins may be one of three types: alpha globulins, beta globulins, and gamma globulins. Alpha and beta globulins are made in the **liver** and transport **fat-soluble vitamins** and **lipids** in the **blood**. Gamma globulins are **antibodies** made by **lymphocytes**.

Glomerular Filtrate The water and solutes filtered into **Bowman's capsule** from the capillaries in the **glomerulus**. Also see **nephron**.

Glomerular Filtration Rate (GFR) The volume of filtrate produced each minute by the two **kidneys**. It is an important indicator of renal function. The normal GFR is approximately 125 ml/minute.

Glomerulonephritis Inflammation of the **glomerulus** in the **nephrons** of the **kidney**.

Glomerulus A tiny ball of capillaries found in the **nephron** of the **kidney**. Also see **nephron**.

Glossitis Inflammation of the tongue.

Glucagon A **hormone** produced and secreted by the alpha cells of the **islets of Langerhans** in the **pancreas**. Glucagon raises **blood glucose levels**. When blood glucose levels are low, glucagon stimulates the liver to break down **glycogen** and release **glucose** into the **blood**, and also stimulates the hydrolysis of stored **fat** to release free **fatty acids** into the blood.

Glucocorticoids A group of **hormones** produced and secreted by the adrenal cortex that regulate the **metabolism** of **glucose**, **fat**, and **protein** and suppress the inflammatory response. The most important glucocorticoid is **hydrocortisone**, also called **cortisol**. Hydrocortisone suppresses the **immune system** and has an anti-inflammatory effect. Hydrocortisone also stimulates the breakdown of protein to **amino acids** in the skeletal **muscle** and increases **gluconeogenesis** in the **liver**. **Cortisone** is a synthetic hormone similar to cortisol. When the body is stressed, **corticotropin-releasing factor (CRF)** is made by the **hypothalamus** and travels to the pituitary where it causes the production and secretion of **adrenocorticotropic hormone (ACTH)**. ACTH, the stress hormone, causes the adrenal cortex to make and secrete cortisol.

Glucogenic Amino Acids **Amino acids** that can be used, in whole or in part, to make **glucose**.

Gluconeogenesis The synthesis of **glucose** from deaminated **amino acids**, the **glycerol** part of **fatty acids**, and **lactate**.

Glucose A six-carbon **monosaccharide** (**sugar**) that is the main source of energy for the body. The level of glucose in the **blood** is maintained within certain limits (see Figure G.4).

Figure G.4 Glucose.

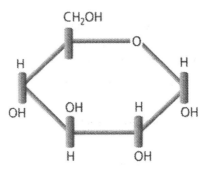

Glutathione Peroxidase A selenium-containing enzyme system that functions as an antioxidant.

NUTRITION AND DISEASE FOCUS: GLUTEN-SENSITIVE ENTEROPATHY (GSE)

A disease in which the gliadin portion of gluten (found in wheat and other grains) causes serious damage to intestinal mucosa, although it is unsure how this occurs. Symptoms include distended stomach, malabsorption, diarrhea, vomiting, and **malnutrition**.

The gliadin portion of the **protein** gluten brings about damage to the intestinal mucosal cells. As the disease progresses, the **villi** of the intestinal mucosa **atrophy** and become flat. There are fewer villi and also sparse microvilli. The end result of this damage is that the surface area for absorption of nutrients decreases by as much as 95 percent.

These mucosal changes lead to malabsorption of nutrients in the **duodenum** and **jejunum**. Nutrients of concern include **iron, vitamin D, vitamin K, calcium, magnesium**, and **folate**. Malabsorption of most **fat** results in loss of kilocalories in the stools and contributes to weight loss and failure to thrive in infants and children. A variety of deficiency symptoms usually occur. Although the intraluminal digestion of proteins is usually normal in GSE, delayed absorption of **amino acids** and **peptides** may occur and thus interfere with protein synthesis in the body. The hypoproteinemia seen in many cases may be partially due to the protein lost from the damaged mucosa. Microcytic or **macrocytic** anemia may result from malabsorption of **folate, vitamin B12**, and/or iron.

The disease appears to be confined largely to Caucasians and is more common in certain European countries than in the United States. It is rare in blacks, Chinese, and Japanese. It is probably more common in women. The prevalence of GSE is higher in adults than children. A familial tendency has been observed in the incidence of GSE.

Also known as *nontropical sprue, celiac sprue,* **celiac disease,** and *gluten-induced sprue* (see Table G.1).

Table G.1   Gluten-Free Diet

	Foods to Omit	Check Food Labels for These
Gluten	All foods containing wheat, oats, barley, or rye as flour or in any other form; salad dressings, gravies, malted beverages, postum, soy sauce, instant puddings, distilled vinegar, beer, ale, some wines, gin, whiskey, vodka.	Flour (unless from sources noted below), modified food starch, monosodium glutamate, hydrolyzed vegetable protein, cereals, malt or cereal extracts, food starch, vegetable starch, vegetable gum, wheat germ, wheat bran, bran, semolina, malt flavoring, distilled vinegar, emulsifiers, stabilizers.

(Corn, rice, soy, arrowroot, tapioca, and potato do not contain gluten so they can be used.)

Glycemic Index   The extent to which a food, when eaten alone, raises the **blood glucose level** in the **blood,** as compared to pure **glucose.**

Glycerol   A trihydroxy **alcohol** that forms the backbone for **triglycerides** or **triacylglycerols.**

Glycogen   The storage form of **glucose** in the body, a polysaccharide. About five to six ounces of glycogen are stored in the **muscle** and two to three ounces in the **liver.** Glycogen is a long, branched-chain structure.

Glycogenesis   The synthesis of **glycogen** from **glucose** in the **liver** and **muscles.**

Glycogen Loading   See **carbohydrate loading.**

Glycogenolysis   The breakdown of stored **glycogen** to **glucose.**

Glycolipid   A **lipid** that contains a **carbohydrate.**

Glycolysis The principal pathway to break down **glucose** and other **sugars**. Glycolysis is a series of ten steps in which glucose is oxidized to two molecules of **pyruvic acid**. The net energy production of glycolysis is 2 **ATP** and 2 **NADH**. In the absence of **oxygen, lactate (lactic acid**) is produced from pyruvate. In the presence of oxygen, pyruvate is converted to **acetyl-coA** and enters the **tricarboxylic** or TCA cycle. Glycolysis occurs in the cytoplasm of the cell. Also called the *Embden-Meyerhoff pathway*. (See Figure G.5.)

Figure G.5 Glycolysis

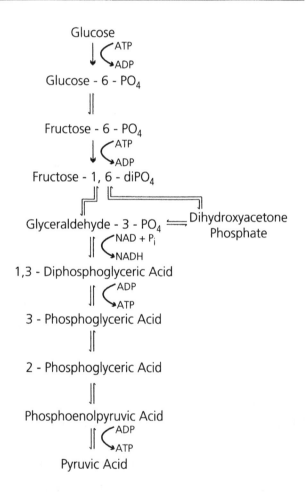

Glycosides A cyclic **sugar** bonded to an **alcohol** with a **glycosidic** bond.

Glycosidic Bond A bond that links **sugars** in their cyclic forms to the **alcohol** (–OH) group of another sugar or an alcohol. Glycosidic bonds link sugars in **polysaccharides** and **oligosaccharides**. (See Figure G.6.)

Figure G.6 Glycosidic bonds.

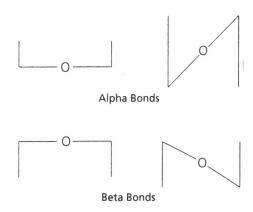

Alpha Bonds

Beta Bonds

Glycosuria **Sugar** in the urine. This is not normal and is often a sign of uncontrolled **diabetes mellitus** or the onset of diabetes mellitus.

Goiter Enlargement of the **thyroid gland**. Goiter may be due to a deficiency of **iodine** (called **endemic** goiter) or other causes. **Hypothyroidism** is associated with endemic goiter.

Gonadotropic Hormones The two **hormones** made in the anterior **pituitary**: **follicle-stimulating hormone (FSH)** and **luteinizing hormone (LH)**. FSH stimulates the growth of ovarian follicles in females and the production of sperm in the male testes. Luteinizing hormone stimulates **ovulation** and the transformation of the ovulated ovarian follicle into an **endrocrine** structure called a **corpus luteum**. LH also influences **mammary gland** secretion of milk. In males, LH stimulates the secretion of male sex **hormones** in the testes.

Gout A form of arthritis in which uric acid crystals are deposited in the **joints**.

Gram A unit of weight or mass in the metric system. There are 28.35 grams in 1 ounce.

Grants A sum of money that is given by a foundation, company, or other organization (called the grantor), that is used by the recipient (called the grantee) for an agreed-upon purpose such as research (see Table G.2).

Table G.2 Basic Elements of a Grant Proposal

1. Cover letter	A letter provides a summary of the project, a pledge of support, some background on the organization seeking the grant, and the contact person and phone number.
2. Cover page	This page lists appropriate grantor and grantee information including addresses, dates, contacts, etc.
3. Table of contents	This page lists the contents of the rest of the proposal.
4. Summary	A summary of the project.
5. Need statement	A statement explaining and documenting the problem and need for the project.
6. Background information	A profile of the grantee's organization.
7. Project goal	A description of the major goal of the project that is hopefully linked to the goals of the grantor.
8. Objectives	The steps to be taken to meet the goals.
9. Activities	These include all procedures and methods to be used.
10. Timetable	The dates of completion for each activity.
11. Personnel	Lists names, titles, and background of every person to be involved in the project, as well as how each will contribute.
12. Evaluation	Includes internal and external evaluation plans.
13. Dissemination	Explains how the results of the project will be disseminated.
14. Budget	A complete listing of expense items and how each was calculated.
15. Future funding	Explains how the project might continue after grantor funding is used up.
16. Attachments	

Granulocytopenia Lower than normal number of granulocytes (types of white blood cells or **leukocytes**) in the **blood**.

Granulocytosis Higher than normal number of granulocytes (a classification of **white blood cells**) in the **blood** that may be due to infection or inflammation. See also **leukocytes.**

Graphics Illustrative materials used to enliven a text. Examples of graphics include tables, charts, graphs, line art figures, photographs, and diagrams.

GRAS See **generally regarded as safe.**

Grave's Disease A condition marked by enlargement of the **thyroid's** glandular cells, overproduction of thyroxine, an increased metabolic rate, and increased heart rate. About half the cases also have bulging of the eyes (called exophthalmos) because of swelling. Grave's disease may be an immunological disorder. Treatment often consists of antithyroid drugs that reduce how much **hormone** is made.

Grazing Eating frequent small meals or snacks during the day.

Grievance Procedures A formal organizational procedure that employees can follow when they feel they have been treated unfairly by management. Grievance procedures often allow an employee the opportunity to present his/her case in a meeting called a **hearing.**

Growth Chart A grid that allows comparison of a child's height and weight to national percentiles. For example, if a girl is in the 90 percentile height for age, it means that, out of 100 girls her age, she is taller than 89 and shorter than 10. These are commonly used by physicians as an indicator of the child's overall health and adequacy of **calorie** intake for children up to 18 years of age. Also called **growth grid.**

Growth Hormone A **hormone** produced and secreted by the posterior **pituitary** that stimulates growth by helping **amino acids** into the body's cells and helping cells make **proteins**. Growth hormone also increases **blood glucose levels**. Also called **somatotropin.**

Growth Spurt A period of rapid growth.

Guanosine Triphosphate (GTP) A high energy phosphate-containing compound involved in some **metabolic pathways**, such as protein synthesis, similar to **ATP.**

Gynecology A branch of medicine that deals with the study and treatment of the female reproductive system. Gynecology is almost always studied and practiced with **obstetrics.**

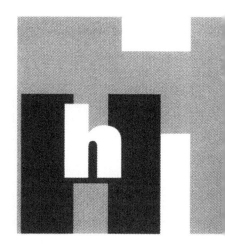

Half Life The time required for half the amount of a substance such as a drug, to disappear from the blood.

Halo Effect The tendency to extend the perception of one outstanding quality of a person to the whole person. For example, if a dietetic assistant has excellent interactions with patients, the **supervisor** may think he/she must do her entire job to high standards.

Hazard Analysis Critical Control Point (HACCP) An evaluation system to identify, monitor, and control contamination (**foodborne illness**) risks in foodservice establishments. HACCP looks closely at the various food handling processes to prevent disease from occurring. The seven steps in a HACCP system are:

1. Identify potentially hazardous foods.

    -   Review the menu and recipes.

    -   Observe employees making recipes.

    -   Measure temperatures.

    -   Test foods.

2. Identify critical control points (CCP).

    A CCP is a point, step, or procedure in the product-handling process where controls can be applied and a food safety hazard can be prevented, elimi-nated, or reduced to acceptable levels. A critical control point is the *kill* step in which the bacteria are killed by cooking, or the *control* step that prevents or slows their growth, such as proper chilled storage or hot holding.

- Critical Items: Personal hygiene

                        Time/temperature

                        Cooking, cooling, reheating, holding

                        Preparation ahead of time

                        Cross-contamination

3. Set up control procedures (standards, criteria) for critical control points.

Each standard should be something that can be immediately monitored—by measurement or observation. Standards should be as specific as possible, using time and temperature as appropriate.

4. Monitor critical control points.

5. Establish corrective action.

6. Set up a record-keeping system.

7. Verify that the system is working.

PRACTICAL NUTRITION FOCUS: HEALTHY MENUS

A menu with nutritious options available to guests who want them.

Planning Menu Items Low in Fat, Saturated Fat, and Cholesterol

Breakfast

- Offer fresh and canned fruits and juices.

- Almost all cold and hot cereals are great choices. Granola cereals tend to be high in **fat** unless labeled as reduced fat.

- Most breads are low in fat except for croissants, brioche, cheese breads, and many biscuits. Bagels, low-fat muffins, and baguettes are good choices.

- Have reduced-fat **margarine** and light cream cheese available to spread on bagels or toast.

- Serve chicken filets, poultry sausages, low-fat ham slices, or fish as leaner sources of **protein** than the traditional bacon and pork sausage.

- Offer egg substitutes for scrambled eggs and other egg-based items. Egg substitutes taste better when herbs, flavorings, and/or vegetables are cooked with them. Instead of egg substitutes, you can offer to make scrambled eggs and omelets by mixing one whole egg to two egg whites.

- Serve an omelet with blanched vegetables such as chopped broccoli or spinach and low-fat cheese instead of regular cheese.

- As a spread or topping on pancakes and waffles, offer sauces combining low-fat or nonfat yogurt with a fruit puree.

- Serve a breakfast buffet with loads of fruits, low-fat dairy products, and cereals.

Appetizer and Soup

- Offer juices and fresh sliced fruits. Fresh sliced fruits can be served with a yogurt dressing flavored with fruit juices.

- Offer raw vegetables with dips using low-fat yogurt, low-fat cottage cheese, or ricotta cheese as the base, rather than dips using sour cream, cheeses, cream, or cream cheese. Try hummus, a chickpea-based dip or salsa, made from tomatoes, onions, hot peppers, garlic, and herbs.

- Offer grilled chicken, broiled Buffalo-style chicken wings, or steamed seafood such as shrimp.

- Dish up baked potato skins (rather than frying them) and baked corn tortillas for tortilla chips. Sprinkle with grated cheese, garlic, onion, or chili powder.

- Feature soups that use stock as the base and vegetables and grains as the ingredients. Dried beans, peas, and lentils make great soups when cooked and pureed, without using cream or high-fat thickeners such as roux.

Salads

- Offer salads with lots of vegetables and fruits.

- Use only small amounts, if any, of bacon, meat, cheese, eggs, or croutons. Choose cooked beans and peas or low-fat cheeses.

- Offer reduced calorie or nonfat salad dressings. Place on the side when desired.

- Make tuna fish salad and other similar salads with low-fat mayonnaise.

- Use cooked salad dressing that contains little fat for Waldorf and other salads. It has a tarter flavor than mayonnaise.

Breads

- Most breads are low in fat and **saturated fat**. Breads with more fat include biscuits, cheese breads, croissants, popovers, brioche, corn bread, and many commercial crackers (although some of these are available or can be made with less fat).

Entrees

- Serve combination dishes with small amounts of meat, poultry, or seafood with whole-grains such as rice, legumes, vegetables, and/or fruits.
- Offer moderate portions of broiled, baked, stir-fried, or poached seafood, white-meat poultry without skin, and lean cuts of meat (see Table H.1).

Table H.1 Lean Cuts of Meat

Beef

Top round (roasted for roast beef, cut into cubes for kebabs, marinated to make London Broil)

Eye of round (roasted for roast beef or braised for pot roast)

Tip round (cut into cubes for kebabs)

Strip loin steak (broiled to make New York Strip Steak, Club Steak, or other name)

Top sirloin butt steak (broiled to make Sirloin Steak, also cut into cubes for kebabs, marinated to make London Broil)

Flank steak (marinated and broiled to make London Broil)

Tenderloin steak (broiled to make Filet Mignon)

Pork (Each cut has less than 9 grams of fat per 3-ounce cooked serving)

Boneless loin roast

Boneless rib roast

Center rib chop

Center loin chop

Top loin chop

Sirloin roast

Table H.1 Lean Cuts of Meat (continued)

Pork

Boneless sirloin chop

Tenderloin

Veal

Almost all cuts are low in fat

Lamb

Sirloin roast

Shank half of leg roast

Loin chops

Blade chops

Foreshank

- Offer hamburger, meat loaf, or other ground beef dishes made with low-fat ground beef.

- Feature one or more meatless entrees, such as vegetarian burgers. Vegetarian burgers either try to imitate a beef burger (usually through using soy products) or are real veggie burgers (they are made of vegetables, especially mushrooms).

- For sauced entrees (or side dishes), feature sauces thickened with flour, cornstarch, or vegetable purees. Salsas, chutneys, relishes, and coulis also work well.

- Offer sandwiches made with roasted turkey, chicken, water-pack tuna fish salad, lean roast beef made from the round, or a spicy bean or lentil spread.

- For sandwich spreads, use reduced-calorie mayonnaise, French or Russian-style salad dressing, mustard, ketchup, barbeque sauce, or salsa.

- Feature lots of different vegetables in sandwiches.

Side Dishes

- Most side dishes of vegetables, grains, and pasta are good choices as long as little fat is added during preparation.

- Serve grilled potato halves instead of french fries, as well as other grilled vegetables.

Desserts

- Offer fruit-based desserts such as apple cobbler.

- Spotlight sorbets, sherbets, frozen yogurt, and ice milk. All contain less fat than ice cream.

- Feature desserts made from fat-free egg whites such as angel food cake and meringues. Serve with a fruit sauce.

- Offer puddings made with skim milk.

- Serve low-fat cookies such as ladyfingers, biscotti, gingerbread, and fruit bars.

Beverages

- Offer 1 percent or skim milk.

Planning Menu Items High in Complex Carbohydrates

Breakfast

- Offer fruit in many different ways because fruit is the most requested breakfast food for guests concerned about eating a nutritious breakfast.

- Serve freshly made fruit and vegetable juices, such as carrot and apple juice.

- Feature whole-grain and multigrain toast, muffins (bran muffins are high in **fiber**), bagels, breads and rolls, and even pancakes, French toast, waffles, and crepes.

- Offer different varieties of cooked and cold cereals, especially whole-grain cereals containing whole-wheat, oats, or other whole-grain. Cereals with bran contain much fiber. Be sure to have fresh fruit for a topping as well as raisins and other dried fruits.

Appetizer and Soup

- Select soups rich in split peas, beans, lentils, vegetables, grains, or pasta. In the summer, feature a cold fruit soup.

- Serve soups with high-fiber crackers such as rye krisps, whole-wheat melba toast, or others made with whole-grains and/or bran.

Salads

- Most salads are good sources of **complex carbohydrates**.

- Feature pasta salads with lots of fresh vegetables and/or fruits.

- Dish up salads with grains, such as bulgur or wild rice, dried fruits and small amounts of nuts or seeds.

Breads

- Breads are great for complex carbohdyrates. Feature whole-grain breads such as oat bread and whole-wheat parkerhouse rolls.

- In bread baskets, be sure to include a fiber-rich muffin or biscuit containing whole-grains, bran, nuts, fruits, or vegetables such as pumpkin.

Entrees

- Dish up pasta dishes, preferably using whole-wheat pasta for more fiber.

- Feature a main dish using grains, such as quinoa mexican style, or legumes, such as lentil tacos.

- Spotlight a veggie whole-wheat pizza.

- On sandwiches, offer toppings such as lettuce, tomatoes, sprouts, cucumbers, onions, hot peppers, green pepper rings, and mushrooms. Use whole-grain breads, rolls, or tortillas.

Side Dishes

- Feature a variety of vegetables and fruits (keep skins on)—they are all good sources of complex carbohydrates.

- Dish up side dishes using grains, such as brown rice, and cooked or canned dry beans and peas.

- Spotlight potatoes in all their cooked forms.

Desserts

- For desserts, offer:

  - Fruits in any form.
  - Cakes or cookies using whole-grain flours, nuts, fruits, or vegetables, such as oatmeal raisin bars or carrot pineapple cake.

- Rice pudding (use brown rice and add cherries), tapioca pudding, or bread pudding.

- Fruit-filled cobblers and tarts with whole-grains, such as oats, used in the cobbler topping or tart shell.

- Fruit toppings on cakes.

Planning Menu Items Low in Refined Sugar

Breakfast

- Offer 100 percent fruit juices. Products labeled as fruit drinks or fruit beverages contain added sugars and often contain little juice.

- In addition to pure fruit juices, have fresh fruits and canned fruits packed in their own juice available.

- Offer unsweetened breakfast cereals. For each four grams listed under "Sugars" on a cereal box label, there is one teaspoon of sugar. For less sugar, choose cereals with less than four grams of sugar per serving, unless the sugar comes from a dried fruit such as raisins.

- Jams, jellies, and pancake syrup contain much refined sugar. Have available low-sugar jams and jellies or fruit spreads made from 100 percent fruit. Other toppings for toast or pancakes include sliced or chopped fresh fruit, unsweetened applesauce, or other unsweetened fruit sauce.

Appetizers and Soup

- Most appetizers and soups are low in refined sugar.

Salads

- Most salads are not high in sugar, except for those made with regular gelatin. Gelatin mixes using **aspartame** or another sugar substitute are sugar-free.

Breads

- Most breads are low in refined sugar.

Entrees

- Most entrees are low in refined sugar.

Side Dishes

- Most side dishes are low in refined sugar.

Desserts

- Spotlight fruits in desserts. Fresh fruit can be baked (as in baked apples), poached (as in poached pears), broiled, or made into compote. Select fruits packed in their own juice rather than fruits packed in light or heavy syrup. One-half cup of fruit canned in heavy syrup contains about four teaspoons of sugar.

- Have sugarless puddings available.

- Offer a baked good sweetened mostly with fruits, such as fruit bars.

Beverages

- Offer bottled waters, sugar-free soft drinks, fruit and vegetable juices, and unsweetened iced tea.

- Have sugar substitutes available for beverages.

Planning Menu Items Low in Sodium

General

- Decrease or replace **salt** in recipes by using vegetables, herbs, spices, and flavorings.

- Offer salt-free seasoning blends and lemon wedges.

Breakfast

- Any fruits and juices are naturally low in **sodium**. Canned tomato or vegetable juice is high in sodium unless labeled low sodium.

- Serve hot cereals, pancakes, french toast, and waffles without adding salt during preparation. Garnish with fruit toppings.

- Toast, bagels, and muffins contain moderate amounts of sodium.

Appetizer and Soup

- Offer unsalted crackers, chips, and pretzels.

- Feature a low-sodium soup made without commercial bases or salt. Use made-from-scratch stocks and use herbs and spices for seasoning.

Salads

- Most salad ingredients are low in sodium, except for bacon, bacon bits, and croutons (unless homemade with little or no salt).

- Offer homemade salad dressings low in sodium.

Breads

- Salt is a necessary ingredient in breads. Breads contain a moderate amount of sodium.

Entrees

- Offer fresh meat, poultry, or seafood instead of canned, cured, smoked or salty meat, poultry, or seafood (such as ham, corned beef, smoked turkey, dried cod, and most luncheon meats). Cheeses are high in sodium so use small amounts in sandwiches.

- Feature freshly-made entrees instead of processed or prepared foods.

- Offer freshly prepared salsas and other low-sodium sauces.

- Feature a homemade low-sodium pasta sauce.

- Instead of high-sodium accompaniments to sandwiches such as pickles, olives, and potato chips, serve fresh vegetables, cole slaw made with reduced-calorie mayonnaise, or another healthful salad.

Side Dishes

- Offer fresh or frozen vegetables instead of canned or pickled products; season with lemon juice, flavored vinegars, herbs, or spices.

Desserts

- Offer fruits, sorbets, sherbets, frozen yogurt, and homemade baked goods made with moderate amounts of sodium (avoid self-rising flour—it's high in sodium).

Healthy People 2000 A report from the U.S. Department of Health and Human Services, Public Health Services designed to improve health promotion and disease prevention efforts. Objectives listed in this report aim for specific, measurable changes in what Americans eat, as well as increased accessibility to healthier foods and encouraging healthy choices in areas other than nutrition.

The full name of the report is *Healthy People 2000: National Health Promotion and Disease Prevention Objectives.*

To enhance meeting the goals set in this document, model standards were developed by a partnership of governmental agencies and private sector organizations. The third edition of the model standards is titled *Healthy Communities 2000: Model Standards. Guidelines for Community Attainment of the Year 2000 National Health Objectives.* It is the guide for local implementation of **Healthy People 2000** (see Tables H.2 and H.3).

Table H.2 Priority Areas for Healthy People 2000

Health Promotion

1. Physical Activity and Fitness

2. Nutrition

3. Tobacco

4. Alcohol and Other Drugs

5. Family Planning

6. Mental Health and Mental Disorders

7. Violent and Abusive Behavior

8. Educational and Community-Based Programs

Health Protection

9. Unintentional Injuries

10. Occupational Safety and Health

11. Environmental Health

12. Food and Drug Safety

13. Oral Health

Preventive Services

14. Maternal and Infant Health

15. Heart Disease and Stroke

Table H.2   Priority Areas for Healthy People 2000 (continued)

16. Cancer

17. Diabetes and Chronic Disabling Conditions

18. HIV Infection

19. Sexually Transmitted Diseases

20. Immunization and Infectious Diseases

21. Clinical Preventive Services

Surveillance and Data Systems

22. Surveillance and Data Systems

Table H.3 Steps for Putting Model Standards to Use

- Assess and determine the role of one's health agency.

- Assess the lead health agency's organizational capacity.

- Develop an agency plan to build the necessary organizational capacity.

- Assess the community's organizational and power structures.

- Organize the community to build a stronger constituency for public health and establish a partnership for public health.

- Assess the health needs and available community resources.

- Determine local priorities.

- Select outcome and process objectives that are compatible with local priorities and the *Healthy People 2000 Objectives*.

- Develop communitywide intervention strategies.

- Develop and implement a plan of action.

- Monitor and evaluate the effort on a continuing basis.

Source: Healthy Communities 2000: Model Standards. Guidelines for Community Attainment of the Year 2000 National Health Objectives (3rd ed.). Washington, DC: American Public Health Association 1991.

PRACTICAL NUTRITION FOCUS: HEALTHY RECIPES

The following tips and hints on modifying recipe ingredients to make them healthier are listed by menu category for ease of use.

Breakfast

- Substitute light cream cheese for regular cream cheese as a spread. Nonfat cream cheese is available but it is not an acceptable spread unless mixed with fruit. Substitute whipped **margarine** in place of butter as a spread. (These substitutes can all be mixed with fruit purees, jellies, jams, syrups, or honey to taste delicious with even less **fat**.) Other low-fat spreads include jam, jelly, preserves, marmalade, fruit butters (they don't include butter—only fruit), and honey.

- Use egg substitutes to make scrambled eggs and omelets. Most egg substitutes are made from egg whites, gums, and coloring to make them look and taste like real eggs. They still contain varying amounts of fat. Or substitute two egg whites and one whole egg for two whole eggs.

- Fill omelets with vegetables and low-fat cheese instead of full-fat cheese.

- Substitute lean smoked ham, Canadian bacon, grilled chicken, poultry sausages, or fish for bacon and pork sausage.

- Fruit can be a topping for cereals, pancakes, waffles, and the like.

- Cut the fat in hash browns by using a **vegetable oil** cooking spray instead of fat.

Appetizers

- Instead of sour cream for dips, substitute nonfat plain yogurt or sour cream made with less or no fat. Or use a noncreamy dip such as salsa, which can be made from a variety of fruits and vegetables, or dips based on pureed beans, peas, or lentil, such as spicy black bean dip. Reduced calorie or fat-free salad dressings, such as peppercorn ranch, also work well as dips.

- Substitute grilled meats, poultry, and seafood for fried versions.

Soups

- To thicken soups, see the discussion about thickeners under **Sauces**.

- Substitute defatted stocks for regular stocks.

- Use vegetables, pasta, whole grains, and legumes instead of fatty meats.

- Instead of using cream or whole milk to make cream soups, substitute evapo-rated skim milk, nonfat buttermilk, low-fat milk, or skim milk. Cooked vegetable purees, such as mashed potatoes, can be used for thickening. When finished with a dollop of cream on top or a dash of wine, a low-fat cream soup can be quite delicious.

- Add rich ingredients through garnishes such as small amounts of shredded cheeses, croutons, sour cream, or filled pasta shapes to add splashes of color, texture, and flavor.

Salads

- Use small amounts of bacon bits, croutons, regular cheeses, and hard-boiled eggs. Instead use homemade croutons made with little fat, low-fat cheeses, and cooked beans, peas, and lentils.

- Substitute low-fat or no-fat commercial salad dressings or salsa for regular salad dressings.

- When making your own dressings, select small amounts of flavorful oils such as extra virgin olive oil, peanut oil, sesame oil, or walnut oil.

- Use flavorful vinegars, such as raspberry or rice vinegar, that require less oil to make a great salad dressing. Try using only two tablespoons of oil per cup of dressing.

- Substitute nonfat yogurts, blenderized low-fat cottage cheese, or low-fat sour cream for cream or sour cream in creamy salad dressings.

- Substitute equal amounts of nonfat plain yogurt and low-fat mayonnaise or try using cooked salad dressing in place of regular mayonnaise in cold salads such as chicken or potato salad.

Breads

- Substitute yeast breads and rolls (preferably whole grain) in place of biscuits, cheese breads, croissants, popovers, brioche, and corn bread. Low-fat recipes are available to make cheese breads, popovers, and corn bread.

- Instead of butter or margarine as spreads on bread, see the lower-fat spreads mentioned under **Breakfast**.

Entrees and Sandwiches

- Substitute lean cuts of beef, pork, and lamb for higher-fat cuts. When appropriate, use smaller portions.

- Substitute whole grains, legumes, vegetables, and/or fruits for some of the meat or poultry in entrees.

- For mixed dishes that include ground beef or pork, substitute two cups of cooked beans for each pound of ground meat. You can also substitute low-fat ground beef or ground chicken or turkey. You can also replace some of the ground meat with fillers such as grains (rolled oats), vegetables (onion, bell peppers), dried fruits (such as currants).

- Substitute vegetable oils for butter and tropical oils (that is, palm, palm kernel, and coconut oil) in cooking. If some butter flavor is needed, mix whipped butter with an equal amount of vegetable oil. Or use small amounts of flavorful oils (such as walnut oil or extra-virgin olive oil) or infused oils.

- Use a yeast bread dough instead of a pie crust for pot pies.

- For regular cheeses, substitute ones lower in fat or use small amounts of a strong-flavored cheese as a garnish to give a great appearance and add flavor (see Table H.4).

Table H.4   Guide to Cheeses

Low in Fat (0–3 grams fat/ounce)	Medium Fat (4 –5 grams fat/ounce)
Cottage cheese, dry curd, 1/4 cup	Light cream cheese (1 ounce = 2 tablespoons)
Cottage cheese, 1/4 cup, 1 percent	Grated Parmesan cheese (1 ounce = 3 tablespoons)
Cottage cheese, 1/4 cup, 2 percent	Mozzarella, part skim
Sap Sago (a hard aged cheese made from skim milk)	Ricotta, 1/4 cup, part skim
Pot cheese (also known as bakers' cheese or farmers' cheese)	String cheese, part skim
Some special low-fat brands of cheese	Some reduced-fat brands of cheese

Table H.4 Guide to Cheeses (continued)

High Fat (6–7 grams fat/ounce)	Very High Fat (8–10 grams fat/ounce)
American cheese food	American cheese
Brie	Blue cheese
Camembert	Brick
Edam	Cheddar
Feta	Colby
Gouda	Cream cheese (1 ounce = 2 tablespoons)
Jarlsberg	Fontina
Limburger	Gruyere
Mozzarella, whole milk	Longhorn
Provolone	Monterey Jack
Romano (1 ounce = 3 tablespoons)	Muenster
Swiss	Port du Salut
Swiss cheese food	Ricotta (1/4 cup), whole milk
	Roquefort

- A naturally fat-free cheese, called fromage blanc, is a wonderful substitute for whole-milk fresh cheeses like ricotta and cottage cheese. Fromage blanc is made by heating buttermilk until the curd begins to separate, then draining the curd.

- Instead of using bread crumbs for breading, crush some whole-grain cereal or crackers and mix with appropriate seasonings.

- Sweeten dishes with unsweetened fruit juice concentrates or fruit purees.

- Substitute roasted, broiled, or grilled lean meats and poultry for cold cuts and hot dogs at lunch time. Mashed, cooked beans, peas, or lentils, when mixed with spices and low-calorie salad dressing, make a tasty sandwich spread for pita bread or tortillas.

- Substitute mustard, ketchup, barbecue sauce, relish, salsa, low-fat or fat-free mayonnaise or salad dressing for butter or margarine on sandwich bread. Also add colorful, crunchy vegetables such as red-tipped leaf lettuce, tomatoes, cucumbers, and bean sprouts (see Table H.5).

Table H.5 Guide to Condiments

Condiment*	Calories	Fat (grams)	Saturated Fat (grams)	Cholesterol (milligrams)
Spreads				
Butter	102	11	7	31
Stick margarine	101	11	2	0
Soft tub	101	11	2	0
Imitation, about 40 percent fat	50	6	1	0
Cream cheese	50	5	3	16
Light cream cheese	35	2.5	2	8
Mayonnaise	99	11	1	51
Low fat	25	1	0	0
Lowfat plain yogurt	9	0	0	1
Nonfat plain yogurt	8	0	0	0
Sweeteners				
Jam/jelly/preserves	52	0	0	0
Honey	65	0	0	0
Apple butter	33	0	0	0
Sauces				
Barbecue	16	0	0	0
Soy	11	0	0	0
Salsa	8	0	0	0
Tartar	70	8	NA	5
Teriyaki	15	0	0	0
Worcestershire	11	0	0	0
Salad Dressings				
Blue cheese	77	8	1.5	0
French	67	6	1.5	0
Reduced calorie	22	1	0	0

Table H.5 Guide to Condiments (continued)

Condiment*	Calories	Fat (grams)	Saturated Fat (grams)	Cholesterol (milligrams)
Italian	69	7	1	0
Reduced calorie	16	1.5	0	0
Russian	76	8	1	0
Reduced calorie	23	1	0	0
Thousand Island	59	6	1	0
Reduced calorie	24	1.5	0	2
Other				
Ketchup	15	0	0	0
Mustard, yellow	15	0	0	0
Pickle relish	20	0	0	0

*Serving size is 1 tablespoon unless otherwise noted.

Source: United States Department of Agriculture

- Instead of pepperoni and sausage on pizzas, heap on vegetables such as broccoli, mushrooms, and green peppers.

- Tenderize tough meats without using commercial tenderizers (they are high in sodium)—marinate the meat instead.

Side Dishes

- Use herbs, spices, garlic, small amounts of toasted nuts or seeds, low-sodium soy sauce, and the like instead of butter or margarine to flavor vegetables and other side dishes.

- On baked potatoes, substitute nonfat or reduced-fat sour cream or plain nonfat yogurt for regular sour cream. Mix with herbs, spices, or vegetables for flavor.

- Mash potatoes with light sour cream, evaporated skim milk, or nonfat buttermilk instead of butter and whole milk.

- Use flavorful rices, such as Basmati rice, instead of long-grain white rice.

- Add grains to vegetable dishes, such as brown rice with stir-fried vegetables.

Sauces

- Instead of thickening with roux (fat and flour) or liaison (egg yolks and cream), healthy thickening agents include the following.

  - Flour. When flour is mixed with a cold liquid such as water, it is called a slurry. When flour is used as a thickener, it must be completely cooked to remove its starchy flavor.

  - Cornstarch. Like flour, cornstarch must first be mixed with a cold liquid before it can be used to thicken. Cornstarch produces a translucent product that doesn't hold up well during long cooking or holding periods.

  - Arrowroot. Although it is an expensive thickener, arrowroot has many advantages. It thickens at lower temperature than other thickeners, it has no starchy taste, and it makes a shiny sauce.

  - Purees of cooked vegetables. Cooked vegetable purees are good thickeners for soups and stews, but can be chosen carefully to thicken sauces too. Use a little olive oil to finish these sauces and give them flavor.

- Instead of using thickening agents, the juices from cooked meat, poultry, or seafood can be reduced, meaning the juices are boiled or simmered until its volume is decreased. At this point its flavors will be quite concentrated. Fat is removed from the juices by chilling the liquid in the refrigerator then removing the congealed (solid) fat, chilling the liquid with ice cubes if time is short and then removing the ice cubes on which the fat is sticking, or using special fat-off ladles or fat-separator pitchers. In a fat-separator pitcher, the spout is at the bottom because the fat will float to the top, allowing you to pour out fat-free juices.

- So who says a sauce has to be a traditional white sauce, brown sauce, or the like? The hottest new sauce in the United States is salsa. Traditional salsa comes from Mexico and is made from tomatoes, onion, chili peppers, garlic, and possibly other ingredients. Salsas can be made from a limitless combination of fruits, vegetables, and/or beans and peas, such as roasted corn and black bean salsa.

- Other vegetable and fruit sauces like salsa include chutneys, relishes, and coulis. They have the following in common: they are made from fruits and/or vegetables, they have primarily a sweet, tart, and/or spicy flavor, and they are used as condiments to complement the main dish.

- If a sauce calls for sour cream, use low-fat or nonfat sour cream or substitute skim-milk ricotta cheese, low-fat cottage cheese, or plain nonfat yogurt.

When cooking with yogurt, use only low heat. High temperatures may cause it to separate and curdle. To prevent this, blend one tablespoon of cornstarch (or two tablespoons of flour) with a cup of yogurt before cooking. If over-mixed, yogurt becomes too thin so be sure not to overstir it.

- Instead of cream, use skim milk or evaporated skim milk.

Desserts

- Substitute frozen yogurt and ice milk for regular ice cream.

- Substitute whipped evaporated skim milk for whipped cream. To do so, whip cold evaporated skim milk with chilled beaters in a chilled bowl. Fold in vanilla and/or cinnamon for flavor.

- Substitute 1 percent or skim milk for whole milk when making puddings or custards. Add a spice, such as cinnamon or nutmeg, to increase the flavor.

- Baked, stewed, or poached fruits are good substitutes for sweet desserts.

- Use fresh sliced fruits and fruit sauces instead of frosting on cakes or other desserts.

Beverages

- Substitute skim and 1 percent milk for regular milk.

- In milkshakes, substitute ice milk or frozen yogurt for ice cream and skim or 1 percent milk for regular milk.

- Add fruit, such as bananas, to milkshakes to make a fruit smoothie.

Baking

The best low-fat baked goods are those in which the originals do not rely on vast amounts of fat and the low-fat version uses some fat as well as flavoring ingredients to make up for the loss of flavor. Modifying baking recipes is trickier than other types of recipes because slight differences in proportions of ingredients (or procedures) can make big differences in the baked good. That's why bakers prefer to call their recipes by another name: *formulas*.

Most baking requires several of these ingredients: flour, sugar, fat, eggs, water or milk, and leavenings. When modifying baking recipes, keep in mind what functions each of these perform in baking.

- Substitute vegetable oil cooking spray or vegetable oil for shortening when preparing pans. Then, flour the pans just as you normally would.

- Substitute whole-wheat pastry flour for one-third of the all-purpose flour called for in a baking recipe. Avoid using any whole-wheat flours in sponge or fine-grained layer cakes because the whole-wheat product is too heavy. Experiment with other whole-grain flours such as barley, rye, and oat by substituting it for part of the wheat flour in a recipe.

- Try using a new whole-wheat flour called *white whole-wheat flour*. It is made from a variety of wheat with the same nutritional value as regular whole-wheat but with a much lighter taste. Milled from hard-white winter wheat, it lacks the strong, almost bitter, flavor associated with the types of wheat used for classic whole-wheat flour. White wheat, nicknamed *sweet wheat* by the farmers who grow it, is a lighter-colored, sweeter-tasting wheat, that can be substituted for all-purpose flour in baking recipes.

- Substitute a low-fat crumb topping or a few decorative dough pieces for the top crust on pies.

- Substitute phyllo dough for the traditional pie crust. Instead of using melted fat to separate the phyllo dough sheets, use a butter-flavored oil cooking spray. Phyllo dough can also be substituted for puffed pastry dough to make desserts such as strudels.

- Meringue shells, made with egg whites and sugar, make excellent crusts for a variety of fruit and other fillings.

- Instead of the traditional high-fat pie crust, make a graham cracker crust. Use less melted margarine or butter to make crumb crusts and add water and honey to help the shell keep its shape and taste good.

- Substitute jams, jellies, fruit spreads, fruit sauces, or powdered sugars for cake frostings.

- When making baked alaska, substitute angel food cake for the sponge cake and substitute ice milk, frozen yogurt, sherbet, or sorbet for the regular ice cream.

- Substitute coconut extract for grated coconut and top the baked good with some toasted coconut.

- Reduce the amount of toasted nuts and seeds.

- Substitute three tablespoons of cocoa powder plus one tablespoon (or less) of vegetable oil for each ounce of baking chocolate. Cocoa powder has excellent flavor and much less fat and **saturated fat** than baking chocolate.

- Substitute skim or 1 percent milk for regular milk.

- Substitute equal portions 1 percent milk and evaporated skim milk for light cream.

- Substitute low-fat or nonfat yogurt for sour cream or heavy cream.

- Substitute one whole egg and two egg whites for every two whole eggs. Using just egg whites gives the baked good a rubbery texture.

- Substitute stick margarine for butter. Avoid using margarines, such as reduced-fat, that list water as the first ingredient. Because of their high water content, they do not perform the same, or as well as, regular fats in baking.

- When a recipe calls for melted butter or melted shortening, substitute oil. Oil can also be used when making soft, moist, bar cookies. When creaming fat and sugar, such as in making cakes, substitute an oil (such as canola oil) for half the solid fat. The texture will be a little more dense but acceptable.

- Substitute half the volume or weight of fat called for with prune puree. Amazingly enough, pureed prunes have been shown to be a good fat substitute. Their flavor is quite subtle, just a fruity nuance, when pureed and baked into a cake. Prunes work best in baked goods with strong flavors, such as brownies and peanut butter cookies. Once worked into a batter, the prunes have only a light tan color so they work well in any baked good that doesn't have to be white. The type of sugar in fruit attracts and holds moisture well so baked goods stay fresh longer. The natural sugar in pureed prunes also reduces the amount of refined sugar needed to sweeten the baked good.

- Light cream can be used in place of regular cream cheese in many baked goods, but don't substitute nonfat cream cheese in baking or frostings because it falls apart.

- Reduce refined sugar in recipes by one-fourth to as much as one-third (use about one-quarter cup sugar per cup of flour) and use sweet spices and extracts to make up for the flavor loss.

- To add flavor, texture, color, and nutritional value, try adding fruits to baked goods.

- Reduce the salt in recipes, except breads, by one-half.

Seasonings and Flavorings

Seasonings and flavorings are very important in modified recipes as they help replace missing ingredients such as fat and salt in hopes of satisfying the taste buds. Seasonings are used to bring out flavor present in a dish, whereas flavorings add a new flavor to a dish or modify the original flavor. The difference between them is one of degree. Flavored vinegars, flavored oils, and certain alcoholic beverages are used successfully as flavorings in certain dishes.

Heart A hollow, muscular **organ** that pumps **blood** through the body. Shaped like an egg, it lies in the center of the chest where the breastbone and rib cage protect it. The **myocardium**, a thin layer of tissue, lines the inside and covers the outside (see Figure H.1).

Figure H.1 Blood Flow through the Heart

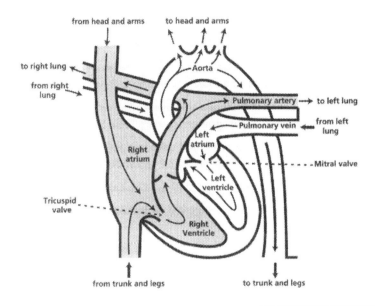

The heart has two upper chambers (each is called an **atrium**) and two lower chambers (each is called a ventricle). **Valves** connect the upper and lower chambers of the heart. Each valve lets blood flow in only one direction.

The heart is actually a double pump: the right side sends blood to the lungs for **oxygen** and the left side pumps blood to the rest of the body. Blood passes through the heart in a specific order.

1. The **veins** bring oxygen-poor blood to the right atrium. The blood then passes through a valve (tricuspid valve) to the right ventricle which pumps the blood to the lungs via the **pulmonary artery**. Once in the lungs, the blood picks up oxygen and releases its **carbon dioxide**.

2. The oxygen-rich blood now returns to the left atrium via the **pulmonary vein**. The blood flows through the **mitral valve** to the left ventricle which is the strongest part of the heart. The left ventricle pumps the blood through the aortic valve and into the **aorta**, which branches to carry blood all around the body.

The heart has three layers: **pericardium** (the outer lining), **myocardium** (the heart muscle), and **endocardium** (the inner lining).

Heart Attack See **myocardial infarction**.

Heartburn A painful burning sensation in the **esophagus** caused by the contents of the **stomach**, which are acidic, flowing back into the lower esophagus. Heartburn is often caused by a **hiatal hernia**, and can also be due to **obesity** or pregnancy. See also **hiatal hernia**.

Heart Disease Any disease that affects the **heart** or **blood** vessels. The appropriate term is **cardiovascular disease**. See **cardiovascular disease**.

Heart Murmur An extra **heart** sound. Heart murmurs are normally caused by a defect in a heart **valve** or a disease that affects the heart's normal pumping.

Height/Weight Tables Tables that show ideal or desirable weight for men and women. See also **anthropometrics**. (See Table H.6.)

Hematocrit Percentage of **red blood cells** in a volume of blood. A percentage of 42 percent means that there are 42 ml of red blood cells in 100 ml of blood.

Hematopoiesis The production and development of **blood** cells.

Heme An **iron**-containing red pigment in **hemeglobin** that carries **oxygen** to the body's cells.

Heme Iron The predominant form of **iron** in animal foods. Heme iron is absorbed and used twice as readily as iron in plant foods, called **nonheme iron**. Animal foods also contain some nonheme iron.

Hemochromatosis A common genetic disease in which individuals absorb about twice as much **iron** from their food and supplements as other people. When **blood** iron levels rise above normal over a period of time, excess iron can damage the **liver** and other **organs**, and there is a question of its relationship to **heart disease** and **cancer**.

Hemodialysis See **dialysis**.

Hemoglobin A conjugated **protein** in **red blood cells** made up of two parts: **heme** and globin. Heme is an **iron**-containing red pigment that carries **oxygen**. Globin is the protein part. Hemoglobin enables the red blood cell to carry oxygen. Hemoglobin is measured in grams/100 ml of **blood**.

Table H.6 Metropolitan Life Insurance 1983 Height and Weight Tables

Height (in shoes)*	Men, Weight in Pounds (indoor clothing)			Height (in shoes)*	Women, Weight in Pounds (indoor clothing)		
	Small Frame	Medium Frame	Large Frame		Small Frame	Medium Frame	Large Frame
5'2"	128–134	131–141	138–150	4'10"	102–111	109–121	118–131
5'3"	130–136	133–143	140–153	4'11"	103–113	111–123	120–134
5'4"	132–138	135–145	142–156	5'	104–115	113–126	122–137
5'5"	134–140	137–148	144–160	5'1"	106–118	115–129	125–140
5'6"	136–142	139–151	146–164	5'2"	108–121	118–132	128–143
5'7"	138–145	142–154	149–168	5'3"	111–124	121–135	131–147
5'8"	140–148	145–157	152–172	5'4"	114–127	124–138	134–151
5'9"	142–151	148–160	155–176	5'5"	117–130	127–141	137–155
5'10"	144–154	151–163	158–180	5'6"	120–133	130–144	140–159
5'11"	146–157	154–166	161–184	5'7"	123–136	133–147	142–163
6'	149–160	157–170	164–188	5'8"	126–139	136–150	146–167
6'1"	152–164	160–174	168–192	5'9"	129–142	139–153	149–170
6'2"	155–168	164–178	172–197	5'10"	132–145	142–156	152–173

Table H.6 Metropolitan Life Insurance 1983 Height and Weight Tables (continued)

Men, Weight in Pounds (indoor clothing)				Women, Weight in Pounds (indoor clothing)			
Height (in shoes)*	Small Frame	Medium Frame	Large Frame	Height (in shoes)*	Small Frame	Medium Frame	Large Frame
6'3"	158–172	167–182	176–202	5'11"	135–148	145–159	155–176
6'4"	162–176	171–187	181–207	6'	138–151	148–162	158–179

*Height for both men and women includes 1" heel. Body weight for women includes 5 pounds of indoor clothing; for men it includes 5 pounds of indoor clothing

Height/Weight Table in 1995 Dietary Guidelines for Americans

Height*	Healthy Weight in pounds**	Height*	Healthy Weight in pounds**
4'10"	91–119	5'5"	114–150
4'11"	94–124	5'6"	118–155
5'0"	97–128	5'7"	121–160
5'1"	101–132	5'8"	125–164
5'2"	104–137	5'9"	129–169
5'3"	107–141	5'10"	132–174
5'4"	111–146	5'11"	136–179
		6'0"	140–184
		6'1"	144–189
		6'2"	148–195
		6'3"	152–200
		6'4"	156–205
		6'5"	160–211
		6'6"	164–216

*Without shoes

**Without clothes. The higher weights apply to people with more muscle and bone, such as many men.

Source: Report of the Dietary Guidelines Advisory Committee on the Dietary Guidelines for Americans, 1995, pages 23–24.

Hemolysis Destruction of **red blood cells.**

Hemolytic Anemia A type of **anemia** involving the premature destruction of **red blood cells.** See also **anemia.**

Hemophilia A group of inherited bleeding disorders in which one of the factors needed for **blood clotting** is missing, resulting in prolonged **coagulation** time. The severity of hemophilia depends on the extent to which the factor is lacking.

Hemopoiesis The formation of **erythrocytes** (**red blood cells**).

Hemorrhoids Enlarged varicose **veins** in the rectal region.

Hemostasis Cessation of bleeding.

Hepatitis Inflammation of the **liver.** Because it is caused by a virus, it is called *viral hepatitis.* There are three forms of viral hepatitis: hepatitis A virus, hepatitis B virus, and hepatitis C virus.

Heparin A **polysaccharide** made by some cells in the circulatory system that is a powerful anticoagulant (it inhibits **blood clotting**).

Hepatic Encephalopathy A condition that most often develops from advanced **cirrhosis** in which toxic substances (ammonia and aromatic **amino acids**) accumulate in the **blood** due to **liver** failure. These toxic substances affect the brain and **nervous system.** Symptoms include confusion, altered consciousness, inappropriate behaviors, and asterixis. **Diet therapy** includes low protein, branched-chain amino acid formulas, and sufficient **calories, vitamins,** and **minerals.** Fluid intake is carefully controlled because of the commonly accompanying conditions of **ascites** and **edema.** See also **cirrhosis.**

Hernia A condition in which an **organ,** or part of an organ, protrudes through the wall of the body chamber in which the organ is contained.

Heteropolysaccharides **Polysaccharides** that contain more than one type of **monosaccharide** and other substances. Pectin and **heparin** are examples of heteropolysaccharides.

Hiatal Hernia A condition in which part of the **stomach** protrudes through the esophageal opening in the **diaphragm.** Hiatal hernia is often associated with **obesity** and losing weight can alleviate symptoms.

High Blood Pressure See **hypertension.**

High-Density Lipoprotein (HDL) A **lipoprotein** that contains much protein and travels throughout the body picking up **cholesterol.** It is thought that the HDLs carry cholesterol back to the **liver** for disposal. Thus HDLs help remove cholesterol from the **blood,** preventing the buildup of cholesterol in the walls of **arteries.** See also **cholesterol.**

High Fructose Corn Syrup Corn syrup that has been treated with an **enzyme** that converts part of the **glucose** it contains to **fructose** to make it sweeter.

Hilum The part of an **organ** through which **blood** vessels and **nerves** enter and leave.

Hind Milk The breast milk stored in the milk-producing cells of the **mammary gland**. Once suckling causes **oxytocin** to be produced, the milk-producing cells contract and release the hind milk. See also **fore milk**.

Holoenzyme An **enzyme** with its cofactor.

Home-Delivered Meals Program Meals for older adults that are delivered to the home and funded by **Title III-C** of the Older Americans Act. Participants in this program must be over 60 years old and unable to prepare their own meals. Meals, often including a hot lunch and cold supper, are normally delivered Monday through Friday. Some programs also provide some type of weekend meal services. Also see **senior nutrition programs**.

Homeless Persons Individuals who lack a permanent home. The ability to be healthy and well fed is diminished when living on the streets. Many homeless people are not getting regular, nutritious meals and therefore are at risk for hunger, **malnutrition**, weight loss, and sickness.

Homeostasis The tendency of the body to maintain a constant, stable state.

Homopolysaccharides **Polysaccharides** that contain only one type of **monosaccharide**. **Starch** and **glycogen** are homopolysacchardies.

Hormone Messengers that travel in the **blood** to target tissues where they bind to receptor **proteins** on the target tissue's cells. When the hormone combines with its receptor protein, a sequence of changes takes place in the target cells. **Hormones** are made by **endocrine glands** such as the islet cells of the **pancreas**.

Hourly Employees Employees who are paid by the hour and are not exempt from federal and state wage and hour laws.

Hunger The physical need to eat.

Human Chorionic Gonadotropin (HCG) A **hormone** produced by the **placenta** during the first three months of pregnancy. HCG causes the fertilized egg to release **estrogen** and **progesterone**, which are important to prepare the **uterus** to accept the **embryo**. About the third month, the placenta takes over producing estrogen and progesterone.

Human Resource (HR) Management The strategic and operational management of activities to enhance the performance of the human resources in an organization. Typical activities of human resource management include recruiting and selecting staff, reviewing accident reports, resolving employee grievances, and setting up compensation (salary and benefits) programs.

Humoral Immunity An **immune response** in which B **lymphocytes** transform into cells, called **plasma cells**, that produce large amounts of **antibodies**.

Hunger **Malnutrition** as measured by anthropometric and clinical tests and the inability to obtain an adequate amount of food even if the shortage is not prolonged enough to cause health problems (as defined by the President's Task Force on Food Assistance, 1984). The issue of hunger may also be referred to as **food insecurity**.

Hydrocephalus A disease state marked by accumulation of fluid in the spaces of the brain.

Hydrochloric Acid (HCl) A compound of **hydrogen** and chlorine that is produced by the muscosal cells of the **stomach** and is the main constituent of gastric juice. Hydrochloric acid aids in **protein** digestion (it converts **pepsinogen** into its active form), destroys harmful bacteria, and increases the ability of **calcium** and **iron** to be absorbed.

Hydrogenation The process by which liquid **vegetable oils** are converted into solid **fats** by the use of heat, **hydrogen**, and certain metal catalysts. Oils are partially hydrogenated to make shortening and most **margarines**. See also **trans-fatty acids**.

Hydrolysis The process in which a compound is split into smaller compounds by the addition of **water**.

Hydrophilic **Water** soluble.

Hydrophobic **Water** insoluble.

Hydroxyapatite **Calcium** and **phosphate** compound found in the matrix of **bones** and teeth that give structural strength.

Hygroscopic Able to hold and absorb **water**.

Hyperbilirubinemia Excessive amount of **bilirubin** in the **blood**.

Hypercalcemia High levels of **calcium** in the **blood**.

Hypercholesterolemia High **blood cholesterol**. A high blood cholesterol level means that you have more cholesterol in your bloodstream than your body needs. The higher your blood cholesterol level, the greater your risk or chance of developing **coronary heart disease**—the most common form of heart diseases. Anyone can develop high blood cholesterol, no matter what his or her age, gender, race, or ethnic background. High blood cholesterol has no warning signs. A predisposition to high blood cholesterol levels can be inherited (then it's called *familial hypercholesterolemia*). See also **cholesterol** and **atherosclerosis.**

Hyperemesis Gravidarum An abnormal condition of pregnancy marked by severe vomiting, electrolyte imbalance, and weight loss. Treatment includes hospitalization.

Hyperkalemia A high **serum potassium** level.

Hyperlipidemia High level of lipids in the **blood.**

Hypernatremia High blood level of **sodium.**

Hyperplasia An increase in tissue size due to an increase in cell numbers. See also **hypertrophy.**

Hyperparathyroidism Overactivity of the parathyroid gland that results in over production of **parathyroid hormone (PTH)**. PTH is secreted in response to low **blood calcium** levels and it mobilizes calcium from the bones into the blood.

NUTRITION AND DISEASE FOCUS: HYPERTENSION

High blood pressure. Blood pressure is measured using the familiar inflatable cuff and the stethoscope. The blood pressure reading is reported in two numbers such as 120/80. The top number is the systolic blood pressure, which is the pressure exerted against the **artery** walls when the **heart** contracts. The bottom number is the diastolic blood pressure, which is the lowest pressure remaining in the arteries between heartbeats when the heart is at rest. A systolic reading above 140, or a diastolic reading of 90 or more, or both, on repeated occasions indicates high blood pressure. Optimal blood pressure is a systolic reading below 120 and a diastolic below 80 (see Tables H.7, H.8, and H.9).

High blood pressure is a concern because it is one of the major risk factors for **coronary heart disease,** and the most important risk factor for the cerebrovascular diseases, such as **stroke.** It is also a concern because there are often no symptoms. As many as 50 million Americans have elevated blood pressure or are taking antihypertensive medication.

Lifestyle changes for controlling hypertension include those listed in Table H.8. If they can't control hypertension well enough, a drug may be selected and used.

Hypertension sometimes can occur secondary to another medical problem such as a tumor of the **adrenal gland** or **kidney** abnormality. This type of hypertension is called **secondary hypertension.** Most cases of hypertension are not due to another medical condition, so they are called **primary hypertension.** The cause of primary hypertension is not known. See also **sodium.**

Table H.7 Classification of Blood Pressure for Adults Age 18 Years and Older*

Category	Systolic mm Hg	Diastolic mm Hg
Normal	<130	<85
High normal	130–139	85–89
Hypertension**		
STAGE 1 (Mild)	140–159	90–99
STAGE 2 (Moderate)	160–179	100–109
STAGE 3 (Severe)	180–209	110–119
STAGE 4 (Very Severe)	≥210	≥120

* Not taking antihypertensive drugs and not acutely ill. When systolic and diastolic pressure fall into different categories, the higher category should be selected to classify the individual's blood pressure status. For instance, 160/92 should be classified as Stage 2, and 180/120 should be classified as Stage 4.

** Based on the average of two or more readings taken at each of two or more visits following an initial screening.

Source: The Fifth Report of the Joint National Committee on Detection, Evaluation, and Treatment of High Blood, Pressure, National Institutse of Health and National Heart, Lung, and Blood Institute, 1994, NIH Publication No. 93-1088.

Table H.8 Lifestyle Modifications for Hypertension Control and/or Overall Cardiovascular Risk

• Lose weight if overweight.

• Limit alcohol intake to no more than 1 ounce of ethanol per day (24 ounces of beer, 8 ounces of wine, or 2 ounces of 100 proof whiskey).

• Exercise (aerobic) regularly.

• Reduce sodium intake to less than 100 mmol per day (<2.3 grams of sodium or <6 grams of sodium chloride).

• Maintain adequate dietary potassium, calcium, and magnesium intake.

Table H.8 Lifestyle Modifications for Hypertension Control and/or Overall Cardiovascular Risk (continued)

- Stop smoking and reduce dietary saturated fat and cholesterol intake for overall cardiovascular health. Reducing fat intake also helps reduce caloric intake—important for control of weight and Type II diabetes.

Source: The Fifth Report of the Joint National Committee on Detection, Evaluation, and Treatment of High Blood Pressure, National Institutes of Health and National Heart, Lung, and Blood Institute, 1994, NIH Publication No. 93–1088.

Table H.9 Recommendations for Follow-up Based on Initial Set of Blood Pressure Measurements for Adults Age 18 and Older

Initial Screening Blood Pressure (mm Hg)*

Systolic	Diastolic	Follow-up Recommended**
<130	<85	Recheck in 2 years
130–139	85–89	Recheck in 1 year
140–159	90–99	Confirm within 2 months
160–179	100–109	Evaluate or refer to source of care within 1 month
180–209	110–119	Evaluate or refer to source of care within 1 week
≥210	≥120	Evaluate or refer to source of care immediately

* If the systolic and diastolic categories are different, follow recommendation for the shorter time follow–up (e.g., 160/85 mm Hg should be evaluated or referred to source of care within 1 month).

**The scheduling of follow-up should be modified by reliable information about past blood pressure measurements, other cardiovascular risk factors, or target-organ disease.

Source: *The Fifth Report of the Joint National Committee on Detection, Evaluation, and Treatment of High Blood Pressure*, National Institutes of Health and National Heart, Lung, and Blood Institute, 1994, NIH Publication No. 93-1088.

See Figure H.2 for more information about the treatment of hypertension.

Figure H.2 Treatment of Hypertension

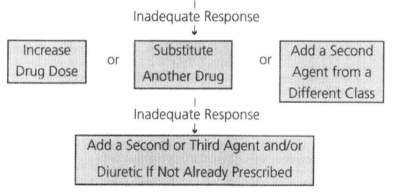

Lifestyle Modifications:
Weight Reduction
Moderation of Alcohol Intake
Regular Physical Activity
Reduction of Sodium
Smoking Cessation

Inadequate Response

Continue Lifestyle Modifications

Initial Pharmacological Selection:

Diuretics or Beta-Blockers are preferred because a reduction in morbidity and mortality has been demonstrated.

ACE inhibitors, Calcium antagonists, Alpha-receptor blockers, and the Alpha-beta blocker have not been tested nor shown to reduce morbidity and mortality

Inadequate Response

Increase Drug Dose   or   Substitute Another Drug   or   Add a Second Agent from a Different Class

Inadequate Response

Add a Second or Third Agent and/or Diuretic If Not Already Prescribed

* Response means achieved goal blood pressure, or patient is making considerable progress towards this goal.

Hyperthyroidism Overactivity of the **thyroid gland** in which too much **thyroxine** is secreted. The most common form of hyperthyroidism is **Grave's disease,** also called **toxic goiter** or **thyrotoxicosis.** See also **Grave's disease.**

Hypertrophy Growth of a tissue due to an increase in the size of its cells. See also **hyperplasia.**

Hypochromia Reduction in hemoglobin in **red blood cells.**

Hypogeusia A diminished ability to taste.

Hypoglycemia Low **blood sugar** levels.

Hypokalemia A low **serum potassium** level.

Hyponatremia A low **blood sodium** level.

Hypothalamus A small **gland** in the brain next to the **pituitary.** The hypothalamus is connected with parts of the **nervous system** and functions as an autonomic nervous center because of its role in speeding up or slowing down certain body functions. The principal functions of the hypothalamus are:

1. Cardiovascular regulation

2. Body-temperature regulation

3. Water and electrolyte balance

4. Regulation of hunger and some gastrointestinal activities

5. Regulation of sleeping and wakefulness

6. Emotional responses

7. Stimulates secretion of a number of **hormones** from the anterior **pituitary**

8. Produces two hormones, **antidiuretic hormone** and **oxytocin,** that are secreted by the posterior pituitary.

See also **antidiuretic hormone** and **oxytocin.**

Hypothesis In **research,** a provisional theory set forth to explain some phenomena. The hypothesis is tested in specific research projects.

Hypothyroidism Underactivity of the **thyroid gland** that may be due to endemic **goiter,** thyroidectomy, or other causes. The symptoms of hypothyroidism include fatigue and sluggishness. In children, hypothyroidism can cause **cretinism.** In adults, it can produce **myxedema.** See also **cretinism** and **myxedema.**

Hypovolemia Low **blood** volume.

Hypoxia A condition in which not enough **oxygen** is in the cells. Mild hypoxia results in increased **heart** and respiratory rates, dizziness, and confusion. Treatment may consist of ventilator therapy, oxygen therapy, and drugs to stimulate the **heart** and lungs.

Hysterectomy Surgical removal of the **uterus**.

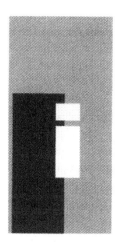

Iatrogenic An abnormal physical or mental condition induced in a patient due to hospital practices or physician treatment. For example, iatrogenic **malnutrition** may be caused by a patient being **NPO** (nothing by mouth) for more than 10 days.

Idiopathic A disease without a recognizable cause.

Ileocecal Sphincter The ring of **muscle** between the **ileum** of the **small intestine** and the **cecum**.

Ileum The final section of the **small intestine** before the **large intestine** starts.

Ileus Intestinal obstruction. Ileus may be due to the failure of **peristalsis** to continue propelling the contents down the intestines, a **tumor**, or abnormal twisting of the intestine.

Immune Response The body's reaction to foreign particles and bodies.

Immune System All the structures and processes of the body that defend the body against foreign organisms such as bacteria and viruses. The immune system includes:

1. The lymphoid **organs: spleen, thymus,** and **lymph** nodes.

2. **Lymphoctyes** (a type of **white blood cell**), **macrophages,** and **antibodies** (**proteins** that bind antigens).

When invading pathogens, such as bacteria, cross the **skin** into the body, nonspecific defense mechanisms, such as **phagocytosis** and fever, go to work. **Neutrophils** and **monocytes** (both **white blood cells**), as well as **macrophages** act to engulf and destroy (phagocytize) foreign bodies. Mild to moderate fevers may provide protection against bacteria.

When nonspecific defense systems are not enough to destroy the foreign bodies, the next line of defense is referred to as specific or acquired **immune response**. The specific **immune response** includes the two major types of lymphocytes: **B cells** and **T cells**. B cells are involved in what is called **humoral immunity**. T cells are involved in what is called **cell-mediated immunity**.

B cells are made in the **bone** marrow stem cells and then travel to **lymph** tissues. When a B cell encounters a specific **antigen**, the B cell transforms into a cell, called a **plasma cell**, that produces large amounts of **antibodies** during its brief life span of five to seven days. The antibodies made by plasma cells are called **immunoglobulins**, such as IgG and IgE. Immunoglobulins travel in the **blood** to where they are needed to react with and neutralize antigens. The resulting antigen-antibody complexes activate a series of nine proteins, called **complement**, that destroy the antigens.

Like B cells, T cells are made in the bone marrow stem cells, but T cells must first be activated in the **thymus** before traveling to lymph tissues. Whereas B cells fight bacteria and some viruses by secreting antibodies into the blood and lymph, T cells do not secrete antibodies but must get close to cells to destroy them. T cells attack mostly cells infected with viruses or fungi, cancerous cells, or transplanted cells. **Killer**, or cytotoxic, **T lymphocytes** destroy specific cells that are identified by the antigens on their surfaces. Other T cells secrete a number of **polypeptides** to contribute to cell-mediated immunity. These polypeptides are called **lymphokines** such as **interferons** and **interleukins**. Interferons are antiviral proteins. Interleukins stimulate the growth of T cells and activate **immune responses**. Lymphokines promote the action of lymphocytes and macrophages. Two other types of T lymphocytes, helper T lymphocytes and suppressor T lymphocytes, act to regulate the activities of the B cells and killer T cells.

Immunocompetence   The capacity to have an **immune response**.

Immunoglobulins   A type of gamma **globulin** (a **plasma protein**) made by plasma cells of the **immune system** that acts as **antibodies**. Immunoglobulins travel·in the **blood** to where they are needed to react with and neutralize **antigens**. Some immunoglobulin antibodies are IgA, IgG, IgM, IgD, and IgE (see Table I.1).

Table I.1   The Immunoglobulins

Immunoglobulin	Function
IgG	Main form of antibodies, more IgG are produced after immunizations.

Table I.1 The Immunoglobulins (continued)

Immunoglobulin	Function
IgA	Main antibody in external secretions such as saliva and breast milk.
IgE	Involved in allergic reactions.
IgM and IgD	Before immunization, function as antigen receptors on the surface of lymphocytes.

Immunology The study of the **immune system**.

Impetigo A **skin** disease caused by bacteria that is marked by crusted-over **lesions** and pustules.

Incidence A measure of disease frequency. Incidence measure the number of new cases of a disease over a given period.

Income Statement A financial format used by businesses to show sales, cost of sales, gross profit, expenses, and net profit (see Table I.2).

Table I.2 The Graduate Restaurant Statement of Income
for the Year Ended December 31, 19XX

SALES		
Food	$276,250.00	
Beverage	48,750.00	
Total Sales		$325,000.00
COST OF SALES		
Food	$ 96,687.00	
Beverages	12,188.00	
Total Cost of Sales		$108,875.00
GROSS PROFIT		$216,125.00
CONTROLLABLE EXPENSES		
Salaries and Wages	$ 65,000.00	
Employee Benefits	16,250.00	
Other Controllable Expenses	48,750.00	
Total Controllable Expenses		$130,000.00
INCOME BEFORE OCCUPANCY COSTS,		
INTEREST, DEPRECIATION, AND		
INCOME TAXES		86,125.00
OCCUPANCY COSTS		27,500.00

Table I.2   The Graduate Restaurant Statement of Income
for the Year Ended December 31, 19XX (continued)

INCOME BEFORE INTEREST,	
DEPRECIATION, AND INCOME TAXES	$ 58,625.00
INTEREST EXPENSE	5,000.00
DEPRECIATION	16,250.00
RESTAURANT PROFIT	$ 37,375.00*

*The Graduate Restaurant is also a subchapter S corporation. Therefore, the restaurant profit is reported as income by Jim Young on his personal income tax return.

Source: Dittmer, Paul and Griffin, Gerald. 1994. *Principles of Food, Beverage, and Labor Cost Control* (5th ed.). New York: Van Nostrand Reinhold. Reprinted with permission.

Incomplete Proteins   Food **proteins** that contain at least one limiting **amino acid**.

Independent Variable   In **research**, the variable that is manipulated to see its effect on the **dependent variable**.

Infant Mortality   The number of deaths during the first year of life per 1,000 live births.

Infarction   A localized area of dead tissue. See also **myocardial infarction**.

Inferential Statistics   See **statistics**.

NUTRITION AND DISEASE FOCUS:
INFLAMMATORY BOWEL DISEASE (IBD)

Two conditions with similar symptoms and clinical management: **Crohn's disease** and **ulcerative colitis**. They are grouped together because they have similar symptoms (such as **diarrhea,** abdominal pain, and **anorexia**) and are treated similarly. Crohn's disease can occur anywhere in the intestines and **rectum**. Ulcerative colitis is limited to the **colon** and rectum. In Crohn's disease, the **lesion** can go through the entire intestinal wall; whereas in ulcerative colitis, the lesion confines itself to the mucosal and submucosal layers of the intestine. Dietary treatment revolves around a diet high in **protein** (due to protein losses from the mucosal lesions and poor intake) and energy (due to weight loss commonly seen). **Fiber** is generally limited during times when healing is taking place. Extra **vitamins** and **minerals** need to be supplied in foods and/or supplemental form. See also **Crohn's disease** and **ulcerative colitis**.

Informal Leader   The individual who, by virtue of having the support of other employees, is in charge.

Informed Consent In **research** and medication, the right of the patient to know what exactly will and can happen during a procedure, research study, etc., so they can decide whether or not to participate.

Ingestion Taking food into the mouth.

Insensible Water Loss Water loss through the **skin**, respiration (breathing), and perspiration.

Insulin A **hormone** produced and secreted by the beta cells of the **islet cells of Langerhans** in the **pancreas**. When **blood sugar** levels are high, insulin is secreted and helps **glucose** enter the cells of the body. Insulin also promotes the storage of **glucose** as **glycogen** or **fat**.

Integumentary System The **skin**, hair, nails, and **glands** in the skin (**sweat glands** and sebaceous glands). Skin has many functions. It guards against excessive loss of **water**, **salts**, **heat**, and invasions by pathogens and their toxins. Sweat glands in the skin help cool the body and sebaceous glands lubricate the skin and prevent hair from becoming brittle. **Nerve** fibers under the skin help to register sensations such as pain, temperature, and touch. The skin has three layers.

1. Epidermis—the outermost thin membrane layer.

2. Corium or dermis—the middle layer made of fibrous connective tissue, **blood** and blood vessels, nerve fibers, hair follicles, and skin glands.

3. Subcutaneous tissue—the innermost layer of skin containing much fat.

Interferons Antiviral **proteins** made by **T lymphocytes** that also fight **tumors**.

Interleukins Proteins made by **T lymphocytes** that stimulate the growth of **T cells** and activate **immune responses**.

Internal Respiration Gas exchange (**oxygen** and **carbon dioxide**) at the cellular level.

International Unit (IU) A measure of **fat-soluble vitamin** activity.

Interrater Reliability The consistency between two or more ratings made by different raters.

Interrupted Time-Series Design A type of **research** design in which single subjects or groups of subjects are measured several times before and after some experimental manipulation. This type of study allows for some control for history.

Interstitial Fluid The fluid in the spaces between tissues.

Intervention A planned action intended to achieve a specific outcome. For example, nutrition intervention of an underweight **cancer** patient may include high-**calorie** food selections and small, frequent meals.

Interstitial Fluid The fluid that surrounds the body's cells. Interstitial fluid originates as fluid from **blood plasma** that normally passes out of the capillary walls due to the hydrostatic pressure of the blood.

Interviewing The gathering of information. Expert interviewing requires training and experience.

Intima The innermost part of the **blood** vessel wall.

Intracellular Fluid All the fluids inside of the body's cells.

Intravenous Pyelogram (IVP) A test using x-rays that evaluates renal function and the urinary system. A contrast medium is injected into a **vein** where it travels to the **kidney** and is filtered into the urine. X-rays are taken that show the dye as it travels through the kidney, into the **ureter** to the **bladder**, and then to the **urethra**. Abnormalities, such as **cysts**, **tumors**, and **calculi** may be seen.

Intrinsic Factor A **protein** secreted by cells in the **stomach** that is necessary for the absorption of **vitamin B12**. See also **vitamin B12**.

NUTRIENT FOCUS: IODINE

A trace **mineral** needed in extremely small amounts for the normal functioning of the **thyroid gland**. The thyroid gland is located in the neck and is responsible for producing two important **hormones** that maintain a normal level of **metabolism** in the body and are essential for normal growth and development, and **bone** and **protein** synthesis. Iodine is necessary for these hormones to be produced.

Iodine is not found in many foods: mostly saltwater fish and grains grown in soil rich in iodide (they were once covered by the oceans so the central U.S. tends to contain little iodine in the soil). Iodized **salt** was introduced in 1924 to combat iodine deficiencies. Iodine also finds its way accidentally into milk (cows receive drugs containing iodine and dairy equipment is sterilized with iodine-containing compounds), baked goods through iodine-containing compounds used in processing, and foods that have certain food colorings. Because iodine can be toxic at high levels, some industries are trying to cut back on its use.

Ion A charged atom that has lost or gained electrons and no longer has the same number of electrons as **protons**. Positive ions are called **cations** and negative ions are called **anions**.

Iris The colored part of the eye.

NUTRIENT FOCUS: IRON

A trace **mineral** that is an important part of **hemoglobin,** a part of **red blood cells** that carries **oxygen** to the cells. Oxygen is needed by the cell to break down **glucose** to produce energy. Iron is also part of myoglobin, a **protein** found in **muscles** that stores and carries oxygen. Iron works with many **enzymes** in energy metabolism and is needed to make new cells and some **hormones** and **neurotransmitters.**

Liver is an excellent source of iron. Other sources are meats, enriched breads and cereals, egg yolk, seafood, green leafy vegetables, legumes, and dried fruits (see Table I.3).

Table I.3   Some Good Sources of Iron

- Meats—beef, pork, lamb, and liver and other organ meats*

- Poultry—chicken, duck, and turkey, especially dark meat; liver*

- Fish—shellfish, like clams, mussels, and oysters; sardines; anchovies; and other fish

- Leafy greens of the cabbage family, such as broccoli, kale, turnip greens, collards

- Legumes, such as lima beans and green peas; dry beans and peas, such as pinto beans, black-eyed peas, and canned baked beans

- Yeast-leavened whole-wheat bread and rolls

- Iron-enriched white bread, pasta, rice, and cereals; read the labels

*Some foods in this group are high in fat, cholesterol, or both. Choose lean, lower fat, lower cholesterol foods most often. Read the labels.

The ability of the body to absorb and use iron from different foods varies from three percent for some vegetables to 35 percent from red meat. The average is about 15 percent. The predominant form of iron in animal foods, called **heme iron,** is absorbed and used twice as readily as iron in plant foods, called *nonheme iron.* Animal foods also contain some nonheme iron. The presence of **vitamin C** in a meal increases nonheme iron absorption, as does consuming meat, poultry, and fish. Some foods actually decrease iron consumption: coffee, tea, phytic acid in whole grains, oxalic acid in some vegetables, and **calcium** supplements. The body increases or decreases iron absorption according to need. The body absorbs iron more efficiently when iron stores are low and during growth spurts or pregnancy. Some iron is stored in the **bone** marrow and in the liver. See also **iron-deficiency anemia** and **hemochromatosis**.

NUTRITION AND DISEASE FOCUS: IRON-DEFICIENCY ANEMIA

A condition in which the size and number of **red blood cells** are reduced. This condition may result from inadequate intake of **iron** or from **blood** loss. Symptoms of iron-deficiency anemia include fatigue, pallor, irritability, and lethargy. Iron-deficiency anemia is a real concern in the United States, more so for women than men. It is also a concern for infants and children. Children with iron-deficiency anemia act like they have behavioral problems (short attention span, restless) when in reality they need more iron in their diet. Supplemental iron is given (in the ferrous form).

Iron Overload See **hemochromatosis**.

Irradiation Exposing foods to gamma rays to kill microorganisms. Food irradiation is regulated by the **Food and Drug Administration**.

Irritable Bowel Syndrome A group of gastrointestinal symptoms associated with stress. Symptoms often include stomach pain, bloating, **diarrhea**, and constipation, but no inflammation of the intestine. Diet therapy includes avoiding foods that are not tolerated well or cause gas, increasing **fiber**, reducing **fat**, and avoiding large meals. Also called **spastic colon**.

Islets of Langerhans Specialized endocrine cells in the **pancreas** that produce two **hormones: insulin** and **glucagon**. The alpha cells of the islet cells make glucagon and the beta cells make insulin. Insulin and glucagon work opposite each other. When **blood sugar** levels are high, insulin is secreted and helps **glucose** enter the cells of the body. Insulin also promotes the storage of glucose as **glycogen** or **fat**. Whereas insulin lowers blood glucose, glucagon raises blood glucose levels. When **blood glucose levels** are low, glucagon stimulates the **liver** to break down glycogen and release glucose into the blood, and also stimulates the hydrolysis of stored fat to release free **fatty acids** into the blood. See also **pancreas**.

Isoenzyme **Enzymes**, usually located in different **organs**, that catalyze the same reaction but have one or several different **amino acids**. Also called **isozyme**.

Isotonic A solution with the same ionic concentration as another solution.

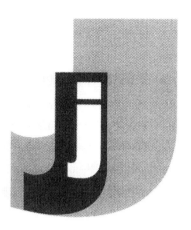

Jaundice A yellow color in the **skin** that is due to high levels of **bilirubin** in the body.

Jejunum The second portion of the **small intestine** between the **duodenum** and the **ileum**. The jejunum is about eight feet long.

Job A group of positions with common duties and responsibilities, such as cook or clinical dietitian.

Job Analysis Determination of the content of a given job by breaking it down into units (work sequences) and identifying the tasks that make up each unit.

Job Description A written statement of the duties performed and responsibilities involved in a given **job** classification (see Figure J.1).

Job Design Organizing tasks, duties, and responsibilities into a unit of work and **jobs.**

Job Enrichment Rearrangement of a given **job** to increase responsibility for one's own work and to provide opportunity for achievement, recognition, learning, and growth.

Job Evaluation The process of examining the responsibilities and difficulties of each **job** in order to determine which jobs are worth more than others.

Job Loading Adding more work to a **job** without increasing interest, challenge, or reward.

Job Posting A policy of advertising open positions within the organization for employees to see.

Job Rotation The process of shifting a person to various **positions** within a job classification.

Job Setting The conditions under which the **job** is to be done, such as physical conditions and contact with others.

Figure J.1 Job Description

POSITION TITLE: Clinical Dietician

REPORTS TO: Chief Clinical Dietician

DEPARTMENT: Food & Nutrition Serv.   COST CENTER CODE: 500

DATE: April, 1996   POSITION CODE: 353

Hours of Work: 8:00 A.M. – 4:30 P.M.   9:30 A.M. – 6:00 P.M. every sixth weekend.

Summary of Duties:

Assumes the responsibility for the nutritional care rendered to all patients on assigned floors, clinics and/or dialysis unit.

Monitors and evaluates nutritional concerns utilizing mechanical, biochemical, and anthropometric data.

Obtains and evaluates diet histories/24 hour recalls when necessary.

Utilizes information contained within the medical record from progress notes made by other allied health professionals.

Designs a nutritional care plan for each patient and utilizes this when providing care. (Uses basic or comprehensive form as appropriate).

Interprets physician's diet orders and modifies the diet according to the order.

Participates in planning general and modified diets and makes recommendations for diet order changes.

Conducts meal rounds daily on half of assigned floors or as designated.

Monitors daily progress of patient tolerance to diet.

Provides assistance to patients with menu selections, when appropriate.

Checks menu selections to insure accuracy and adequacy of patient's menu choices, in absence of diet technician.

Plans nourishments and between meal feedings.

Instructs patients and families as directed by physicians' orders.

Responds to nutrition consults upon request by physicians with 24-hour notice.

Makes recommendations and assists in the supervision of enteral and parenteral nutrition.

Performs nutrient intake studies and utilizes other tools for assessments of patient's intakes.

Figure J.1 Job Description (continued)

Records patient's nutrition care plan and progress in the medical record using SOAP method of charting, when appropriate.

Directly supervises the nutritional care delivered by the Dietetic Technician when assigned to the same floor.

Assists in the development and implementation of quality assurance audits for clinical area.

Develops Policies and Procedures applicable to patient care.

Assists in the maintenance and updating of clinical library and nutrition information files.

Participates in professional related activities within the Department, Medical Center and community, as well as ADA sponsored activities.

Performs other related duties as assigned by Management.

Job Specification A list of the qualifications needed to perform a given **job.**

Job Title The name of the **job,** such as cook or dietetic assistant.

Joint A place where bones come together.

Joint Commission on Accreditation of Healthcare Organizations (JCAHO) A nongovernmental professional association that evaluates healthcare organizations, including most hospitals in the U.S. and also many nursing facilities.

Just-Cause Termination When an employee is terminated because his/her offense affected the specific work he/she did or the operation as a whole in a detrimental way.

Juxtaglomerular Apparatus Region in each **nephron** where the **afferent arteriole** and **distal convoluted tubule** are in contact. The juxtaglomerular apparatus is responsible for sensing the **sodium** content of the **blood.**

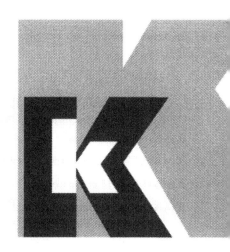

Keratin A hard **protein** substance found in the **skin**, hair, and nails.

Keto Acid Organic **acids** that result from deamination of the **amino acid**. Ketogenic keto acids go on to make **fats**. Glycogenic keto acids go on to make **carbohydrates**.

Ketoacidosis See **acidosis**.

Ketogenic Amino Acids Those **amino acids** whose carbon skeletons are used to make **acetyl coA** and/or **acetoacetyl CoA**.

Ketone A group of organic compounds formed when an alkyl group is positioned on each of the two remaining carbon bonds of a carbonyl group. The carbonyl group is not on a terminal carbon atom (see Figure K.1).

Figure K.1 Ketone

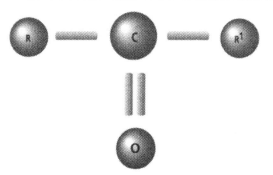

Ketone Bodies A group of organic compounds including **acetone**, **acetoacetic acid**, and B-hydroxybutyric acid, that occur as intermediate products of **fat metabolism**. When fat is burned for energy without any **carbohydrate** present (as can occur during starvation or a complication of **diabetes mellitus**), the process is incomplete and ketone bodies are produced. An excessive level of ketone bodies in the blood and urine (called **ketosis**) can cause the blood to become too acidic. Ketosis can cause **dehydration** and eventually leads to a fatal coma.

Ketose A **monosaccharide** with a **ketone** carbonyl group.

Ketosis See **ketone bodies**.

Kidney Major **organ** of the **urinary system** that maintains the proper balance of **water, salts, electrolytes,** and **acids** in the body fluids; removes nitrogenous wastes in the form of **urea**; and forms **urine**. The kidneys also have an **endocrine** function: they secrete **renin**, a substance involved in regulation of **blood pressure**, and an active form of **vitamin D**. The outer region of the kidney is the renal cortex; the inner portion of the kidney is called the renal medulla; the calyces and renal pelvis serve to collect urine and transport it to the **ureter**. The **hilum** is the place on the kidney through which blood vessels (the renal **artery** and renal **vein**) and **nerves** enter and leave. The kidneys lie on each side of the vertebral column, high in the abdominal cavity. Each kidney is shaped like a lima bean and is about four inches long and two to three inches wide. Also see **nephron.** (See Figure K.2.)

Figure K.2 Kidney

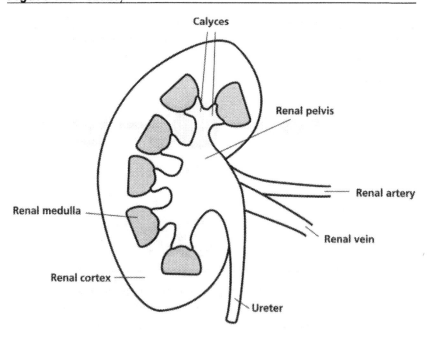

Kidney Stone Abnormal stones that develop and often lodge in the **ureter**, **urinary bladder**, or renal pelvis. Kidney stones are often made of **uric acid** or **calcium salts**. Why they occur is not totally understood. The latest treatment for kidney stones is lithotripsy, in which shock waves are focused on stones so they are pulverized and leave the body painlessly.

Killer T Lymphocytes T **lymphocytes** that destroy specific cells such as **tumor** cells and bacteria. See also **immune system**.

Kilocalorie A unit of energy. The energy in food is measured in kilocalories. One kilocalorie represents the amount of heat needed to raise 1000 g of water 1 degree Celsius. In nutrition, it is common to shorten the word kilocalorie to **calorie**.

Kinetic Energy Energy released from storage in the body (such as stored in **ATP**), used to move **muscles** and for other bodily activities.

Kwashiorkor A type of **protein**-energy **malnutrition** characterized by retarded growth and development, a protruding **abdomen** due to **edema** (swelling), peeling **skin**, a loss of normal hair color, irritability, and sadness. Kwashiorkor is associated with poor **protein** intake and late weaning.

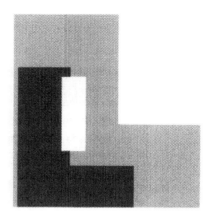

Labor Contract The written conditions of employment that are negotiated between management and a union.

Laboratory Tests Tests involving materials, fluids, or tissues obtained from patients. Laboratory tests, also called *biochemical tests,* can be very helpful in assessing a patient's nutrition status. Following are some of the laboratory tests with nutritional significance.

1. **Serum** albumin—Fifty to sixty percent of all the **protein** in the **blood** is albumin. Serum albumin is a good indicator of nutrition status, particularly protein status, but it takes time for it to change. Therefore a patient with a low serum albumin (less than 3.5 **grams**) has been in poor nutrition status for some time. Serum albumin decreases in trauma, severe infection, or protein-**calorie malnutrition**.

2. Serum **transferrin**—Like albumin, transferrin is a protein found in the blood. Transferrin carries **iron** to where **red blood cells** are made. Serum transferrin levels are considered a more sensitive indicator of protein deficiency than albumin because transferrin levels change quicker in response to changes in nutrition status. Levels lower than 170 milligrams/ 100 milliliters is indicative of undernutrition.

3. Total **lymphocyte** count (TLC)—Lymphocytes are **white blood cells** involved in fighting infection, so lymphocyte counts are a good indicator of immunocompetence. Low TLC may indicate that malnutrition exists since they are an indicator of protein stores. Certain drugs also decrease total lymphocyte count. A TLC less than 1500 cells/cubic millimeter may indicate nutritional concerns.

4. **Hematocrit** and **hemoglobin**—Hematocrit is the percent of red blood cells found in blood. The normal hematocrit in men is 39 to 49 percent, and is 33 to 44 percent in females. Hemoglobin is the **oxygen**-carrying pigment of the red blood cells. A low hemoglobin level may indicate iron-deficiency anemia. Normal values for hemoglobin are 12–16 grams/100 milliliters for women and 14–18 grams/100 milliliters for men.

5. Blood **glucose**—Elevated **blood glucose levels** may indicate **diabetes**. A normal range for fasting blood sugar is 70 to 110 milligrams glucose/100 milliliters.

Examples of laboratory tests with nutritional significance include **cholesterol, triglycerides,** and **potassium.**

Lactation The process of producing and secreting milk in the **mammary gland.** When an infant breast feeds, the **fore milk** is readily available. Once suckling causes **oxytocin,** a hormone, to be produced, the milk-producing cells contract and release the **hind milk.** Oxytocin therefore is needed for the milk-ejection reflex, also called **milk letdown,** in lactating women. See also **mammary gland, fore milk,** and **hind milk.**

Lactase A **brush border enzyme** in the **duodenum** that splits lactase into its components: **glucose** and **galactose.**

Lactiferous Ducts Ducts that carry milk within the breast from where the milk is made to where it is stored and secreted. See also **mammary gland.**

Lactoferrin An iron-binding **protein** in human milk.

Lactose A **disaccharide** found in milk and milk products that is made of **glucose** and **galactose** (see Figure L.1).

Figure L.1 Lactose

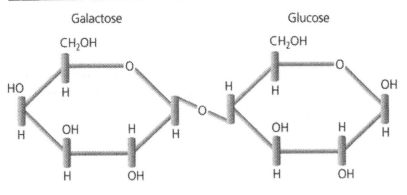

Lactose Intolerance An inability to digest lactose because of a deficiency or insufficient lactase. Symptoms include bloating, gas, and diarrhea.

Lacto-Ovovegetarian A **vegetarian eating** style in which the individual does not eat meat, poultry, or fish but does consume animal products in the form of eggs (ovo) and milk and milk products. Lacto-ovovegetarians are the largest group of vegetarians. See also **vegetarian eating**.

Lactovegetarian A **vegetarian eating** style in which the individual does not eat meat, poultry, or fish but does consume animal products in the form of milk and milk products.

Lanugo Downy, soft hair covering many parts of the body.

Large Intestine The part of the **gastrointestinal tract** between the **small intestine** and the **rectum**. The large intestine is about 2 1/2 inches wide and 5 feet long. The large intestine, also called the **colon**, consists of the ascending, transverse, descending, and **sigmoid colon**. The sigmoid colon leads into the rectum, where feces is stored until elimination.

The large intestine has no digestive functions, although it does absorb **water** and some **minerals**. In addition, the large intestine stores the waste products of **digestion** and forms and expels feces through the **anus**, which opens to allow elimination. See also **digestive enzymes**. (See Figure L.2.)

Figure L.2 Large Intestine

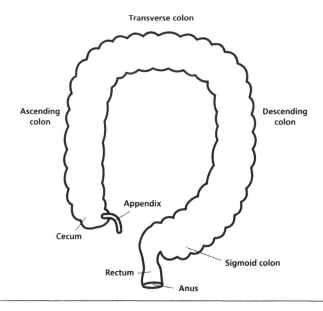

Larynx The tube between the **pharynx** and trachea (windpipe that goes into the lungs) that houses the vocal cords. The larynx has two functions: to produce sounds and to prevent food from entering the trachea and lungs during swallowing (along with the **epiglottis**). Also called the **voicebox**. See also **epiglottis**.

Leadership The process of influencing the activities of an organized group toward willingly attaining specified purposes or goals. There are many ways to define leadership. For example, it can be defined in terms of individual traits, behaviors, influence over other people, and **interaction** patterns. Bennis and Nanus (1985) proposed that "managers are people who do things right and leaders are people who do the right thing." In other words, managers use more technical skills to do their **job** correctly, whereas leaders envision which work needs to be done and develop trusting relationships with staff and supportive work environments in which to achieve goals and success. Transformational leadership refers to leadership in which there is a collective purpose between the leader and followers (see Table L.1). See also **management**.

Leading The process by which managers interact with subordinates to get certain plans and projects accomplished, as well as how managers determine and maintain an organization's culture.

Table L.1 Leadership Assessment Tool

Directions: Answer each question realistically using the following scale.

1. I do this always or most of the time.
2. I do this occasionally.
3. I do this seldom or never.

PERSONAL QUALITIES

SELF-CONFIDENT

_____ 1. I believe in myself

CONSISTENT/COMMITTED

_____ 2. I stay focused on the vision.

_____ 3. I keep my word and keep my commitments.

UPBEAT/POSITIVE

_____ 4. I am a positive thinker.

_____ 5. I am an optimist — my glass is half full.

Table L.1 Leadership Assessment Tool (continued)

HONEST/OPEN

_____ **6.** I am upfront and honest with others.

_____ **7.** I do not get defensive in conversation.

INTEGRITY

_____ **8.** I honor my commitments and promises.

FUNNY

_____ **9.** I use my sense of humor.

_____ **10.** I love to laugh at myself.

RISK-TAKING

_____ **11.** I take calculated risks when appropriate.

_____ **12.** I let myself and others make mistakes.

CREATIVE/DIVERGENT & ABSTRACT THINKER

_____ **13.** I encourage and try to look at things in new and different ways.

INTELLIGENT/ COMPETENT

_____ **14.** I am knowledgeable and competent in my field.

_____ **15.** I can make the complex simple.

_____ **16.** I am a life-long learner.

WIN/WIN ORIENTATION

_____ **17.** In interactions with others, I want everyone to be a winner.

ETHICAL

_____ **18.** I maintain appropriate ethical standards for an educator.

ORGANIZED

_____ **19.** My work and paperwork is well-organized.

LOOKS TO FUTURE

_____ **20.** I keep an eye and ear to trends in my field.

_____ **21.** I try to implement newer thinking in my job.

Table L.1   Leadership Assessment Tool (continued)

CONGRUENT

_____ **22.** I walk the talk.

FLEXIBLE

_____ **23.** I keep an open mind.

_____ **24.** I can change my mind and change my plans when appropriate.

VISION

ORGANIZATIONAL VISION

_____ **25.** I participate in writing/revising our organizational mission statement yearly.

PERSONAL VISION

_____ **26.** I write and revise my personal mission statement yearly.

MANAGING RELATIONSHIPS

SUPPORTING

_____ **27.** I seek first to understand, then to be understood.

_____ **28.** I genuinely show acceptance and positive regard to staff and colleagues.

_____ **29.** I refrain from rudeness and treat others diplomatically and politely.

_____ **30.** I maintain the self-respect of all individuals.

_____ **31.** I help others when needed.

DEVELOPING/MENTORING

_____ **32.** I believe developing and mentoring others is part and parcel of being a professional, and that this will enhance, not detract, from my career.

_____ **33.** I actively develop and act as a mentor.

EMPOWERING

_____ **34.** I actively empower staff to do their jobs the way they see fit.

RECOGNIZING & REWARDING

_____ **35.** I use a variety of techniques to recognize and reward staff for their achievements and contributions.

Table L.1 Leadership Assessment Tool (continued)

_____ **36.** I provide fair, specific, and timely recognition and rewards.

_____ **37.** I recognize and reward more than just the top performers.

_____ **38.** I use recognition and rewards that are desirable to the recipients.

MANAGING CONFLICT & CHANGE

_____ **39.** I see conflict as an opportunity to grow.

_____ **40.** I mediate conflicts and encourage constructive resolution of conflicts.

_____ **41.** I work on building and maintaining cooperative staff relationships.

_____ **42.** I realize that people generally don't resist change, but being changed.

TEAMBUILDING

_____ **43.** I understand the teambuilding process.

_____ **44.** I model teambuilding skills.

_____ **45.** I encourage staff to work as teams.

NETWORKING

_____ **46.** I actively network with people both within and outside of the college.

_____ **47.** I keep in touch with members of my network.

_____ **48.** I am good at remembering names.

MANAGING THE WORK

PLANNING

_____ **49.** With input, I help establish clear priorities and goals for our program.

ORGANIZING

_____ **50.** With input, I organize the work.

DECISION-MAKING

_____ **51.** I do much information gathering and get much input before making decisions.

_____ **52.** I build commitment for my decisions.

_____ **53.** I develop creative solutions.

Table L.1 Leadership Assessment Tool (continued)

PROBLEM-SOLVING

_____ **54.** I identify problems and take responsibility for them.

_____ **55.** I use the problem-solving process including trying creative solutions.

CLARIFYING ROLES & OBJECTIVES

_____ **56.** My employees know what is expected of them.

_____ **57.** Staff know their scope of authority.

INFORMING

_____ **58.** I interact with and inform my colleagues and employees.

_____ **59.** I keep my supervisor informed about what I am doing.

_____ **60.** I prepare meeting agendas for all meetings I conduct.

_____ **61.** I keep employees informed about policies, procedures, and all changes.

MONITORING

_____ **62.** I monitor the performance of staff.

_____ **63.** I meet regularly with staff.

_____ **64.** I periodically walk around to talk with people.

_____ **65.** I keep an open door for staff.

MANAGING TIME

_____ **66.** I set daily priorities and do first things first.

_____ **67.** I set time every day for physical exercise and reading.

DELEGATING

_____ **68.** I delegate appropriate tasks.

_____ **69.** I delegate authority and retain responsibility.

Lean Body Mass The part of the body that is not **fat**. Lean body mass includes **muscle, bone, organs, skin**, connective tissue, and other tissues.

Lecithin A **phospholipid** that is part of the cell membrane structure. Lecithin is like a **triglyceride** in that it has two **fatty acids** (both **polyunsaturated**) but the third position is not a fatty acid but **choline**. Lecithin lets substances through the cell membrane, especially **fats** and **water**. Lecithin is made by the **liver** and also found in foods, such as eggs. Lecithin is used as a food additive for its ability to be an emulsifier.

Lecithin Cholesterol Acyltransferase (LCAT) An **enzyme** that transfers a **fatty acid** from **lecithin** to free **cholesterol**, producing cholesterol **ester**.

Lesion An area of damaged tissue. Common lesions include cysts (sac filled with a solid or liquid), **ulcers** (open sores), fissures (splits), and polyps (growths).

Let-Down Reflex See **lactation**.

Leukemia Any of four different types of a cancerous disease of the **bone** marrow. In leukemia, there are abnormal numbers and forms of immature **white blood cells** in the **blood** and bone marrow. Leukemia is seen in both children and adults. The cause is not known but may be due to something toxic to bone marrow, such as radiation. Treatment includes bone marrow transplants, chemotherapy, antibiotics to prevent infections, and blood transfusions.

Leukocytes White blood cells or WBCs. WBCs are larger than **red blood cells** but not as numerous. Whereas there is only one type of red blood cell, there are five types of leukocytes, classified by whether or not they contain granules (small particles) in the **cytoplasm**.

Granulocytes

> **Basophils**—Releases the anticoagulant **heparin**.
>
> **Eosinophils**—Function in the allergic response to detoxify foreign substances. Secretes **enzymes** that break down **blood** clots.
>
> **Neutrophils**—Act as **phagocytes** to destroy bacteria at sites of infection.

Agranulocytes

> **Lymphocytes**—Found in **lymph** nodes and bloodstream where they make **antibodies** to destroy **antigens** and attack foreign bodies.
>
> **Monocytes**—Phagocytic cells that dispose of bacteria, dead cells, and other tissue debris.

Life Expectancy The average number of years a person is expected to live in a given society.

Limiting Amino Acid An **essential amino acid** in a dietary **protein** that is present in an insufficient amount to meet the body's needs.

Line Functions The functions involved in producing goods and services.

Linear Growth Height.

Linoleic Acid An **essential fatty acid**.

Lipase A group of **fat**-splitting **enzymes** that help in **digestion**. Lipases split **fatty acids** from their **glycerol base**. Lipase is made both by the **small intestine** and the **pancreas**. See also **digestive enzymes**.

Lipids A group of fatty substances, including **triglycerides** (**fats** and oils), sterols (**cholesterol**), and **phospholipids** (**lecithin**), that are present in **blood** and body tissues. Chemically, lipids are biological molecules that are insoluble in water but soluble in organic solvents. See also **fat, triglyceride, lecithin,** and **cholesterol**.

Lipogenesis The synthesis of **fatty acids**. Lipogenesis takes place in the cytosol of **liver** cells. **Acetyl coA** provides the carbon atoms for new fatty acids.

Lipolysis The breaking down of **fats**.

Lipoprotein Lipase An **enzyme** that breaks down **triglycerides** in the **blood** into **fatty acids** and **glycerol** so they can be absorbed into the body's cells.

Lipoproteins Protein-coated packages that carry **fat** and **cholesterol** through the bloodstream and **lymph**. They are classified according to their density.

1. Chylomicron

2. Very low-density lipoproteins (VLDL)

3. Low-density lipoproteins (LDL)

4. High-density lipoproteins (HDL)

See also **chylomicron, very low-density lipoprotein, low-density lipoprotein,** and **high-density lipoprotein**.

Lithotripsy A treatment for a **calculus** in which shock waves are focused on stones so they are pulverized and leave the body painlessly.

Liver The biggest **organ** of the body that regulates the chemical composition of the **blood** in many ways and produces and secretes **bile**. The liver is in the right upper quadrant of the **abdomen**, located just under the **diaphragm**. The liver has two major and two minor lobes.

Bile is made by the hepatocytes (liver cells) and is carried away from the liver in the hepatic ducts to the common hepatic duct. The common hepatic duct connects to the cystic duct which leads to the **gallbladder**. The gallbladder stores and concentrates bile until food is in the **stomach** and **duodenum**. Then the gallbladder contracts and bile travels down the cystic duct to the **common bile duct** to the duodenum. The pancreatic duct joins the common bile duct just before the common bile duct empties into the duodenum.

Absorbed nutrients flow via the hepatic portal system from the intestines to the liver, thereby giving the liver the opportunity to store, use, or repackage these nutrients for delivery to the tissues (see Table L.2 and Figure L.3).

Table L.2   Functions of the Liver

Carbohydrate metabolism	Converts blood glucose to liver glycogen (glycogenesis) and fat. Makes glucose from glycogen (glycogenolysis) and from amino acids and fat (gluconeogenesis). Helps regulate blood glucose levels.
Lipid metabolism	Makes triglycerides and cholesterol. Excretes cholesterol via bile.
Protein metabolism	Makes all blood plasma proteins except for immunoglobulins. Makes blood clotting factors.
Bile	Makes and secretes bile.
Detoxification	Removes drugs, hormones, and other molecules by excretion in the bile, phagocytosis by liver cells, or chemically converting to a less toxic substance.

Liver Function Tests (LFTs)   A series of laboratory tests that screen for **liver** disorders including **SGOT, SGPT, ALK** and **bilirubin.** See also **SGOT, SGPT, ALK,** and serum **bilirubin.**

Lobule   A subdivision of a larger lobe.

Loop of Henle   One of the renal tubules in the **nephron** or funtional unit of the **kidney.** Also see **nephron.**

Long Bones   **Bones** found in legs and arms.

Longitudinal Design   A research design in which subjects are followed over time.

Long-Term Care   Institutions meeting the needs of individuals who can no longer care for themselves. Nursing facilities are an example.

Low Birthweight Baby   A newborn who weighs less than 5 1/2 pounds. These babies are at higher risk for disease and experience more difficulties surviving the first year. Often the mother of a low birthweight baby has a history of poor nutrition status before and/or during pregnancy. Other factors associated with low birthweight are smoking, **alcohol** use, drug use, and certain disease conditions.

Low-Density Lipoprotein (LDL) The **lipoprotein** that transports much of the **cholesterol** found in the **blood** to the body's cells. LDLs are made from **very low-density lipoproteins**. Certain cells (especially in the **liver**) have the ability to absorb the entire LDL particle. The LDLs not absorbed by cells are somehow involved in depositing cholesterol on the inner blood vessel wall, causing hardening and narrowing of the **arteries**. The more LDL-cholesterol you have in your blood, the greater your risk of **heart disease**. See also **very low-density lipoproteins** and **cholesterol**.

Lumen A space or channel within an **organ**.

Luteinizing Hormone (LH) A **hormone** produced by the **pituitary gland** after the onset of menstruation that, along with **follicle stimulating hormone**, stimulates the development of the **ovum** (egg cell) and **ovulation**. LH also induces the development of the **corpus luteum** and its production of **estrogen** and **progesterone**. The high levels of estrogen and progesterone during pregnancy shut down the production of FSH so ovulation cannot occur. In males, LH stimulates the secretion of male sex hormones in the testes.

Lymph A clear fluid found in the lymph vessels. Lymph contains **water**, **salts**, **sugar**, metabolic wastes, some **protein**, and **lymphocytes** and **monocytes** (both are **white blood cells**). Lymph is formed from interstitial or tissue fluid that surrounds the body's cells. Some of this fluid enters into lymph vessels and is returned to the venous blood at certain sites. Lymph nodes, a small mass of lymph tissues, serve to cleanse the lymph before going back into blood vessels.

Lymphatic System A system made up of **lymph**, lymphatic vessels, and lymph nodes that serves a number of functions. Lymph, a clear fluid, enters into lymph vessels from the interstitial or tissue fluid and is returned to the venous blood at certain sites. Lymph nodes, a small mass of lymph tissues, serve to cleanse the lymph before going back into blood vessels.

Lymph capillaries are thin-walled vessels that begin at the spaces around cells. Lymph capillaries merge into larger lymphatic vessels called **lymph vessels**. Lymph vessels have thicker walls than the capillaries and, like **veins**, have valves to help return the lymph and prevent the lymph from flowing backwards. Lymph vessels all move toward the thoracic cavity and empty into the right lymphatic duct and the thoracic duct, which then empty into the subclavian veins in the neck.

The lymphatic system has several functions.

1. Lymph vessels return the interstitial fluid to the bloodstream.

2. The lymphoid **organs**, the **spleen** and the **thymus**, have important functions. The spleen, although not an essential organ in the adult, filters the **blood** of

bacteria and other foreign materials, activates **lymphocytes** as it filters the blood, destroys old **red blood cells,** and stores blood. If the spleen is removed or not functioning, other organs, such as the **liver** and lymph nodes, take over its functions. The thymus is important in the **immune system,** particularly in children. The thymus changes undifferentiated lymphocytes into **T lymphocytes**.

3. Lymph nodes produce lymphocytes and filter foreign bodies and debris from the lymph with the help of **macrophages.**

4. Lymphatic vessels in the intestines absorb **fats** from the **small intestine** and transport them to the bloodstream.

Lymphocytes A type of **leukocyte (white blood cell)** found in the **lymph** nodes and bloodstream where they make **antibodies** to destroy **antigens** and attack foreign bodies. Lymphoctyes are found in human milk. A low Total Lymphocyte Count (TLC—a type of **laboratory test**) may indicate that **malnutrition** exists since they are an indicator of **protein** stores. Certain drugs also decrease total lymphocyte count. A TLC less than 1500 cells/cubic millimeter may indicate nutritional concerns.

Lymphokines Polypeptides secreted by **T lymphocytes** that contribute to cell-mediated immunity. Lymphokines are not **antibodies.** Examples of lymphokines include **interferons** and **interleukins**. See also **immune system, interferons**, and **interleukins.**

Lymphoma A **cancer** of the lymphoid tissue.

Lysozyme An bactericidal **enzyme** found in a number of body fluids such as tears and saliva.

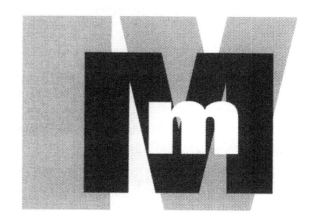

Macrocytic Anemia A type of **anemia** characterized by unusually large **red blood cells**.

Macrocytosis **Red blood cells** that are larger than normal size.

Macronutrients The three nutrients that supply energy: **carbohydrate**, **lipid** (**fat**), and **protein**. They are called macronutrients because of their large molecular size and also because they are needed in larger quantities than the **vitamins** and **minerals**, which are referred to as **micronutrients**.

Macrophages Large phagocytic cells of the **immune system** that engulf and destroy bacteria, viruses, and other foreign bodies. Macrophages are present in the **lymph** nodes, **spleen**, **liver**, lungs, brain, and **bone** marrow where they break down worn-out **red blood cells** into its **heme** and **protein** portions. The **iron** is removed from the heme to be recycled and the heme then decomposes into a dark green pigment, **bilirubin**. Bilirubin is then excreted by the **liver** into the bile.

NUTRIENT FOCUS: MAGNESIUM

A major **mineral** found in all body tissues, with about 60 percent in the **bones** and the remainder in the soft tissues, such as **muscles**, and in the blood. It is essential to many **enzyme** systems responsible for energy conversions in the body and other functions. Magnesium is used in building bones and teeth and works with other minerals to contract the **heart** and **smooth muscles**. Magnesium also has a role in making **protein**. Magnesium is a part of the green pigment called chlorophyll found in plants, so good sources include green leafy vegetables, potatoes, nuts (especially almonds and cashews), seeds, whole-grain cereals, and legumes such as soybeans. Seafood is also a good source. Meat and dairy products supply small amounts.

We probably take in less than the **RDA** but deficiency symptoms are rare.

Magnetic Resonance Imaging (MRI) A way of producing images of the body by means of a strong magnetic field and low-energy radio waves. For this test, the patient is placed into a cylindrical magnetic resonance machine that can take images in all three planes of the body: frontal, sagittal, and transverse.

Major Minerals See **minerals.**

Malnutrition Lack of proper **nutrition.** Malnutrition may be due to excessive amounts of food energy or nutrients (called overnutrition) or inadequate food energy or nutrients (called undernutrition). Undernutrition may be indicated by physical signs, such as a swollen face, or abnormal laboratory values, such as **serum albumin** below 3.5 g/dl.

Maltase A **brush border enzyme** in the **duodenum** that splits **maltose** into **glucose.**

Maltose A **disaccharide** made of two **glucose** units bonded together (see Figure M.1).

Figure M.1 Maltose

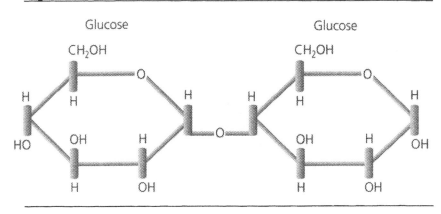

Mammary Gland Glands in female breasts that make milk. Each mammary gland is made of 15 to 20 lobes that have their own individual drainage pathway to the outside. Each lobe is separated into lobules that contain the glandular **alveoli** that produce and secrete milk. The alveoli secrete milk into a series of mammary ducts, which converge to form **lactiferous ducts.** Milk is stored in the lactiferous sinus until it drains to the tip of the nipple.

Management The process of managing or being responsible for meeting certain organizational goals, policies, and practices. Managerial activities typically include **planning, organizing, staffing, leading, controlling, coordinating,** and **representing.** Some managerial success factors include analytical thought, forecasting, multiple focus, organizational knowledge, priority setting, and risk taking. Three levels of management **jobs** can be distinguished: **supervisor**, middle, and top. See also **supervisor**.

Management by Wandering Around (MBWA) Spending a significant part of your day talking to your employees, your guests, your peers, while listening, **coaching**, and trouble-shooting.

Management Dietitian A dietitian who oversees foodservice operations or clinical management. Management dietitians work in healthcare facilities, **college and university foodservices**, school foodservices, **business and industry foodservices**, and other settings.

Managerial Activities Activities that managers perform: **planning, organizing, staffing, leading, controlling, coordinating**, and **representing**. See also **planning, organizing, staffing, leading, controlling, coordinating**, and **representing**.

Managerial Skills The three types of skills a manager needs: technical, human relations, and conceptual.

Manganese A **trace mineral** needed for **bone** formation and as part of many **enzymes** involved in energy **metabolism** and the metabolism of **carbohydrate, fats**, and **protein**. Manganese is found in many foods, especially whole grains, dried beans, nuts, and leafy vegetables. A deficiency is unknown.

Mannitol A **sugar alcohol**.

Marasmus A type of **protein-energy malnutrition** characterized by gross underweight, no **fat** stores, and wasting away of **muscles**. Marasmus is usually associated with severe food shortage, prolonged semistarvation, or early weaning.

PRACTICAL NUTRITION FOCUS: MARGARINE

A **fat** made from **vegetable oils**, **water**, milk or milk solids, flavorings, coloring, emulsifiers, preservatives, and **vitamins**. The mixture is heated and blended, then firmed by exposure to **hydrogen** gas at very high temperatures, a process known as **hydrogenation**. The firmer the margarine, the greater the degree of hydrogenation and the longer its shelf life. Like butter, margarine is 80 percent water and they both supply the same amount of fat, but margarine's fat is much higher in **polyunsaturates** than butter, which is high in **saturates**. Butter also contains much **cholesterol**. There are a variety of margarines available.

- Stick margarine—These are made by hydrogenating plant oils and adding water, milk solids, flavoring, and coloring to make a product similar to butter.

- Soft tub margarine—These have a higher content of polyunsaturated **fatty acids** than stick margarines so they melt at lower temperatures and are easier to spread.

- Whipped margarine—Stick margarines that have been whipped. It contains more air and therefore fewer **calories** per tablespoon (don't substitute it for regular butter or margarine in recipes—it contains a lot of air and water).

- Liquid margarine—These are packaged in squeeze bottles in which the margarine is truly liquid, even in the refrigerator.

- Margarine spread—These are soft margarines with water added. They contain about 50 to 75 percent fat.

- Light margarine—More water is added to this product, which contains about 40 to 60 percent fat.

- Diet margarine—Has about 40 percent fat and therefore more air and water than margarine spreads and light margarine.

- Fat-free margarine—If you are wondering how they make a margarine fat free, here's the answer: gelatin. Gelatin is what is used in Promise Ultra Fat Free™ and Promise Extra Light™ margarines. Rice starch is also used in the fat-free version.

Check out these tips for buying margarine.

- Read the margarine label for **calories**, calories from fat, and fat grams, and compare labels of different products.

- If the margarine you choose has water as the first ingredient, don't use it for cooking or baking as it won't get the same results as a regular margarine.

- Pick a margarine that meets your needs in terms of fat and taste.

Marketing Ascertaining the needs and wants of the consumer, creating the product-service mix that satisfies these needs and wants, and promoting and selling the product-service mix in order to generate a level of income satisfactory to the management and stockholders of the organization (Reid, 1989).

Marketing Cycle A cycle encompassing the following steps.

- Ascertaining the needs and wants of the consumer

- Creating the product-service mix that satisfies these needs and wants

- Promoting and selling the product-service mix in order to generate a level of income satisfactory to the management and stockholders of the organization. (Reid, Robert. 1989. *Hospitality Marketing Management* New York: Van Nostrand Reinhold.)

Mastication Chewing food and mixing it with saliva.

Mastitis Infection of the breast. Mastitis is usually caused by a bacterial infection and is most common during the first two months of breast-feeding. Symptoms include swelling, redness, fever, and pain. Mastitis is generally treated with **antibiotics** and breast-feeding can often continue.

Maturation The process of becoming physically and mentally mature.

Meals-on-Wheels See **Home-Delivered Meals Program**.

Mean The average of a group of numbers.

Mean Cell Hemoglobin (MCH) A laboratory test that measures the **hemoglobin** content of each individual **red blood cell**. MCH is expressed as micromicrograms or picograms of hemoglobin per red blood cell.

Mean Cell Hemoglobin Concentration (MCHC) A laboratory test that measures the concentration of **hemoglobin** in grams per 100 ml of **red blood cells**. MCHC is the average concentration of hemoglobin per red blood cell.

Mean Cell Volume (MCV) A laboratory test that describes the **red blood cells** in terms of individual cell size. Cell size is expressed as microcubic millimeters per red cell.

Median The middle value in a group of numbers, with half of the group of numbers above and half below.

Medical Nutrition Therapy (MNT) A process of assessing a patient's nutritional status and treating it via **diet therapy**, **counseling**, or the use of nutritional support. MNT is necessary to maintain quality of care and is an integral part of disease prevention, treatment, and recovery. MNT also saves money.

Medical Terminology Words common to the medical field. Medical terminology uses many prefixes, suffixes, and words that maintain the same meaning while being used in a wide variety of words.

a-	without, from
aden-, adeno-	gland
-algia	pain
amyl-	starch
andr-, andro-	man or male
angio-	vessel
ap-, apo-	detached

arteri-, arterio-	**artery**
arthr-, arthro-	**joint**
-ase	**enzyme**
athero-	**plaque**, fatty substance
azot-	nitrogen
bili-	gall, **bile**
-blast	immature form
brady-	slow
calc-	**calcium**
carcino-	**malignant tumor**
cardi-, cardio-	**heart**
celi-	**abdomen**
cheil-	lip
chol-, chole-	bile, gall
cholecyst-	**gallbladder**
chondr-, chondrio-	cartilage
chrom-, chromo-	color, colored
col-, colo-	**colon**
cyan-, cyano-	blue
cyst-, cysto-	**urinary bladder**
cyt-, cyto-	cell
dent-, denti-	tooth
derm-	**skin**
duoden-	**duodenum**
dys-	difficult, painful
ect-, ecto-	outside, external
-ectomy	removal or excision of
-emia	in the **blood**
encephal-	brain
endo-, ent-, ento-	within
enter-, entero-	intestine, usually **small intestine**
erythr-, erythro-	red
eu-	well, good

gastri-, gastri-, gastro-	**stomach**
glomerul-	**glomerulus**
gloss-	tongue
gluco-	**sugar**
gyn-, gyneco-	women or female
hem-, hemat-	blood
hepat-, hepato-	**liver**
hist-, histo-	tissue
homeo-	the same
hydr-, hydro-	water
hyp-, hypo-	under, deficient
hyper-	above, excessive
hyster-, hystero-	**uterus**
ile-, ileo-	**ileum**
inter-	between, among
intra-	within
-itis	inflammation of
jejun-, jejuno-	**jejunum**
kilo-	1000 times
labi-	lip
lact-, lacti-, lacto-	milk
leuc-, leuk-	white
lingu-, linguo-	tongue
lip-, lipo-	**lipid, fat**
lith-, litho-	stone
-lysis	destruction
mal-	bad, badly
mega-, megalo-	large
metallo-	containing metal
mono-	one
morph-, morpho-	shape
my-, myo-	**muscle**
myel-, myelo-	marrow, spinal cord

nas-, naso-	nose
necr-, necro-	dead
nephr-, nephro-	**kidney**
neur-, neuro-	**nerve**
noct-	night
-ol	**alcohol**
-oma	tumor
ophthalm-, ophthalmo–	eye, eyeball
ost-, oste-, osteo-	**bone**
-ose	sugar
-osis	action, process, result
ot-	ear
ox-	**oxygen**
para-	beside
path-, patho-	disease
ped-	child, foot
-penia	lack of
phleb-, phlebo-	**vein**
pneum-, pneumo-	lung
-poiesis	production
poly-	many, much
post-	after
pre-	before
proct-, procto	**anus** and **rectum**
prot-, proto-	first
pulmo-, pulmon-	lung
-prandial	meal
pyel-, pyelo-	pelvis
pyo-	pus
pyr-	fever
rect-, recto-	rectum
reni-, reno-	kidney
rhin-, rhino-	nose

-rrhagia	rupture, excessive fluid discharge
scler-, sclero-	hard
-scopy	viewing
-soma, somat-, somato-	body
-stasis	slowing or stopping of
steat-	fat
stomat-	mouth
-stomy	surgical opening
sub-	under, below
super-	over
tachy-	fast
thromb-, thrombo-	blood clot
tox-, toxi-	poison
-trophy	growth
ure-, urea-, urin-	urine
valvul-, valvulo-	**valve**
vas-, vaso-, vasculo-	blood vessel
ven-, veni-, veno-	vein
xer-	dry

Medulla Inner region. For example, the renal medulla is the inner part of the **kidney**.

Megadose When referring to supplement intake, taking 10 times the **RDA** of a **vitamin** or **mineral**.

Megaloblastic Anemia A form of **anemia** characterized by large immature **red blood cells** that is caused by a deficiency of **folate** or **vitamin B12**.

Melanin A dark pigment made by melanocytes in the **epidermis** (**skin**). Melanin is also the pigment of the hair.

Melanoma A malignant **skin tumor**.

Menarche The time when menstruation (also called menses) starts in young females.

Menaquinone A form of **vitamin K** made by intestinal bacteria and absorbed into the body.

Mentoring A relationship in which more experienced manager/professionals help individuals in the early stages of careers.

PRACTICAL NUTRITION FOCUS: MENU PLANNING OVER THE LIFESPAN

Menu Planning for Pregnancy and Lactation

1. Offer a varied and balanced selection of nutrient-dense foods. Because energy needs increase less than nutrient needs, empty calories are rarely an acceptable choice.

2. In addition to traditional meat entrees, have some entrees based on legumes and/or grains and dairy products. Beans, peas, rice, pasta, and cheese can be used in many entrees.

3. Be sure to offer dairy products made with skim or low-fat milk.

4. Use a variety of whole-grain and enriched breads, rolls, cereals, rice, pasta, and other grains in menus.

5. Use assorted fruits and vegetables in all areas of the menu, including appetizers, salads, entrees, side dishes, and desserts.

6. Be sure to have good sources of problem nutrients: **fiber, vitamin B6, folate, vitamin D, iron, calcium, magnesium,** and **zinc.**

7. Be sure to use iodized **salt.**

8. Keep in mind how many extra servings from the meat/meat alternate group and dairy group are needed for pregnant and lactating women. (See Table M.1).

Table M.1   Food Guide Pyramid Servings During Pregnancy and Lactation

Food Group	Minimum Number of servings	Servings Needed During Pregnancy	Lactation
Meat, Poultry, Fish, and Alternates	2	3	3
Milk and Dairy Products	2	3	4
Fruits	2	2	2
Vegetables	3	3	3
Breads, Cereals, Grains	6	6	7

Menu Planning for Infants

For the first four to six months, breast milk or formula are the only food given to babies. Foods are generally introduced as follows. Keep in mind that the order of introducing different types and textures of foods is tied to the baby's developmental stages.

- **4–6 months:**   Iron-fortified baby cereals

- **5–7 months:**   Strained/pureed vegetables and fruits

- **7–9 months:**   Strained or soft **protein** foods (meat, chicken, fish, cheese, yogurt, beans, egg yolk)

    Finger foods such as crackers

    Fruit juice

- **9–12 months:**   Soft, chopped foods (finely chopped at first)

    Breads and grain products

- **12 months:**   Cut-up table foods

    Whole milk

    Whole eggs

Menu Planning for Preschoolers

1. Offer simply prepared foods and avoid casseroles or any foods that are mixed together, as children need to identify what they are eating.

2. Offer at least one colorful food, such as carrot sticks.

3. Preschoolers like nutritious foods in all food groups but are often reluctant to eat vegetables. Part of this problem may be due to the difficulty involved in getting them into a spoon or onto a fork. Vegetables are more likely to be accepted if served raw and cut up as a finger food; however, if serving celery, be sure to take off the strings. When serving cooked vegetables, serve them undercooked so they are a little crunchy. Brightly-colored mild-flavored vegetables such as peas and corn are more popular with kids.

4. Provide at least one soft or moist food that is easy to chew at each meal. A crisp or chewy food is important, too, to develop chewing skills.

5. Avoid strong-flavored and highly salted foods because children have more taste buds than adults so these foods taste too strong to them.

6. Preschoolers love **carbohydrate** foods, including cereals, breads, and crackers, as they are easy to hold and chew.

7. Smooth-textured foods such as pea soup or mashed potatoes should not have any lumps because children find this unusual.

8. Before the age of four, at which time the skills to cut up food start to develop, food needs to be served in bite-sized pieces that are either eaten as finger foods or with a spoon or fork. For example, cut meat into strips or use ground meat, cut fruit into wedges or slices, and serve pieces of raw vegetables instead of a mixed salad. Other good finger foods include cheese cut into sticks, wedges of hard-boiled eggs, dry ready-to-eat cereal, fish sticks, arrow-root biscuits, and graham crackers.

9. Serve foods warm, not hot. A child's mouth is more sensitive to hot and cold than an adult's. Also, little children need little plates, utensils, and cups, as well as seats that allow them to reach the table comfortably.

10. Cut-up fruit and vegetables make good snacks. Also let the preschooler spread peanut butter on crackers or use a spoon to eat yogurt. Snacks are important to preschoolers because they need to eat more often than adults.

11. Before four years old, minimize choking hazards by doing the following:

    Slice hotdogs in quarters lengthwise.

    Shred hard raw vegetables and fruits.

    Remove pits from apples, cherries, plums, peaches, and so on.

    Cut grapes in half lengthwise.

    Spread peanut butter thinly.

    Chop nuts and seeds finely.

    Check to make sure fish being served is really boneless.

    Avoid popcorn and hard candies.

12. Children learn to like new foods by being presented with them repeatedly.

Menu Planning for School-Age Children

1. Serve a wide variety of foods, including children's favorites: tuna fish, pizza (use vegetable toppings), macaroni and cheese, hamburgers (use lean beef combined with ground turkey breast), hot dogs (use ones that are lower in fat), and peanut butter.

2. Good snack choices are important, as children do not always have the desire or the time to sit down and eat. Snacks can include fresh fruits and vegetables, dried fruits, fruit juices, breads, cold cereals, popcorn (without excessive fat), pretzels, tortillas, muffins, milk, yogurt, cheese, pudding, sliced lean meats and poultry, and peanut butter.

3. Balance menu items that are higher in fat with those containing less fat.

4. Pay attention to serving sizes.

5. The most common nutritional problem of children is **iron-deficiency anemia**. Offer iron-rich foods such as meat in hamburgers or roast beef sandwiches, peanut butter, baked beans, chili, dried fruits, and fortified dry cereals.

6. As children grow, they need to eat more high-fiber foods, such as fruits, vegetables, beans and peas, and whole-grain foods. Whereas adults need at least 25 grams of fiber daily, children need an amount equal to or greater than their age plus five grams/day. In other words, a 12-year old child would need 17 grams of fiber daily.

Menu Planning for Adolescents

1. Emphasize **complex carbohydrates** such as assorted breads, rolls, cereals, fruits, vegetables, potatoes, pasta, rice, and dried beans and peas. These foods supply **calories** along with needed nutrients. Whole-grain products are preferred.

2. Offer well-trimmed lean beef, poultry, and fish. Don't think that just because these adolescents need more calories that fatty meats are in order. Their fat calories should be less **saturated**.

3. Low-fat and skim milk need to be offered at all meals. Females are more likely to need to select the skim milk than males. Other forms of calcium also need to be available, such as pizza, macaroni and cheese and other entrees using cheese, yogurt, frozen yogurt, ice milk, puddings, and custards made with skim milk.

4. Offer **margarine** because many adolescents probably are used to eating it at home.

5. Have nutritious choices available to hungry adolescents on the run looking for a snack. Nutritious snack choices could include fresh fruit, muffins and other quickbreads, crackers or rolls with low-fat cheese or peanut butter, pita pocket stuffed with vegetables, yogurt or cottage cheese with fruit, or fig bars.

6. Emphasize quick and nutritious breakfasts, such as whole-grain pancakes or waffles with fruit, juices, whole-grain toast or muffin with low-fat cheese, cereal topped with fresh fruits, or a bagel with peanut butter.

7. The nutrients most often lacking in adolescent diets are iron, folate, and calcium. Significant iron sources include meats, poultry, fish, eggs, legumes, and dried fruits. **Vitamin C** helps the iron from legumes and dried fruits to be absorbed. Folate is found in leafy green vegetables, orange juice, and beans and peas. Calcium may be lacking for those who have an inadequate intake of milk and other dairy products. If teenagers frequently drink soft drinks instead of milk, they may not have enough calcium in their diets to support **bone** growth.

Menu Planning for the Later Years

1. Meals need to be moderate in size. Older adults frequently complain when given too much food because they hate to see waste, so offering moderate portions is desirable. Restaurants perhaps can reduce their entree serving size by 15 to 25 percent.

2. Emphasize complex carbohydrate and high-fiber foods such as fruits, vegetables, grains, and beans. Older people requiring softer diets may have problems chewing some high-fiber foods. High-fiber foods that are soft in texture include cooked beans and peas, bran cereals soaked in milk, canned prunes and pears, and cooked vegetables such as potatoes, corn, green peas, and winter squash.

3. Moderate the use of fat. Many seniors don't like to see their entree swimming in a pool of butter. Use lean meats, poultry, or fish and sauces prepared with vegetable or fruit purees. Have low-fat dairy products available such as skim milk.

4. Offer adequate but not too much protein. Use a variety of both animal and vegetable sources. Providing protein on a budget such as in a nursing home need not be a problem. Lower-cost protein sources include beans and peas, cottage cheese, macaroni and cheese, eggs, liver, dried skim milk, chicken, and ground beef.

5. Moderate the use of salt. Many seniors are on low-sodium diets and they know a salty soup when they taste it so avoid highly salted soups, sauces, and other dishes. It is better to let them season the way they want.

6. Use herbs and spices to make foods flavorful. Seniors are looking for tasty foods just like anyone else, and they may need them more than ever!

7. Offer a variety of foods including traditional menu items and also cooking from other countries and regions of the United States.

8. Fluid intake is critical, so offer a variety of beverages. Diminished sensitivity to **dehydration** may cause older adults to drink less fluid than needed by the body so special attention must be paid to fluids, particularly for those who need assistance to eat and drink. Beverages, such as water, milk, juice, coffee, or tea, and foods such as soup contribute to fluid intake.

9. Intake of the following **vitamins** and **minerals** may be inadequate in older adults and need to be considered when menu planning: **vitamin A,** vitamin D, calcium, and zinc. Meat, dairy products, and vegetables can provide these nutrients.

10. If chewing is a problem, softer foods can be chosen to provide a well-balanced diet. Following are some guidelines for soft diets.

   • Use tender meats, and if necessary, chop or grind them. Ground meats can be used in soups, stews, and casseroles. Cooked beans and peas, soft cheeses, and eggs are additional softer protein sources.

   • Cook vegetables thoroughly and dice or chop by hand if necessary after cooking.

   • Serve mashed potatoes or rice, with gravy if desired.

   • Salads are possible if chopped.

   • Soft fruits such as fresh or canned bananas, berries, peaches, pears, or melon, as well as applesauce, are some possible choices.

   • Soft breads and rolls can be made even softer by dipping them briefly in milk.

   • Puddings and custard are good dessert choices.

   • Many foods that are not soft can easily be chopped by hand or blended in a blender or food processor to allow a wider variety of foods.

Mesentery A double fold of peritoneal membrane (the serous membranes of the abdominal cavity) that attaches each abdominal **organ** to the abdominal wall.

Metabolic Pathway A series of reactions that chemically convert one substance in the body to another.

Metabolism All the chemical reactions occurring in your body that sustain life.

Metabolite Any intermediate compound made during the catabolism of a substance, such as an **amino acid** or **triglyceride**.

Meta-Analysis The process of combining results of independent experiments for the purpose of quantifying their findings using a common measure. Meta-analysis therefore integrates the findings of many studies.

Metalloenzyme An **enzyme** that contains metal atoms.

Metastasis The process by which **tumor** cells spread from one part of the body to another.

MFP Factor A factor found in meat, fish, and poultry that enhances the absorption of **nonheme iron**. See also **iron**.

Micelle An aggregate, or clump, of molecules that takes a spherical shape in water. Inside the micelle are the nonpolar ends of the molecules. On the surface of the micelle are the polar ends of the molecules. In digestion, **bile salts** act as micelles to emulsify or split up **fat** globules.

Microbes See **microorganisms**.

Microcephaly When the size of the head is small in relationship to the rest of the body.

Microcytosis **Red blood cells** that are smaller than normal size.

Micronutrients The two groups of nutrients that do not supply energy but are needed to regulate and control body processes: **vitamins** and **minerals**. They are called micronutrients because only small amounts of them are necessary.

Microorganisms Bacteria, viruses, and other organisms that are invisible to the eye. Most microorganisms do not cause disease.

Micturition Urination.

Mid-Upper-Arm Circumference (MAC) See **anthropometrics**.

Mid-Upper-Arm Muscle Circumference (MAMC) See **anthropometrics**.

Mild Obesity See **obesity**.

Milligram A unit of weight or mass in the metric system. There are 1000 milligrams in a **gram**.

Mineralocorticoids A group of **hormones** produced and secreted by the adrenal cortex that regulate the balance of **sodium** and **potassium** in the **blood**. The most important mineralocorticoid is **aldosterone**. Aldosterone increases sodium **reabsorption** and potassium excretion by the **kidney**. Aldosterone is secreted in response to high blood potassium levels.

Minerals Naturally occurring, inorganic chemical elements that form a class of nutrients. Some minerals are needed in relatively large amounts in the diet—over 100 **milligrams** daily. These minerals are called **major minerals** and include **calcium, chloride, magnesium, phosphorus, potassium, sodium,** and **sulfur.** Other minerals, called **trace minerals** or **trace elements,** are needed in smaller amounts—less than 100 milligrams daily. The trace minerals include **chromium, cobalt, copper,** fluoride, **iodine, iron, manganese, molybdenum, selenium,** and **zinc.**

Mitochondria (Singular: mitochondrion) Organelles found in the cytoplasm of the cell that serve as sites for the production of most of the cell's energy. Mitochondria are nicknamed the "powerhouse" of the cell.

Mitral Valve The **valve** in the **heart** found between the left atrium and left ventricle. The mitral valve lets **blood** flow from the left atrium into the left ventricle.

Mitral Valve Prolapse (MVP) A condition in which one or both of the flaps (also called cusps) of the **mitral valve** bulge (prolapse) upward. This may result in the backflow of a small amount of **blood** into the atrium during ventricular contraction. MVP is the most frequently diagnosed deformity of the heart's valves, occurring in 6 to 10 percent of young women and 4 percent of young men. Only a small percentage of individuals with MVP have symptoms such as chest pain, fatigue, dizziness, lightheadedness, shortness of breath, or anxiety. Having MVP increases the risk of ineffective **endocarditis,** a potentially life-threatening inflammation of the **endocardium** (the membrane that lines the heart's chambers). People with MVP need to take prescribed antibiotics before and after dental and some surgical procedures to prevent endocarditis. Also called **floppy-valve syndrome** or **Barlow's syndrome.**

Modeling A process by which **clients** learn behaviors from observing the counselor/teacher and then try the behaviors themselves.

Moderate Diet A diet that avoids excessive amounts of **calories** or any particular food or nutrient.

Modified Diet A particular selection of food chosen to treat a disease, correct a nutritional deficiency, change body weight, allow rest to the body or an **organ,** or act as a supplement to medical or surgical care. Modified diets were first called special diets because special foods were often prepared for patients. As dietitians spent more time modifying the hospital menu rather than preparing special foods, the newer term of modified diets caught on.

Moderate Obesity See **obesity.**

Molybdenum A **trace mineral** that is a part of a number of **enzymes**. It appears in legumes, whole grains, nuts, and organ meats. Deficiency does not seem to be a problem.

Monocytes A type of **leukocyte (white blood cells)** that acts as a **phagocyte** to dispose of bacteria, dead cells, and other tissue debris.

Monoglyceride A **triglyceride** with only one **fatty acid**. Monoglycerides are produced when **fats** are digested in the **gastrointestinal tract**.

Monosaccharides Single **sugars** including **glucose, fructose,** and **galactose**. The monosaccharides are the building blocks of sugars and starches.

Monounsaturated Fat A monounsaturated **triglyceride** containing at least one **monounsaturated fatty acid**. Monounsaturated fats are found in greatest amounts in foods from plants, including olive, peanut, and canola oils.

Monounsaturated Fatty Acid A **fatty acid** that contains only one (*mono*- means one) double bond in the chain.

Morbidity The prevalence of a disease in a population. Morbidity statistics are given in two ways.

1. Incidence rate—the number of new cases of the disease, divided by the number in the at-risk population over time.

2. Prevalence rate—the number of existing cases of the disease divided by the number in the total population at a point in time.

Morning Sickness Symptoms, especially nausea and vomiting, that occur in some women during the first half of pregnancy. Morning sickness is really a misnomer; the symptoms can occur any time of the day. Morning sickness may be due to an increase in one or more of the 30 **hormones** that increase during pregnancy. Gastrointestinal distress, ranging from **constipation** to **diarrhea**, also accompany the nausea and vomiting. Each woman experiences it a little bit differently. Morning sickness lasts for an average of 17 weeks and, for some unlucky women, it lasts until delivery. A major health concern with morning sickness is that it can cause **dehydration**, which in turn causes nausea.

Dietary advice in the past has concentrated on small, **carbohydrate**-rich meals and tea and crackers. For many women, this dietary advice doesn't work. Recent advice says to eat whatever food you feel you can keep down, even when it means a food that isn't terribly nutritious such as potato chips. The logic behind this recommendation is that your tastes change when you are sick and you often crave something when you feel ready to eat. It's better to eat that food and keep it down, than to try to eat something that is not appealing and then vomit.

Morphology The study of the shape or form of cells.

Mortality The total number of deaths from a given disease in a population during a specific interval of time, usually one year. Mortality is generally reported as the number of deaths per 100,000 people.

Motor Neurons **Neurons** that conduct impulses out of the **central nervous system** to **muscles, glands,** and **organs.** Also called **efferent neurons.** See also **neuron.**

Multigravida A woman who has been pregnant two or more times.

Multipara A woman who has given birth to two or more living babies.

Multiple Myeloma Malignant **tumor** of the **bone** marrow.

Muscles A tissue responsible for locomotion, moving one part of the body, and moving materials through the body. There are three types of muscle tissue: smooth, cardiac, and skeletal.

1. **Smooth muscle**—the muscle fibers that usually form sheets and wrap around tubes and vessels in the body such as the **digestive tract** and **blood** vessels. We do not have conscious control over smooth muscle. Also called *involuntary* or *visceral muscles.*

2. **Cardiac muscle**—the muscle fibers that make up most of the wall of the **heart**.

3. **Skeletal muscle**—the muscle fibers that move the face, the eyes, and the bones. We have control over the skeletal muscles. Also called *voluntary* or *striated muscle.*

Myasthenia Gravis A neuromuscular disease marked by relapsing weakness of **skeletal muscles** and fatigue. Symptoms begin gradually.

Myelin Sheath The covering of myelin, a fatty substance with some **protein,** surrounding the axons of many **nerve** cells in the body. The myelin sheath accelerates **nerve** impulses and also functions as electrical insulation.

Myocardial Infarction (MI) A sudden, irreversible injury to the **heart** in which cells die because of **oxygen** deprivation, often called a **heart attack.** Most heart attacks are caused by a clot in a **coronary artery** at the site of narrowing and hardening that stops the flow of **blood.** Clots normally form and dissolve in response to injuries in the blood vessels, but in **atherosclerosis** (hardening of the arteries) blood clots appear to form in response to **plaque** when they are not needed. If an area of the heart is supplied by more than one vessel, the heart muscle may live for a period of time even if one vessel becomes blocked. See also **cholesterol.**

Myocardial Ischemia When part of the **heart muscle** is deprived of **blood** flow and **oxygen** to a lesser degree, causing a temporary injury.

Myocarditis Inflammation of the **heart's myocardium** or **muscle** tissue that is associated with a number of conditions such as infections.

Myocardium The middle layer of the heart wall. The myocardium is the **heart muscle** and is the thickest of its layers.

Myoglobin A **protein** found in **muscles** that stores and carries **oxygen**.

Myosin A **protein** that makes up about half of the proteins in **muscles**. Myosin works with actin, another protein, to contract and relax muscles.

Myxedema Advanced **hypothyroidism** in adults in which the **thyroid gland** atrophies and little **thyroxine** is produced. Myxedema causes edema, swelling, and increased **blood** volume and **blood pressure**. The metabolic rate is low and the patient is very fatigued. Treatment is with thyroxine.

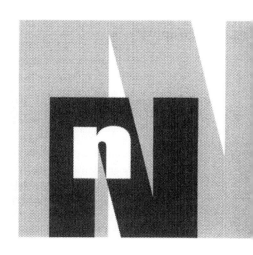

Nasogastric Intubation A medical procedure in which a nasogastric tube is passed through the nose into the **stomach**. The purpose of this procedure is to remove fluid after surgery, to obtain stomach contents for analysis, or to provide means of feeding or giving medication.

National Center for Nutrition and Dietetics (NCND) The public education initiative of The **American Dietetic Association** and its Foundation. NCND is a unique partnership between the public and private sectors working toward promoting the nutritional health of Americans. NCND sponsors National Nutrition Month® and Consumer Nutrition Hot Line and co-sponsors public education programs and conferences.

National Nutrition Monitoring System (NNMS) See **nutrition monitoring.**

Necrosis Cell death due to disease or injury.

Negative Nitrogen Balance A condition in which the body excretes more **protein** than is taken in. Negative nitrogen balance can occur during starvation and certain illnesses.

Neonatal The first four weeks of life.

Neonate An infant during the first four weeks of life.

Neonatology The study and treatment of the newborn child—the infant during the first four weeks of life.

Neoplasm The new and abnormal development of cells. Neoplasms may be harmless (**benign**) or cancerous (**malignant**).

Nephrolithiasis See **kidney stone.**

Nephrologist A physician who diagnoses and treats **kidney** disorders.

Nephron The functional unit of the kidney. Each kidney has more than a million nephrons. The nephrons filter substances from the entering blood, reabsorb needed substances, secrete ions as needed to maintain pH (acid-base) balance, and excrete unnecessary substances in a concentrated form of urine. The nephrons are found primarily in the renal cortex (the outer part of the kidney), with two of its tubules dipping down into the renal medulla (the inner part). The key structures in the nephon are the:

1. **Glomerulus**—a tiny ball of capillaries.

2. **Bowman's or glomerular capsule**—a capsule surrounding the glomerulus.

3. **Renal tubules**—tubes where urine is formed as water, sugar, salts, and some other substances are reabsorbed back into the bloodstream (see Figure N.1).

Figure N.1 Nephron

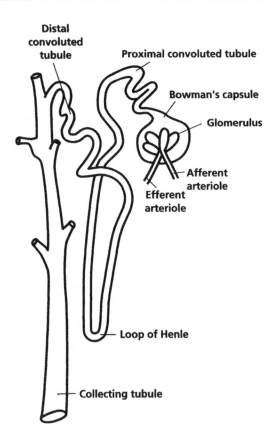

As blood flows through the glomerulus, water and solutes of the blood filter through the capillary walls into Bowman's capsule, forming what is called **glomerular filtrate**, or simply filtrate. Blood cells and **proteins** remain in the blood and are not filtered into the filtrate. The filtrate enters the renal tubules in this order: **proximal convoluted tubule, loop of Henle, distal convoluted tubule**, and **collecting tubule**. In the proximal convoluted tubule, all the **glucose** is reabsorbed and much of the **sodium, potassium, chloride**, and other substances as well. Only about one-quarter of the filtrate remains. Next, the urine is concentrated as it goes through the loop of Henle. In the distal convoluted tubule, hydrogen ions are secreted to maintain acid-base balance and sodium and water are conserved through the action of **hormones**. Water is reabsorbed in the collecting tubule.

Nephropathy **Kidney** disease.

Nephrotic Syndrome A clinical condition that includes excessive **protein** loss in the urine (also called *nephrosis*), hypoalbuminemia (low **blood** levels of **albumin**), and **edema** (swelling). Nephrotic syndrome results from **glomerular** injury that allows proteins, such as albumin, to leak through the glomeruli to then become part of the filtrate. See also **renal disease**.

Neuralgia A painful condition that affects the **nervous system**. It can be caused by a number of disorders.

Neural Tube The tissue in the **embryo** that develops into the brain and spinal cord.

Neural Tube Defects A group of defects of the brain and/or spinal cord that are caused by failure of the **neural tube** to close during early pregnancy. Such defects include **spina bifida** and meningocele. See also **spina bifida.**

Neuroglia Cells found in nervous tissue that do not transmit impulses but support and bind **neurons** together.

Neuromotor Nervous impulses to **muscles**.

Neuron The **nerve** cell. Every neuron contains a **cell body, dendrites**, and an **axon**. The cell body contains the nucleus and is the nutritional center of the neuron. Dendrites are thin branches that extend from the cytoplasm of the cell body. They act to receive stimuli and transmit electrical impulses to the cell body. The axon is longer and it conducts impulses away from the cell body. Axons are sometimes called *nerve fibers.*

Neurons are classified according to their structure or function. Sensory, also called **afferent**, neurons conduct impulses from sensory receptors, such as the **skin**, into the **central nervous system**. Motor, also called **efferent**, neurons conduct impulses out of the central nervous to **muscles, glands**, and **organs**.

Association neurons, also called *interneurons*, are located completely inside the central nervous system.

Neuropathy Any diseased condition of the **nervous system**.

Neutropenia Low number of **neutrophils** (a type of **white blood cell** or **leukocyte**) in the **blood**.

Neurotransmitter A chemical messenger released at the end of the **nerve** cell that stimulates or inhibits a second cell, which may be another nerve cell, a **muscle** cell, or a **gland** cell.

Neutrophils A type of **leukocyte** (**white blood cell**) that acts as a **phagocyte** to destroy bacteria at sites of infection. See also **leukocytes**.

Nerve See **neuron**.

Nerve Fibers Another name for **axon**, part of a **nerve** cell. See **neuron**.

Nervous System A complex system of **nerve** cells that controls all of the functions of the body. The nervous system has two parts: the **central nervous system**, made up of the brain and spinal cord; and the **peripheral nervous system**, which conveys impulses to and from the brain and spinal cord. See **central nervous system** and **peripheral nervous system**.

Networking Talking with other people and sharing ideas, information, and resources.

Newborn The infant during the first four weeks of life.

NUTRIENT FOCUS: NIACIN

A **water-soluble vitamin** that plays a key role as a part of a **coenzyme** in energy metabolism. Niacin is needed for the maintenance of healthy **skin** and the normal functioning of the **nervous system** and **digestive tract**.

The main source of niacin is meat, poultry, and fish. Organ meats are quite high in niacin. Whole-grain and enriched breads and cereals are also important sources of niacin. All foods containing complete **protein**, such as those just mentioned and also milk and eggs, are good sources of the precursor of niacin, **tryptophan**. Tryptophan is an **amino acid** present in some of these foods that is converted to niacin. About half the niacin we use is made from tryptophan.

Megadoses of niacin can cause problems. **Nicotinic acid**, a form of niacin, has been prescribed by physicians to lower elevated **blood cholesterol** levels. Unfortunately it has some undesirable side effects. Starting at doses of 100 **milligrams**, typical symptoms include flushing, rashes, tingling, itching, hives, nausea, **diarrhea**, and abdominal discomfort. Flushing of the face, neck, and chest lasts for about 20 minutes after taking a large dose. More serious side effects of large doses include **liver** malfunction, high **blood sugar** levels, and abnormal **heart** rhythm.

Niacin Equivalents The measure of the amount of **niacin** in food that includes how much niacin will be made from **tryptophan**.

Nicotinamide Adenine Dinucleotide (NAD+/NADH) A **nucleotide** that is involved in removal and storage of electrons for oxidation-reduction reactions. **NAD+** can accept a hydrogen ion and two electrons to be reduced to NADH. When NADH is oxidized (the reverse reaction) to NAD+, heat is released. Like **ATP**, NADH is a way to store energy. NAD is derived from the B **vitamin niacin**.

Nicotinamide Adenine Dinucleotide Phosphate (NADP) A **coenzyme** functionally like **NAD** but with an extra phosphate group and a different specificity.

Nicotinic Acid A form of **niacin** prescribed by physicians to lower elevated **blood cholesterol** levels. Unfortunately it has some undesirable side effects. Starting at doses of 100 **milligrams**, typical symptoms include flushing, rashes, tingling, itching, hives, nausea, **diarrhea**, and abdominal discomfort. Flushing of the face, neck, and chest lasts for about 20 minutes after taking a large dose. More serious side effects of large doses include **liver** malfunction, high **blood sugar** levels, and abnormal **heart** rhythm.

Night Blindness A condition due to insufficient **vitamin A** in which it takes longer to adjust to dim lights after seeing a bright flash of light (such as oncoming car headlights) at night. This is an early sign of vitamin A deficiency.

Nitrogen Balance The balance in the body between intake of nitrogen (from **protein**) and output of nitrogen (in **urea** and **creatinine**). One **gram** of nitrogen is excreted for every 6.25 grams of protein.

Nocturia Having to urinate during the night.

Nonexempt Employees Employees who are paid by the hour and are not exempt from federal and state wage and hour laws. Also called **hourly employees**.

Nonheme Iron A form of **iron** found in all plant sources of iron, and also as part of the iron in animal food sources. Nonheme iron is less readily absorbed than **heme iron**.

Nonnutritive Sweetener Sweeteners that contain either no or very few **calories**. Four nonnutritive sweeteners used in the U.S. are **saccharin, aspartame**, and **acesulfame—K**. See **aspartame, acesulfame—K, cyclamate**, and **saccharin**.

Nonverbal Communication Thoughts and ideas that an individual communicates through the use of not only the voice, but also the body, physical distance, or dress. Nonverbal communication is also evident in the arrangement of the furniture in an office and the degree to which surroundings are pleasant. Body language refers specifically to body posture, facial expressions, vocal inflections, and gestures used to communicate attitudes and feelings.

Noradrenaline See **norepinephrine.**

Norepinephrine A **hormone** produced and secreted by the adrenal medulla. Norepinephrine increases **blood pressure** by constricting blood vessels. It also dilates respiratory passageways, increases the respiratory rate, and increases **glycogenolysis** and **lipolysis,** like **epinephrine** but to a lesser degree. Norepinephrine and epinephrine are called the catecholamines. The **catecholamines** work together to mimic the actions of the **sympathetic nervous system** by increasing the heartbeat, respiratory rate, **blood pressure,** and **blood sugar** levels during stress.

Normocytic Normal cell size.

NPO A medical abbreviation for nothing by mouth. A patient who is NPO should not eat or drink.

Nucleosides A **nucleotide** without the phosphate group. See also **nucleotide.**

Nucleotides The building blocks of **deoxyribonucleic acid (DNA)** and **ribonucleic acid (RNA).** Nucleotides contain a **sugar** (either **ribose** or **deoxyribose**), a nitrogenous base, and one or more phosphate groups.

Nulligravida A woman who has never been pregnant.

Nullipara A woman who has not given birth to a living baby.

Nutrient The nourishing substances in food. They provide energy and promote the growth and maintenance of the body. In addition, nutrients regulate the many body processes, such as **heart** rate and **digestion,** and support the body's optimum health and growth. The six groups of nutrients are **carbohydrates, lipids, proteins, vitamins, minerals,** and **water.**

Nutrient Analysis The process of calculating the nutrient content of a recipe, a meal, a day's food intake or longer period of time, using a nutrient database such as **U.S. Department of Agriculture's** Handbook 8.

Nutrient-Dense Foods Foods that contain many **nutrients** for the **calories** that they provide.

Nutrient Density The **nutrient** content of a food expressed in relation to its **calories.**

Nutrient Retention Five factors are responsible for most **nutrient** loss: heat, exposure to the air and light, cooking in water, and baking soda. Because the **fat-soluble vitamins** are insoluble in water, they are fairly stable in cooking. The **water-soluble vitamins** easily leach out of foods during washing or cooking. Of all the **vitamins, vitamin C** is the most fragile and the most easily destroyed during preparation, cooking, or storage. **Oxygen** and high temperatures readily oxidize or destroy vitamin C. **Thiamin** and **folate** are also fragile. Factors that destroy vitamins often spoil the color, flavor, and texture of food as well (see Table N.1).

Table N.1 Tips to Retain Nutrients in Foods

1. Buy food that is fresh and of high quality.

2. Examine fresh fruits and vegetables thoroughly for appropriate color, size, and shape.

3. Store fruits and vegetables in the refrigerator (except green bananas, potatoes, and onions) because they contain **enzymes** that make fruits and vegetables age and lose nutrients. The enzymes are more active at warm temperatures.

4. Foods should not be kept in storage too long as they lose some nutrients during storage. Store canned goods in a cool place. Refrigerated goods should be maintained at a temperature of 45 degrees F or lower, freezer goods at 0 degrees F or lower. Thermometers should be kept in the refrigerator and freezer to monitor temperatures.

5. When storing food, close up tightly to decrease exposure to the air.

6. When washing vegetables, do so quickly and do not soak them.

7. Potatoes and other vegetables that are boiled or baked without being peeled retain many more nutrients than if peeled and cut. In general, the smaller the pieces into which you cut vegetables before cooking them, the higher the vitamin loss because leaching and oxidation are increased by having created more exposed surfaces. Vegetables should not be cut more than necessary.

8. Keep skins on fruits as much as possible because there are more vitamins and minerals under the skin than in the center of the fruit.

9. Steaming, microwaving, and stir-frying are good choices to retain nutrients when cooking vegetables. Each method is fast and uses little or no water. If boiling vegetables, the longer they are cooked and the more water used, the higher the nutrient loss. Cook quickly and use as little water as possible.

10. Frying's high temperature can destroy vitamins in vegetables. For instance, french-fried potatoes lose much of their vitamin C.

11. Never use baking soda with green vegetables to improve appearance as it will cause nutrient loss.

Table N.1 Tips to Retain Nutrients in Foods (continued)

12. Meats that are broiled or roasted retain more B vitamins than meats that are braised or stewed.

13. Use the cooking water from vegetables and the drippings from meats (after skimming off the fat) to prepare soup and gravy.

14. Don't make foods too far ahead of when they will be served.

15. Don't keep milk in glass containers as light destroys the riboflavin.

Nutrition A science that studies **nutrients** in foods and the body and their action, interaction, and balance in relation to health and disease. Nutrition also examines the processes by which an organism ingests, digests, absorbs, transports, utilizes, and excretes food substances. Lastly, nutrition looks at how you select foods and the type of diet you eat. The six groups of nutrients are **carbohydrates**, **lipids**, **proteins**, **vitamins**, **minerals**, and **water**.

Nutrition Assessment An evaluation of a patient's nutrition status using various methods and measures. Nutrition assessments usually include four parts (see Table N.2).

1. **Anthropometric** measurements

2. Biochemical or **laboratory** tests

3. Clinical signs of **malnutrition** (such as dry, brittle hair or underweight and lethargic)

4. **Diet**, medical, and social **history**

Table N.2 Sample Nutrition Assessment of Persons with Type II Diabetes

Factor	Assessments
Clinical data	Obtain height and weight (when patient is wearing light clothing and no shoes)
	Determine a reasonable body weight
	Estimate daily energy needs
	Assess minimum referral data especially medications (type, amount, and timing), and glucose, glycated hemoglobin, and other laboratory data

Table N.2 Samplel Nutrition Assessment of Persons with
Type II Diabetes (continued)

Factor	Assessments
Nutrition history	Determine usual food intake and pattern of intake
	Evaluate energy intake, macronutrient composition (types and amounts), nutrient distribution, other nutritional concerns, frequency and timing of meals
	Obtain weight history, recent weight changes, and weight goals
	Assess appetite and eating or digestion problems
	Determine frequency of and choices in restaurant meals
	Assess alcohol intake
	Determine use of vitamin/mineral or nutrition supplements
Exercise history	Determine activity types and frequency
	Estimate energy expenditure
	Determine limitations that hinder or prevent exercise
	Assess willingness and ability to become more physically active
Psychosocial and economic issues	Assess living situation, cooking facilities, finances, educational background, employment
	Assess ethnic or religious belief considerations
	Assess level of family and social support
	Determine if there are other important issues
Blood glucose monitoring	Assess knowledge of target blood glucose ranges
	Assess blood glucose testing method and frequency of testing

Table N.2 Samplel Nutrition Assessment of Persons with
Type II Diabetes (continued)

Factor	Assessments
Blood glucose monitoring (continued)	Assess blood glucose records for frequency of hyperglycemia and hypoglycemia and number of target range blood glucose values
Knowledge, skill level, attitudes, and motivation	Assess survival or continuing education knowledge level
	Assess basic knowledge level
	Assess attitudes toward nutrition and health and readiness to learn

Source: Monk, Arlene; Barry, Barbara; McClain, Kathryn; Weaver, Tanya; Cooper, Nancy; Franz, Marion J. Practice guidelines for medical nutrition therapy provided by dietitians for persons with non-insulin-dependent diabetes mellitus. Copyright The American Dietetic Association. Reprinted by permission from *Journal of the American Dietetic Association*, Vol. 95: 1003.

The purpose of the nutrition assessment is not only to examine the nutrition status of the patient, but also to look at any factors (social, cultural, or medical) that influence nutrition status. See also **anthropometrics, laboratory tests,** and **diet history.**

Nutrition Care Plan A plan for a patient that includes the following four steps.

1. Identify **nutrition** problems such as **obesity.**

2. For each problem, develop goals that are relevant, measurable, and realistic.

3. For each goal, choose appropriate methods or approaches to reach it.

4. Review and evaluate the care plan on a regular basis.

Nutrition care plans are documented in the patient's records.

Nutrition Care Team The individuals involved with the nutritional care of a patient. The makeup of the nutrition care team will vary depending on the type of facility, the patient population, the facility's philosophy, and staffing.

Nutrition Counseling Helping people who have, or have the potential for, nutrition problems, by making them more knowledgeable about **nutrition,** committed to good nutrition, and able to turn nutrition knowledge into appropriate food choices. There are many counseling theories or models, such as cognitive-behavioral and humanistic. See also **cognitive psychology, behavior modification,** and **client-centered therapy.**

Nutrition Education A process that assists the public in applying knowledge from **nutritional science** and the relationship between diet and health to their food practices. It is a deliberate effort to improve the nutritional well-being of people by assessing the multiple factors that affect food choices, tailoring educational methodologies and messages to the publics being reached, and evaluating results. It can help individuals develop a knowledge base, make a commitment to good nutrition, select nutritionally adequate diets and develop decision-making skills (The American Dietetic Association, 1990). (See Table N.3.)

Table N.3 Why Nutrition Education is Important: A Fact Sheet

Diet and Disease

• Diet and physical activity patterns together account for at least 300,000 deaths in the U.S. each year: only tobacco use contributes to more deaths.[1]

• Diet is a known risk factor for the three leading causes of death–heart disease, cancer, and stroke–as well as for diabetes, high blood pressure, and osteoporosis.[2]

• Researchers have estimated that as many as 35% of cancer deaths may be prevented through dietary changes.[3]

• Annual economic costs to the nation from heart disease and cancer alone exceed $150 billion.[4, 5]

• Early indicators of atherosclerosis, the most common cause of heart disease, often begin in childhood and adolescence and are related to young people's blood cholesterol levels.[6]

Obesity and Overweight

• The number of overweight children and adolescents in the United States has more than doubled in the past 30 years, with most of the increase occurring since the late 1970s.[7]

• Approximately 4.7 million, or 11% of, U.S. youths aged 6–17 are seriously overweight.[7]

• Obese children and adolescents are more likely to become obese adults.[8-10]

• The number of overweight adults has increased dramatically in recent years. Surveys taken between 1976 and 1980 found that one in four U.S. adults was overweight; surveys taken between 1988 and 1991 found that one in three, or approximately 58 million, U.S. adults are overweight.[11]

Table N.3 Why Nutrition Education is Important: A Fact Sheet
(continued)

- Overweight adults are at increased risk for heart disease, high blood pressure stroke, diabetes, some types of cancer, and gallbladder disease.[2]

Diet and Academic Performance

- Skipping breakfast can adversely affect children's performance in problem-solving situations.[12]

- Participation in the School Breakfast Program can improve student standard-ized test scores and reduce rates of absence and tardiness.[13]

- Even moderate undernutrition can have lasting effects on children's cognitive development and school performance.[14]

Eating Behaviors of U.S. Children and Adolescents

- Children and adolescents in the U.S. eat too much fat[15-17], saturated fat[15-17], and sodium.[17-18]

Nutrient	Recommended Intake	Actual Average Intake
Total fat	≤30% of calories	33–34% of calories
Saturated fat	<10% of calories	12–13% of calories
Sodium	2400 mg per day	2998–4633 mg per day

- Children and adolescents eat, on average, only 3.6 servings of fruits and vegetables per day with fried potatoes accounting for a large proportion of the vegetables consumed.[19] Only one in five children eat 5 servings of fruits and vegetables a day as recommended by the National Cancer Insti-tute.[19] 51% of children and adolescents eat less than one serving of fruit per day and 29% eat less than one serving per day of vegetables that are not fried.[19]

- 41% of high school students ate no vegetables and 42% ate no fruits on the day before a survey.

- Average calcium intake for adolescent females is around 800 mg per day, although the Recommended Dietary Allowance for adolescents is 1200 mg per day.[18]

Table N.3 Why Nutrition Education is Important: A Fact Sheet
(continued)

References

1. McGinnis J.M., Foege WH. Actual causes of death in the United States. JAMA 1993;270:2207-12.

2. Public Health Service. The Surgeon General's report on nutrition and health. Washington, D.C.: U.S. Department of Health and Human Services, Public Health Service, 1988: DHHS publication no. (PHS) 88-50210.

3. Doll R., Peto R. The causes of cancer: quantitative estimates of avoidable risks of cancer in the United States today. Oxford: Oxford University Press, 1981.

4. American Heart Association. Heart and stroke facts: 1995 statistical supplement. Dallas: American Heart Association, 1994.

5. American Cancer Society. Cancer facts and figures—1995. Atlanta, GA: American Cancer Society, 1995.

6. National Cholesterol Education Program. Report of the Expert Panel on Blood Cholesterol Levels in Children and Adolescents. National Heart, Lung, and Blood Institute, 1991; NIH Publication No. 91-2732.

7. Troiano R.P., et al. Overweight prevalence and trends for children and adolescents: The National Health Examination Surveys, 1963–1991. Arch Ped Adol Med 1995; 149:1085-91.

8. Casey V.A., et al. Body mass index from childhood to middle age: a 50-y follow-up. Am J Clin Nutr 1992:56:14-18.

9. Ernst N.D., Obarzanek E. Child health and nutrition: Obesity and high blood cholesterol. Prev Med 1994; 23:427-36.

10. Guo S.S., et al. The predictive value of childhood body mass index values for overweight at age 35 y. Am J Clin Nutr 1994; 59:810-9.

11. Kuczmarski R.J., et al. Increasing prevalence of overweight among US adults. JAMA 1994;272:205-11.

12. Pollitt E., Leibel R.L., Greenfield D. Brief fasting, stress, and cognition in children. Am J Clin Nutr 1981; 34:1526-33.

13. Meyers A.F., et al. School breakfast program and school performance. Am J Dis Child 1989;143:1234-39.

14. Center on Hunger, Poverty, and Nutrition Policy. Statement on the link between nutrition and cognitive development in children. Medford, MA: Tufts University School of Nutrition, 1995.

Table N.3 Why Nutrition Education is Important: A Fact Sheet (continued)

15. McDowell M.A., et al. Energy and macronutrient intakes of persons ages 2 months and over in the United States: Third National Health and Nutrition Examination Survey, Phase 1, 1988–91. Advance data from vital and health statistics: no. 255. Hyattsville, MD: National Center for Health Statistics, 1994.

16. Tippett K.S., et al. Food and nutrient intake by individuals in the United States, 1 day, 1989–91. Riverdale, MD: US Dept. of Agriculture, Agricultural Research Service, 1995; nationwide food survey rep. no. 91-2.

17. Devaney B.L., Gordon A.R., Burghardt J.A. Dietary intakes of students. Am J Clin Nutr 1995;61(suppl):205S-12S.

18. Alaimo K., et al. Dietary intake of vitamins, minerals, and fiber of persons ages 2 months and over in the United States: Third National Health and Nutrition Examination Survey, Phase 1, 1988–91. Advance data from vital and health statistics: no 258. Hyattsville, MD: National Center for Health Statistics, 1994.

19. Krebs-Smith S.M., et al. Fruit and vegetable intakes of children and adolescents in the United States. Arch Pediatr Adolescent Medicine 1995; in press.

From: Nutrition: Making a Difference in Schools A Satellite Videoconference. January 25, 1996. Division of Nutrition and The Public Health Training Network of the Centers for Disease Control and Prevention.

Nutrition Education and Training Program (NET)
(See **School Lunch and Breakfast Programs.**)

PRACTICAL NUTRITION FOCUS: NUTRITION LABELING

Under the Nutrition Labeling and Education Act of 1990 and regulations from the **Food and Drug Administration** and the **U.S. Department of Agriculture,** virtually all food labels must now give information about a food's nutritional content. That wasn't always the case. Until 1994, nutrition information was voluntary. Manufacturers had to provide it only when a food contained added **nutrients** or when **nutrition** claims appeared on the label. Nearly 40 percent of products didn't carry nutrition information (see Figure N.2).

Serving size is the first stop when you read the Nutrition Facts. That's because **calorie** and **nutrient** content is given per serving so you need to know the serving size. Just how big is a serving? On the new label, serving sizes are real-life, given in amounts close to what most people really eat. Of course, if you eat more or less than the serving size, you will need to increase or decrease the calories and nutrients on the label.

If you check serving sizes on similar foods, you'll see that they are similar. That means you don't need to be a math whiz to compare two foods. It's easy to see the calorie and nutrient differences between similar servings of canned fruit packed in syrup and in natural juices. The same is true for two brands of packaged macaroni and cheese.

Look for servings in two measurements—common household and metric measures. A serving of applesauce would read one-half cup (114 g). The household measure is easier to understand. But the metric measure gives a more precise idea of the amount—for example, 114 g means 114 **grams**. A gram is a measure of weight; there are 28 grams in 1 ounce. The label helps you get familiar with metrics, too.

The next stop on the Nutrition Facts panel is Calories per Serving. The label tells you the total calories in one serving, as well as the calories from fat.

Figure N.2 Nutrition Label

Nutrition Facts

Serving Size 1 cup (228g)
Servings Per Container 2

Amount Per Serving

Calories 250 Calories from Fat 110

	%Daily Value*
Total Fat 12g	**18%**
Saturated Fat 3g	**15%**
Cholesterol 30mg	**10%**
Sodium 470mg	**20%**
Total Carbohydrate 31g	**10%**
Dietary Fiber 0g	**0%**
Sugars 5g	
Protein 5g	

Vitamin A 4%	•	Vitamin C 2%
Calcium 20%	•	Iron 4%

* Percent Daily Values are based on a 2,000 calorie diet

After calories, nutrients are listed next. Information about some nutrients is required. These nutrients are total **fat, saturated fat, cholesterol, sodium**, total **carbohydrate**, dietary **fiber, sugars, protein, vitamin A, vitamin C, calcium**, and **iron**. Others are listed voluntarily. If foods contain insignificant amounts of a required nutrient, they might be omitted from the label.

Information about other nutrients is required in two cases: if a claim is made about the nutrients on the label, or if the nutrients are added to the food. For example, fortified breakfast cereals must give Nutrition Facts for any added vitamins and minerals.

Nutrient amounts actually are listed in two ways—in the metric amount (such as 3 grams) or as a percentage of the **Daily Value**. Daily Values are a guide to the total nutrient amount you need for a day based on a 2,000 calorie diet. Therefore, the Daily Value may be a little high, a little low, or right on target for you. Percent Daily Values show you how much of the Daily Value is in one serving. For example, in the nutrition label of Figure N.2, the Percent Daily Value for total fat is 18 percent and for dietary fiber is 0 percent. The Daily Value for fat (and also carbohydrate and protein) is based on a diet with 2,000 calories a day. The Daily Value for dietary fiber is 25 grams.

Nutrient Claims

The FDA now has a dictionary for food producers, marketers, and consumers to consult for consistent and uniform definitions on an expanded list of nutrient content claims. "High in calcium," "low fat," "sugar free"—these words and phrases describe the amount of a nutrient in a food, but don't tell exactly how much. They are called nutrient content claims, or simply nutrient claims. Nutrient content claims differ from Nutrition Facts, which list specific nutrient amounts. You need to read them both. Together nutrient content claims and Nutrition Facts help you compare one food with another and choose foods for a healthful diet.

Consider a package of macaroni and cheese. The claim might say "rich in calcium." The Nutrition Facts panel shows that one serving supplies 20 percent of the Daily Value for calcium. Macaroni and cheese really is an excellent calcium source. Of course, when you use nutrient content claims in choosing foods, always check the other nutrients on the Nutrition Facts panel to see how the food fits into your overall diet.

Products must meet strict nutrition requirements before they can carry these claims. Daily Values help define nutrient content claims. For example, to say "high in fiber," a food must provide at least 20 percent of the Daily Value for fiber—that is, 5 grams of fiber per serving. The government strictly defines terms like these: free, low, high, reduce, less, light, fewer, more, and good source (see Table N.4).

Table N.4 Label Dictionary

Just like the Nutrition Facts, nutrient content claims are defined for one serving. For example, that means that a high-fiber cereal has 5 or more grams of fiber *per serving*.

Nutrient Content Claim	Definition (per serving)
Calories	
Calorie free	Less than 5 calories
Low calorie	40 calories or less
Reduced or fewer calories	At least 25% fewer calories*
Light or lite	One-third fewer calories or 50% less fat*
Sugar	
Sugar free	Less than 0.5 gram sugars
Reduced sugar or less sugar	At least 25% less sugars*
No added sugar	No sugars added during processing or packing, including ingredients that contain sugars, such as juice or dry fruit
Fat	
Fat free	Less than 0.5 gram fat
Low fat	3 grams or less of fat
Reduced or less fat	At least 25% less fat*
Light	One-third fewer calories or 50% less fat*
Saturated Fat	
Saturated fat free	Less than 0.5 gram saturated fat
Low saturated fat	1 gram or less saturated fat and no more than 15% of calories from saturated fat
Reduced or less saturated fat	At least 25% less saturated fat*
Cholesterol	
Cholesterol free	Less than 2 milligrams cholesterol and 2 grams or less of saturated fat

Table N.4 Label Dictionary (continued)

Nutrient Content Claim	Definition (per serving)
Low cholesterol	20 milligrams or less cholesterol and 2 grams or less of saturated fat
Reduced or less cholesterol	At least 25% less cholesterol* and 2 grams or less saturated fat

Sodium

Sodium free	Less than 5 milligrams sodium
Very low sodium	35 milligrams or less sodium
Low sodium	140 milligrams or less sodium
Reduced or less sodium	At least 25% less sodium*
Light in sodium	50% less*

Fiber

High fiber	5 grams or more
Good source of fiber	2.5 to 4.9 grams
More or added fiber	At least 2.5 grams more*

Other Claims

High, rich in, excellent source of	20% or more of Daily Value*
Good source, contains, provides	10% to 19% of Daily Value*
More, enriched, fortified, added	10% or more of Daily Value*
Lean**	Less than 10 grams fat, 4.5 grams or less saturated fat, and 95 milligrams cholesterol
Extra lean**	Less than 5 grams fat, 2 grams saturated fat, and 95 milligrams cholesterol

*As compared with a standard serving size of the traditional food

**On meat, poultry, seafood, and game meats

If a food is labeled with a descriptor for a certain nutrient but that food contains other nutrients at levels known to be less healthy, the label would have to bring that to consumers' attention. For example, if a food making a low-sodium claim is also high in fat, the label must state "see back panel for information about fat and other nutrients."

Health Claims

The Nutrition Labeling and Education Act of 1990 provided, for the first time, the specific statutory authority to allow food labels to carry claims about the relationship between the food and specific diseases or health conditions. This was a major shift in labeling philosophy. Until 1984, a food product making such a claim on its label was treated as a drug and considered misbranded unless the claim was backed up by an approved new drug application.

The FDA has examined the scientific evidence on 10 relationships between nutrients and the risks of certain diseases, and has authorized eight such claims; they are the only ones that can be used in a label. The claims may show a link between the following.

- Calcium and **osteoporosis**. A calcium-rich diet is linked to a reduced risk of osteoporosis, a condition in which the **bones** become soft or brittle.

- Fat and **cancer**. A diet low in total fat is linked to a reduced risk of some cancers.

- **Saturated fat** and **cholesterol**, and **heart disease**. A diet low in saturated fat and cholesterol can help reduce the risk of heart disease.

- **Fiber**-containing grain products, fruits, and vegetables, and cancer. A diet rich in high-fiber grain products, fruits, and vegetables can reduce the risk for some cancers.

- Fruits, vegetables, and grain products that contain fiber, and heart disease. A diet rich in fruits, vegetables, and grain products that contain fiber can help reduce the risk for heart disease.

- Sodium and **high blood pressure**. A low-sodium diet may help reduce the risk for heart disease.

- Fruits and vegetables, and some cancers. A low-fat diet rich in fruits and vegetables (foods that are low in fat and may contain dietary fiber, vitamin A, or vitamin C) is linked to a reduced risk of some cancers.

- **Folic acid** and neural tube birth defects. Women who consume 0.4 mg folic acid daily reduce their risk of giving birth to a child affected with a **neural tube defect**.

The wording on health claims can differ. As an example, a claim on a package of macaroni and cheese links calcium and osteoporosis:

> "Regular exercise and a healthy diet with enough calcium helps teen and young adult white and Asian women maintain good bone health and may reduce their risk of osteoporosis later in life."

Regulations for the general requirements for health claims set forth a number of definitions to clarify their meanings. One of the most significant defines the nutrient levels that would disqualify a health claim. Disqualified are those foods that contain more than 13 grams of fat, 4 grams of saturated fat, 60 milligrams of cholesterol, or 480 milligrams of sodium per amount commonly consumed, per labeled serving size, and per 100 grams (about 3 ounces). Also see **Daily Value.**

Nutrition Monitoring Obtaining data about the nutritional intake and status of a population. Some examples of nutrition monitoring activities in the U.S. include the following.

1. Nationwide Food Consumption Surveys (NFCS)—conducted by **U.S. Department of Agriculture** about every ten years since 1935. Current NFCS examine the adequacy of food and nutrient intake of Americans by region and city.

2. National Health and Nutrition Examination Survey (NHANES)—conducted by the Department of Health and Human Services to obtain information on food and nutrient intakes.

3. Ten State Nutrition Survey—conducted from 1968 to 1970 as the first comprehensive survey of nutritional status of a large number of Americans, especially low-income Americans.

The National Nutrition Monitoring and Related Research Act of 1990 required a ten-year plan for obtaining data on food and nutrient consumption; nutrition knowledge, attitudes and behaviors, the food supply, and other aspects. The Interagency Board for Nutrition Monitoring and Related Research, consisting of over 20 different federal agencies, was established to oversee the **National Nutrition Monitoring System (NNMS).** Most of the activities of the NNMS fall into one of these categories: record-based surveillance systems (such as the number of children receiving free meals during the summer) and population surveys designed to obtain nutrition-related information (such as the Nationwide Food Consumption Surveys).

Nutritional Science The body of scientific knowledge on human nutritional requirements for growth, maintenance, health, and reproduction.

Nutrition Screening Initiative A project committed to the promotion of **nutrition** screening and better nutrition care for America's elderly. The Nutrition Screening Initiative is a joint effort of the **American Dietetic Association**, the American Academy of Family Physicians, and the National Council on Aging.

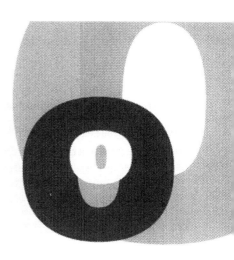

Obesity Body weight of 20 percent or more over desirable weight. Obesity is classified into three categories: mild, moderate, and severe. Mild obesity is 20 to 40 percent, moderate obesity is 41 to 91 percent, and severe obesity is 100 percent or more over desirable weight. To calculate percent of desirable weight, use the following equation.

$$\frac{\text{Actual weight}}{\text{Desirable weight}} \times 100 = \text{Percent of desirable weight}$$

For example, if your actual weight is 120 pounds and your desirable weight is 100 pounds, your percent of desirable weight would be 120 percent. See also **weight management**.

Obstetrics A specialty of medicine concerned with the pregnancy and delivery of the **newborn**.

Occlusion Blockage in a passage of the body, such as an **artery** or **vein**.

Occlusive Vascular Disease Blockage of **arteries** in the lower extremities. Treatment consists of controlling its causes such as atherosclerosis, **hypertension**, and **diabetes**.

Occult Blood **Blood** that is often not visible to the eye and that comes from an unknown place.

Oils A form of **fat**. **Triglycerides** that are liquid at room temperature. Many plant triglycerides are oils. See aslo **vegetable oils**.

Oleic Acid A **monounsaturated fatty acid**.

Olestra See **fat substitutes**.

Olfactory Relating to the sense of smell.

Oligopeptide A **peptide** with 10 or fewer **amino acids**.

Oliguria Lessened ability to make and excrete **urine.**

Oligosaccharides **Carbohydrates** made of 4–10 **monosaccharide** units.

Omega-3 Fatty Acids Fatty acids that have a double bond at the #3 carbon from the methyl end. **Linolenic acid, eicosapentaenoic acid (EPA), and docosahexaenoic acid (DHA)** are the omega-3 fatty acids. EPA and DPA are found in fatty fish and they may help prevent heart disease.

Omega-6 Fatty Acids The **fatty acids linoleic acid** and **arachidonic acid.**

Omnibus Budget Reconciliation Act (OBRA) Federal regulations that require inspection of nursing facilities receiving Medicare and/or Medicaid funds. Inspections focus on how the needs of each resident are being met as well as the quality of services. OBRA also requires that a standard form, Minimum Data Set for Nursing Home Resident Assessment and Care Screening, be filled out within three weeks of a patient's admission. The dietitian fills out Section L, Oral/Nutritional Status, on this form and also writes a care plan in the medical chart. Every 90 days or as significant changes occur, another form, the Quarterly Review form is filled out.

Omnivores Someone who eats both animal and plant foods.

Operant Conditioning A psychological model that states a response followed by a reinforcing stimulus is more likely to occur again. Pleasant reinforcers are called positive reinforcers. Positive reinforcement makes the response more likely to occur again. The concept of positive reinforcement, and other operant conditioning concepts, have influenced how we view teaching and learning. See also **behavior modification.**

Optic Nerve The cranial **nerve** that carries nerve impulses from the retina to the brain.

Oral Cavity Mouth.

Organic Containing carbon.

Organic Foods Foods that have been grown without synthetic pesticides or fertilizers. Organic farmers use, for example, animal and plant manures to increase soil fertility and crop rotation to decrease pest problems. The goal of organic farming is to preserve the natural fertility and productivity of their land. The exact meaning of the term organic has varied from one part of the United States to another. In 1995, the United States instituted national standards for organic foods and agriculture as required by the Organic Foods Production Act. These standards prohibit certain materials, such as mostly synthetic fertilizers, from being used and require certain practices, such as those that make the soil richer. In addition to fruits and vegetables, other organic foods include meat, dairy products, and processed foods.

Organization Chart Diagram of company organization showing levels of management and lines by which **authority** and **responsibility** are transmitted.

Organizing Putting together the money, personnel, equipment, materials, and methods for maximum efficiency to meet an enterprise's goals.

Orientation A new worker's introduction to the **job**.

Orifice An opening.

Organizational Culture The shared values and beliefs within an organization that give members rules for behavior and meaning.

Organs Separate groups of tissues that perform specific functions. Examples include the **heart, liver,** and **kidneys.**

Orthopedist Physicians who treat **bones** and bone disease.

Osmosis The movement of a fluid through a membrane from a solution that has less solute (dissolved substance) to one with more solute, causing the concentration of the solute to equalize. The process of osmosis depends in large part on the osmotic pressure of the two solutions and the permeability of the membrane.

Osseous Tissue Bone tissue.

Ossification **Bone** formation. Bones are formed by the gradual replacement of cartilage and its intercellular substances by **osteoblasts** (immature bone cells) and **minerals** (**calcium** and **phosphorus**). See also **cortical bone, trabecular bone, long bones,** and **short bones.**

Osteoblasts Immature **bone** cells that form bone to replace cartilage during **ossification** (bone formation).

Osteoclasts Large cells that break down bony tissue. Also called *bone phagocytes.*

Osteocytes **Bone** cells.

Osteomalacia A disease due to a **vitamin D** deficiency in adults in which the **bones** of the leg and spine soften and may bend. Osteomalacia may be seen in elderly individuals with poor milk intake and little exposure to the sun.

Osteomyelitis A bacterial infection causing inflammation of the bone and **bone** marrow that usually occurs in children. Osteomyelitis is treated with antibiotics.

NUTRITION AND DISEASE FOCUS: OSTEOPOROSIS

The most common disease affecting **bone** that is characterized by loss of bone density and strength. Osteoporosis is associated with debilitating fractures, especially in people aged 45 and older. It is due to either a failure to build strong bones during the time bones are being built (up to about age 30 to 35) or to a tremendous loss of bone tissue in midlife.

As many as 8 million Americans, 80 percent of them women, now suffer from the condition, with more than 1.5 million osteoporosis-related fractures occurring annually. A little less than half the women over 50 will experience an osteoporosis-related fracture in their lifetime. Another 17 million women are at risk. Luckily, osteoporosis can be prevented, detected, and treated, and it is never too late to do something about it.

The development of osteoporosis is influenced by age, sex, **estrogen** levels, diet, and exercise. For maximum bone health, adequate amounts of **calcium** and **vitamin D** need to be taken in during childhood, adolescence, and adulthood, and exercise is also important.

Outcome The end result of health care **intervention** in terms of the effects on the patient's health status.

Outpatient Nutrition Services Services provided to individuals who are outpatients (living at home and coming to the hospital for care as needed). Outpatient nutrition services often include **nutrition counseling** one-on-one and teaching nutrition topics to groups.

Ovarian Hormones Hormones produced by the **ovaries: estradiol** (an **estrogen**) and **progesterone**. See also **estrogen** and **progesterone**.

Ovaries Female gonads or endocrine glands that produce eggs and **hormones**.

Overweight Body weight between 10 and 19 percent over desirable weight.

Ovulation Release of the ovum (egg cells) from the **ovary**.

Overnutrition Excessive intake of **calories** or **nutrients**, such as megadoses of **vitamins**. Overnutrition can be thought of as **malnutrition**.

Oxalic Acid A substance found in some plant foods such as spinach, beet greens, Swiss chard, sorrel, and parsley that prevents **calcium** from these foods from being absorbed. Oxalic acid is also in tea and cocoa.

Oxidative Phosphorylation The process during which **ATP** is made as a result of the operation of the **electron transport chain**. See also **electron transport chain**.

Oxidized An atom or molecule that loses electrons in a chemical reaction. The atom or molecule that gains the electrons is said to become reduced.

Oxidizing Agent The atom or molecule that accepts electrons from another atom or molecule.

Oxygen A gas that is necessary for human life. Oxygen enters the body through the lungs then travels in the **blood** to the **heart** to be pumped all around the body.

Oxytocin A **hormone** made in the **hypothalamus** and stored and secreted by the posterior **pituitary**. Oxytocin stimulates uterine contractions during labor and maintains labor. Oxytocin also stimulates contractions in the **mammary gland** in response to suckling, resulting in the milk-ejection reflex, also called *milk letdown*, in lactating women.

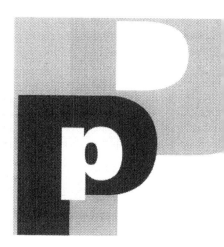

Pacemaker 1) See **sinoatrial node**. 2) A device powered by lithium batteries that can be implanted into the **heart** to establish a normal heart rhythm.

Palate The roof of the mouth.

Palliative Treatment Medical treatment that relieves symptoms, such as pain, but doesn't cure.

Palmar Grasp The ability of a baby from about six months of age to grab things with the palm of the hand.

Pancreas An **organ** located behind the **stomach** that is both an **exocrine** and **endocrine gland**. As an exocrine gland, the pancreas secretes **digestive enzymes** and juices that enter the **duodenum** of the **small intestine**. The pancreas has specialized endocrine cells, called the **islets of Langerhans**, that produce two **hormones: insulin** and **glucagon**. The alpha cells of the islet cells make glucagon and the beta cells make insulin. Insulin and glucagon work opposite each other. When **blood sugar** levels are high, insulin is secreted and helps **glucose** enter the cells of the body. Insulin also promotes the storage of glucose as **glycogen** or **fat**. Whereas insulin lowers blood glucose, glucagon raises **blood glucose levels**. When blood glucose levels are low, glucagon stimulates the **liver** to break down glycogen and release glucose into the blood, and also stimulates the hydrolysis of stored fat to release free **fatty acids** into the blood.

Pancreatitis Inflammation of the **pancreas** in which the pancreatic **enzymes** are blocked from emptying, causing some of these strong enzymes to digest the pancreas itself. Pancreatitis can be either acute or chronic and symptoms include pain, nausea, vomiting, and malabsorption. In chronic patients, weight loss and **malnutrition** are common. Most cases of pancreatitis are associated with either **gallstones** or alcoholism. Dietary treatment includes pancreatic enzyme replacements, **vitamin** and **mineral** supplements, and increased

calories and nutrients to maintain a desirable weight. **Nutrition** support is sometimes necessary.

NUTRIENT FOCUS: PANTOTHENIC ACID

A **water-soluble vitamin** needed to release energy from **carbohydrates, fats,** and **protein.** There is no **RDA** set for this **vitamin** because the specific requirement has not been established yet; instead, an estimated safe and adequate daily dietary intake has been established.

Pantothenic acid is widespread in foods. Good sources include meat, eggs, milk, some vegetables, and legumes.

Papillae Small projections on the tongue that contain **taste buds**. See also **taste** and **taste bud.**

Paradigm A model for practice or behavior.

Parasympathetic Nerves Nerves in the **autonomic nervous system** that control involuntary functions, such as slowing of the **heart**, dilation of visceral **blood** vessels, increased motility of the **gastrointestinal tract**, and stimulation of the **pancreas**. The effects of the parasympathetic nerves are often opposite to the effects of **sympathetic nerves**. See also **autonomic nervous system** and **sympathetic nerves.**

Parathyroid Hormone (PTH) A **hormone** secreted by the **parathyroid glands**. PTH is secreted in response to low **blood calcium** levels. PTH mobilizes calcium from the **bones** into the blood. Also called *parathormone.*

Parenteral Nutrition **Nutrient** feeding directly into a **vein** that is used when the **gastrointestinal tract** can't be used. Parenteral solutions may contain dextrose (**glucose**), **fat, amino acids, electrolytes, vitamins,** or **trace elements**. It may be used when:

- Patients have a nonfunctional gastrointestinal tract.

- Patients have diseases in which nutrients are not being absorbed.

- Patients have high nutrient needs secondary to sepsis, burns, or **cancer.**

- Patients are malnourished and not receiving enough nourishment by other feeding methods.

When a patient receives his or her total nutrient needs via parenteral nutrition, it is called *total parenteral nutrition (TPN).* TPN may use a central or peripheral vein. In *central total parenteral nutrition* (CTPN), a central vein near the **heart** is used because these veins are large in diameter. At other times, a peripheral vein (a vein in the arm or leg) is chosen, and this is called *peripheral parenteral nutrition* (PPN). PPN is used only when short-term support is needed because it cannot provide enough **calories** (under 1000 **calories** per day).

Parotid Gland   One of the **salivary glands** located near the ear. See also **salivary glands**.

Partial Thromboplastin Time (PTT)   A test that measures the presence of **clotting** factors in the clotting process.

Participative Management   A system that includes workers in making decisions that concern them.

Parturition   The act of giving birth.

Pay Grades   Different levels of pay within an organization. **Jobs** with approximately the same job worth are grouped together in a pay grade.

Peak Bone Mass   The maximum **bone** density that can be attained during the time when bones are still forming (the first three decades of life).

Pedagogy   The art and science of teaching.

Pediatrics   The branch of medicine focusing on the growth and care of children.

Peer Review   A process in which **research** studies are reviewed by other researchers and peers prior to publication to ensure that the research is competent and unbiased.

Pellagra   A condition caused by a deficiency of the **vitamin niacin**. The symptoms of pellagra include the four Ds: **diarrhea**, dermatitis, **dementia**, and eventually, death, if untreated.

Pentose Phosphate Pathway   A series of reactions that converts **glucose** to pentoses (**ribose** and **deoxyribose**) and **NADPH**. The **enzymes** that catalyze the pentose phosphate pathway are in the cytoplasm of cells in the **liver**, adrenal cortex, **mammary glands**, and **fat** tissues. Also called the *pentose shunt*.

Pepsin   See **digestive enzymes**.

Pepsinogen   See **digestive enzymes**.

NUTRITION AND DISEASE FOCUS: PEPTIC ULCER DISEASE (PUD)

A **lesion** of the mucous membrane in the lower esophageal, gastric, or duodenal (most common) region. A pain, or gnawing sensation, is normally present. The exact cause is unknown although it may be related to hypersecretion of **hydrochloric acid** and **pepsinogen** in the **stomach**, a bacteria known as

Helicobacter pylori, or the use of a certain class of drugs called nonsteroidal anti-inflammatory drugs such as aspirin that irritates the gastric mucosa. **Diet therapy** includes the following.

1. A well-balanced, individualized diet is important.

2. Small frequent meals have not proven to be more effective than three meals a day so the patient's preference should be considered. Evening snacks are not recommended because they increase gastric secretion during sleep.

3. Caffeinated and decaffeinated beverages, red and black pepper, and chili powder are usually avoided because they stimulate gastric acid secretion. Moderate use may be tolerated by some patients.

4. **Alcohol** should be avoided.

Peptide A polymer of **amino acids** with fewer than 50 amino acids.

Peptide Bond The chemical bonds that connect **amino acids** together in **proteins** and **peptides**. The peptide bond is an amide bond between the amino group of one amino acid and the carboxylic acid group of another amino acid.

Performance Evaluation Periodic review and assessment of an employee's performance during a given period. Also called *performance appraisal* or *performance review.*

Performance Standard Describes the what, how-to, and how-well of a **job**; explains what the employee is to do, how it is to be done, and to what extent.

Pericardium The outer lining of the **heart**.

Pericarditis Inflammation of the **pericardium** or outer lining of the **heart**. Pericarditis may be due to other diseases in the body, **heart attack**, or injury.

Periosteum A fibrous connective tissue covering the outer surface of **bone**.

Peripheral Nervous System (PNS) The part of the **nervous system** outside of the **central nervous system**, meaning outside of the brain and spinal cord. The PNS conveys impulses to and from the brain or spinal cord. The PNS includes the cranial **nerves**, spinal nerves, plexuses, ganglia, and peripheral nerves.

Peristalsis Involuntary wave-like contractions of **muscles** in the wall of the **gastrointestinal tract** that force food through the entire **digestive system**.

Peritoneal Dialysis A form of **dialysis** in which fluid is introduced into the abdominal cavity by a catheter or tube permanently placed in the **abdomen**. The fluid causes wastes in the capillaries to pass out of the **blood** and into the fluid. Fluid with wastes is then removed by the catheter. Peritoneal dialysis may be performed intermittently (called *intermittent peritoneal dialysis—IPD*) with a mechanical device or continuously by the patient without a mechanical device (called *continuous ambulatory peritoneal dialysis—CAPD*).

Pernicious Anemia A type of **anemia** due to a deficiency of **vitamin B12** that is characterized by **macrocytic anemia** and deterioration in the functioning of the **nervous system** that, if untreated, could cause significant and sometimes irreversible damage. The deficiency of vitamin B12 is most likely due to a problem with absorbing the **vitamin**. See also **vitamin B12**.

pH In chemistry, a measure of acidity or alkalinity using a scale from 0 to 14. A pH of 7 is neutral, 1 is very acidic, and 14 is very basic.

Perquisites (Perks) Special benefits for management, usually top management, that are usually noncash items such as a leased car.

Pesticides Chemicals used on crops to protect them from insects, disease, weeds, and fungi.

Phagocytes Cells that can surround, eat, and digest microorganisms, other cells, and cell wastes.

Pharynx Throat. The pharynx is a funnel-shaped passageway about five inches long that connects the mouth (and nasal cavity) to the **esophagus** and trachea (windpipe).

Phenylketonuria (PKU) A birth defect in which a crucial **enzyme** that converts the **amino acid phenylalanine** to **tyrosine**, is lacking. In undiagnosed PKU, phenylalanine builds up in the **blood**, which can be dangerous to the brain, and mental retardation can occur. Most states require screening of babies to detect this treatable disorder. Individuals with PKU must drink a milk substitute that has little or no phenylalanine and carefully choose a low-phenylalanine diet with the help of a dietitian.

Phenylpropanolamine (PPA) An over-the-counter drug found in weight-loss pills, such as Dexatrim™. PPA is a stimulant and is also found in cold medications.

Phlebitis Inflammation of a **vein** that usually develops as a result of trauma or an aftermath of surgery. Phlebitis disrupts normal venous circulation.

Phosphoenolpyruvic Acid (PEP) A high energy phosphate-containing compound that occurs as an intermediary in **carbohydrate metabolism** and can transfer its phosphate group to **ADP** to make **ATP**.

Phospholipid One of three classes of **lipids** that contains **glycerol**, two **fatty acids**, and a phosphate group. Phospholipids are part of every cell. The most important phospholipid is **lecithin** or phosphatidyl-choline, a part of the cell membrane structure. Phospholipids are a part of **lipoproteins**.

NUTRIENT FOCUS: PHOSPHORUS

A major **mineral** used for building **bones** and teeth. Phosphorus circulates in the **blood** and is involved in the release of energy from **fat, protein,** and **carbohydrates** during **metabolism,** and is a part of **DNA** (genetic material) and many **enzymes.** Normal processes of the body produce **acids** and **bases** that can cause major problems in the blood and in the body, such as coma and death, if not buffered (or neutralized) somehow. Phosphorus has the ability to buffer both acids and bases.

Phosphorus is widely distributed in foods and is not likely to be lacking in the diet. Milk and milk products are excellent sources of phosphorus, as they are for **calcium.** Good sources of phosphorus are meat, poultry, fish, eggs, legumes, and whole-grain foods. Fruits and vegetables are generally low in this mineral. Compounds made with phosphorus are used in processed foods, especially soft drinks (phosphoric acid).

Photophobia Sensitivity to light. Photophobia can occur due to certain drugs, viruses, or other reasons.

Photosynthesis A process by which plants and algae make **glucose** and **oxygen** from **carbon dioxide** and **water** using the green pigment chlorophyll to trap the sun's light (energy).

Phylloquinone The form of **vitamin K** found in plants or supplements.

Phytates Compounds present in plant foods, especially whole grains such as whole wheat, that bind with **iron** in the **gastrointestinal tract** and prevent iron from being absorbed.

Phytochemicals Minute compounds found in plants that fight the formation of **cancer.** For instance, broccoli contains a chemical called sulforaphane that seems to initiate increased production of cancer-fighting **enzymes** in the body's cells. Isoflavonoids, found mostly in soy foods, are known as plant **estrogens** or *phytoestrogens* because they are similar to estrogen and interfere with its actions (estogen seems to promote breast tumors). Members of the cabbage family (cabbage, broccoli, cauliflower, mustard greens, kale) also called cruciferous vegetables, contain phytochemicals such as indoles and dithiolthiones. They activate enzymes that destroy carcinogens.

Pica A desire to eat nonfood substances, such as clay or ice.

Pincer Grasp The ability of a baby at about eight months to use his thumb and forefinger together to pick things up.

Pituitary Gland A small **gland** located at the base of the brain. The pituitary gland consists of the anterior lobe (also called the **adenohypophysis**) and the posterior lobe (also called the **neurohypophysis**). Both the anterior and posterior pituitary secrete **hormones**. Hormone secretion is regulated by the **hypothalamus**, a part of the brain that is close to the pituitary gland. The hypothalamus secretes hormones called *releasing* and *inhibiting factors* to stimulate secretion of the hormones from the anterior pituitary. The hormones of the anterior pituitary are:

1. **Adrenocorticotropic hormone (ACTH)**—When the body is stressed, **corticotropin-releasing factor (CRF)** is made by the hypothalamus and travels to the pituitary where it causes the production and secretion of adrenocorticotropic hormone (ACTH). ACTH, the stress hormone, causes the adrenal cortex to make and secrete **cortisol**. Cortisol has an anti-inflammatory effect and stimulates the breakdown of **protein** to **amino acids** in the skeletal **muscle** and increases **gluconeogenesis** in the **liver**.

2. **Follicle-stimulating hormone (FSH)**—This hormone stimulates the growth of ovarian follicles in females and the production of sperm in the male testes.

3. **Luteinizing hormone (LH)**—Luteinizing hormone stimulates **ovulation** and the transformation of the ovulated ovarian follicle into an endrocrine structure called a **corpus luteum**. LH also influences **mammary gland** secretion of milk. In males, LH stimulates the secretion of male sex hormones in the testes. FSH and LH are referred to collectively as the **gonadotropic hormones**.

4. **Growth hormone (GH)**—Growth hormone stimulates growth by helping amino acids into the body's cells and helping cells make proteins. Growth hormone also increases **blood glucose levels**. Also called **somatotropin**.

5. **Thyroid-stimulating hormone (TSH)**—This hormone prompts the **thyroid gland** to make and secrete **thyroxine**.

6. **Prolactin**—Prolactin promotes the growth of breast tissue and stimulates and sustains lactation in the mother postpartum (after birth).

The posterior pituitary secretes two hormones made in the hypothalamus and stored in the pituitary.

1. **Antidiuretic hormone (ADH)**—ADH acts on the distal tubules in the **kidney** to reabsorb water into the bloodstream. Also called **vasopressin**.

2. **Oxytocin**—A hormone that stimulates uterine contractions during labor and maintains labor. Oxytocin also stimulates contractions in the mammary gland

in response to suckling, resulting in the milk-ejection reflex, also called milk letdown, in lactating women.

The pituitary is also called the *hypophysis*.

Placebo A pill or medication with no pharmacological effects. Placebos may be given to control groups in experimental studies.

Placenta The **organ** that develops during the first month of pregnancy that provides for exchange of nutrients and wastes between **fetus** and mother, and secretes the **hormones** necessary to maintain pregnancy. If a mother is not sufficiently nourished during early pregnancy (when she probably doesn't even know she's pregnant), the placenta will not perform properly and the fetus will not get optimal nourishment.

Planning Looking ahead to chart the best courses of future action. See also **strategic action.**

Plaque Deposits in **arteries** that contain **cholesterol, fat,** fibrous scar tissue, **calcium,** and other biological debris. Why plaque deposits are formed and what role fat and cholesterol play in its formation are questions with only partial answers. See also **atherosclerosis.**

Plasma Cell A cell derived from **B cell lymphocytes** that produces and secretes large amounts of **antibodies.** Plasma cells are responsible for **humoral immunity.**

Platelet The smallest **blood** cell. Platelets start the process of blood **clotting** by clumping at the site of injury and releasing **thromboplastin.** Also called **thrombocytes.**

Platelet Count The number of **platelets** per cubic millimeter.

Point of Unsaturation The location of the double bond on **unsaturated fatty acids.**

Policy Statements that set the tone for how a group, department, agency, or a government will operate. Policies give direction for setting goals and priorities, allocating money, program operation, and other aspects. Public policy refers to polices of government, including federal, state, and local.

Polydipsia Increased thirst. This is often seen at the onset of **diabetes mellitus** or in a case of poorly controlled **diabetes.**

Polypeptide A **peptide** with between 10 to 50 **amino acids.**

Polyphagia Increased appetite or hunger. This is often seen at the onset of **diabetes mellitus** or in a case of poorly controlled **diabetes.**

Polysaccharides Carbohydrates, including **starch** and **fiber**, that contain many **monosaccharides**. Also called **complex carbohydrates**.

Potential Energy Energy in storage and ready to be used but not yet released.

Polyunsaturated Fat A polyunsaturated **triglyercide**, also called a **saturated fat**, is made of at least one **polyunsaturated fatty acid**. Polyunsaturated fats are found in greatest amounts in foods from plants, including safflower, sunflower, soybean, corn, cottonseed, and sesame oils.

Polyunsaturated Fatty Acid A **fatty acid** that contains two or more double bonds in the chain.

Polyuria Increased urination. This is often seen at the onset of **diabetes mellitus** or in a case of poorly controlled **diabetes**.

Position The duties and responsibilities performed by one employee.

Positive Nitrogen Balance A condition in which the body excretes less **protein** than is taken in. Positive nitrogen balance occurs during growth and pregnancy.

Positive Regard In **counseling**, the ability of the counselor to value the **client** as a person of worth. Positive regard is shown by the counselor's understanding, nonevaluative stance, warmth, and commitment.

Postpranial Hypoglycemia A type of **hypoglycemia** that occurs generally two to four hours after meals and has symptoms such as quick heartbeats, shakiness, weakness, anxiety, sweating, and dizziness, which mimic anxiety or stress symptoms.

NUTRIENT FOCUS: POTASSIUM

A **mineral** that functions as an **electrolyte** in the body. Potassium, with a positive charge, is found mainly within the cells. As an electrolyte, potassium plays an important role in **water** balance and **acid-base balance** in the body. Water balance means maintaining the proper amount of water in each of the body's three compartments: inside the cells, outside the cells, and in the **blood** vessels. Electrolytes maintain the water balance by moving the water around in the body. Electrolytes also have the ability to **buffer**, or neutralize, various acids and bases in the body.

In the blood, potassium assists in **muscle** contraction, including maintaining a normal heartbeat, and sending **nerve** impulses.

Potassium is distributed widely in foods, both plant and animal. Unprocessed, whole foods such as fruits and vegetables (especially winter squash, potatoes, oranges, and grapefruits), milk, and yogurt are excellent sources of potassium (see Table P.1).

Table P.1   Some Good Sources of Potassium

* Vegetables and fruits in general, especially

  * Potatoes and sweet potatoes

  * Spinach, swiss chard, broccoli, winter squashes, and parsnips

  * Dates, bananas, cantaloupes, mangoes, plantains, dried apricots, raisins, Prunes, orange juice, and grapefruit juice

  * Dry beans, peas, lentils

* Milk and yogurt are good sources of potassium and have less sodium than cheese; cheese has much less potassium and usually has added salt.

A potassium deficiency is very uncommon in healthy people but may result from **dehydration** or from using a certain class of **blood pressure** medications called **diuretics**. Diuretics cause increased **urine** output and some cause an increased excretion of potassium as well. Symptoms of a deficiency include muscle cramps, weakness, nausea, and abnormal **heart** rhythms that can be very dangerous, even fatal.

Power   Capacity to influence the behavior of others.

Prader-Willi Syndrome   A congenital disease marked by a huge appetite, mental retardation, and lack of **muscle** tone.

Prealbumin (PAB)   A plasma **protein** with a short half-life (about two days). PAB is used in assessing nutritional status.

Precompetition Meal   An athlete's meal closest to the time of a competition or athletic event. The functions of this meal include getting the athlete fueled up (both physically and psychologically), helping settle the **stomach**, and preventing hunger. It should be mostly **complex carbohydrates** (because they digest easier and faster and help maintain **blood sugar levels**) and low in **fat**. High-fat foods take longer to digest and can cause sluggishness. Substantial precompetition meals are usually served three to four hours prior to competition in order to allow enough time for the stomach to empty; this avoids cramping and discomfort during the competition. Menus might include the following foods: cereals with low-fat or skim milk topped with fresh fruit, low-fat yogurt with muffins and juice, or one to two eggs with toast and jelly and juice. The meal should include two to three cups of fluid for hydration and typically provides 300 to 1,000 **calories**. Smaller precompetition meals may be served two to three hours before competition. Many athletes have specific "comfort" foods that they enjoy before competition.

Precursor A form of **vitamins** that occurs in foods that must be changed chemically in the body to an active vitamin form.

Pregnancy-Induced Hypertension (PIH) A condition of pregnancy that usually shows symptoms in the **third trimester**. PIH is marked by **hypertension, albuminuria**, and **edema**. In severe cases, called **eclampsia**, convulsions and possibly coma occur. Although the exact cause is not known, pregnant women with PIH often have inadequate diets and little or no prenatal care. A nutritionally balanced diet with adequate **protein, salt, vitamins**, and **minerals** is a cornerstone of treatment.

Press Release A piece written by an organization that is sent out to various news media in hopes that they may pick up the story and use it. The first paragraph often tells the who, what, when, where, and why of the story.

Pressure Sore See **decubitus ulcer**.

Preterm Milk The milk produced by lactating mothers of premature infants.

Prevalence A measure of disease frequency. Prevalence measures the total number of cases of a given disease existing in a population at a specific point in time.

Primary Hypertension **High blood pressure** that is not due to another condition. The cause of primary hypertension is not known. Most cases of **hypertension** are of this type. Also called **essential hypertension**. See also **hypertension**.

Primary Structure The number and sequence of the **amino acids** in the **protein** chain.

Primigravida A woman pregnant for the first time.

Primipara A woman who has given birth once to a living baby.

Problem Solving A special kind of decision making that involves more than a choice between courses of action; it involves identifying the cause of a problem and developing ways to correct or remove the cause. The steps are as follows.

1. Describe the problem.

2. Search out the cause and get the facts.

3. Define the real problem and set objectives.

4. Develop alternative solutions.

5. Decide on the best solution.

6. Implement the decision.

7. Follow up.

Problem-Oriented Medical Recording (POMR) A system of recording information in the medical chart that focuses on the patient's problems, plans for care and for patient education, assessment of progress, and results. Initially a database is developed about the patient and a problem list is drawn up along with appropriate care plans. A *problem* is any condition (health, socioeconomic, personal) the patient presents that the healthcare team will need to treat. The problem list is continually updated and **progress notes** are written into the chart by the physicians and various disciplines (nutrition, physical therapy, etc.).

Using the POMR method, progress notes are usually structured according to the SOAP format.

S–Subjective information: What the patient/patient's family tells you about how the patient/family feels, what the patient wants.

O–Objective information: Results of **laboratory tests**, height/weight, and any other objective information that has direct bearing on the patient's nutrition status and treatment.

A–Assessment: Judgments based on the subjective and objective information.

P–Plan: Recommendations, which usually fall into three categories: obtain more information, treat, and educate.

Writing the progress notes and the care plan is often the responsibility of the dietitian. State regulations vary as to who is responsible for writing progress notes and care plans. State regulations also vary as to how often the progress notes and care plans must be updated. It may be 30 days, 60 days, or another interval of time.

Subjective Information

• Eating habits and patterns

• Food preferences

• **Appetite**

• Reaction/adherence to diet

- Problems chewing or swallowing

- **Food allergies**

- Usual weight

- Changes in eating habits

- Changes in weight

- Previous diets and instructions

- Habits—activity, sleep, bowel

- Use of **vitamin/mineral** supplements

- Use of medications

Examples

1. Patient reports feeling nauseated and wants less food.

2. Patient reports feeling better and is requesting more food.

3. Patient reports difficulty swallowing due to sore mouth; has requested liquids or soft foods only.

Objective Information

- Height

- Actual weight, desirable weight, usual weight

- Diet order

- Pertinent laboratory values

- Nutritional needs: **calories** and **protein**

- Calorie count or food intake information

- Medications (as they pertain to **nutrition**)

- Observed feeding, eating ability

- **Diet history** taken

- Diet instruction given

Examples

1. Patient is blind.

2. Diet order is 4 gm. Na.

3. Patient given diet instruction on Type 1 diet.

Assessment

- Evaluation of weight as it compares to standards and usual past weight

- Evaluation of appropriateness of prescribed diet

- Evaluation of nutrient and drug interactions

- Evaluation of laboratory values

- Evaluation of diet history

- Evaluation of eating/feeding ability

- Evaluation of patient's compliance with diet

- Evaluation of any other problems that are nutritionally related

Examples

1. Patient seems to understand four **gram sodium** diet

2. Diet history shows patient's daily intake of sodium is over 10 grams due to frequent consumption of high sodium foods

3. Patient's low **albumin** indicates significant **malnutrition**

Plan

- Weight goal

- Initiate/recommend supplemental feedings

- Initiate/recommend vitamin/mineral supplements

- Initiate/recommend diet instruction prior to discharge

- Initiate/recommend calorie counts (intake records)

- Request more **laboratory tests**

- Request daily weights

- Referral to other health team members—nutrition clinic, physical therapist, etc

Examples

1. Will provide Ensure™ between meals

2. Will design 1800 calorie diabetic diet with patient

3. Will start calorie count tomorrow AM

Process The actions taken to provide care to patients, such as **counseling** or **diet therapy.**

Processed Foods Foods prepared using a certain procedure: cooking (such as frozen pancakes), freezing (frozen dinners), canning (canned vegetables), dehydrating (dried fruits), milling (white flour), culturing with bacteria (yogurt), or adding **vitamins** and **minerals** (enriched foods). In some cases processing removes and/or adds **nutrients.** See also **fortification** and **enriched foods.**

Productivity A measure of the quantity and quality of work done that takes into account the cost of the resources. Productivity is a ratio of output to input.

Productivity Standard A definition of the acceptable quantity of work an employee is expected to do, such as how many patient charts can be screened.

Progesterone A **hormone** produced by the **corpus luteum** (empty follicle) in the **ovary** and also the **placenta** of pregnant women. Progesterone prepares and maintains the **uterus** during pregnancy. Progesterone also stimulates the development of the milk-producing structures in the breast.

Progressive Discipline A multistage formula for disciplinary action.

Prohormone The precursor of a **hormone.**

Prolactin A **hormone** secreted by the anterior **pituitary gland** that, along with other hormones, promotes the growth of breast tissue and stimulates and sustains lactation in the mother postpartum (meaning after birth).

Promoters Substances, such as **fat**, that advance development of a mutated cell into a **tumor**. Promoters do not initiate **cancer** but enhance its development once initiation has occurred.

Proposal A plan or project being offered for acceptance by another party. Some examples of proposals that dietitians might write include the following.

1. **Grant** proposals are written to organizations that grant money for projects such as **research**.

2. Proposals to provide specific services are written in response to a bid or Request for Proposals (RFP) from an organization.

3. Proposals are also written to get backing to initiate new projects, such as a dietitian doing **nutrition counseling** in a physician's office or a foodservice director in a hospital who wants to start a take-out deli in the hospital's cafeteria.

4. Book proposals describe a book that an author wants a publisher to publish.

The actual format of the proposal will depend on many factors, but any proposal has to do an exceptional job of explaining and selling your project. See also **grants**.

Prophylactic A treatment that is preventive in nature.

Prospective Studies **Research** studies that go forward in time.

Prostaglandins **Hormone**-like substances that are active in almost all tissues. Prostaglandins are made from **polyunsaturated fatty acids**. A prostaglandin is a 20-carbon-long **fatty acid** with a five-membered carbon ring. Prostaglandins are physiologically important in the body.

1. They promote much of the inflammatory response.

2. They inhibit gastric secretions.

3. Some constrict the **blood** vessels and others dilate them.

4. Some promote blood **clotting** and others inhibit **clotting**.

5. They promote **diuresis**.

6. They may cause respiratory distress.

Protected Class Individuals who are in groups identified for protection under equal employment laws and regulations. See also **Equal Employment Opportunity**.

NUTRIENT FOCUS: PROTEIN

A major structural part of animal tissue that is made up of nitrogen-containing **amino acids**. Protein is a **nutrient** that yields four **calories/gram**. Protein is part of most body structures; builds and maintains the body; is a part of many **enzymes**, **hormones**, and **antibodies**; transports substances around the body; maintains fluid balance and **acid-base balance**; and can provide energy for the body.

Tips for nutritious food selection are concerned with the quantity, quality, and variety of protein eaten.

1. **Pick a variety of protein foods to meet your needs.**

2. **Eat enough, but not too much protein.** Assume you need 50 grams of protein daily, and you normally eat 3 ounces of meat, poultry, fish, or cheese for lunch and supper, 1 cup of milk, 2 servings of vegetables, and 4 servings of bread daily. You are already consuming 66 grams of protein, which would increase to 74 if you add 1 more cup of milk. To cut down on your protein, you could switch from eating 3 ounces of animal protein at lunch or supper to a pasta meal, for example, or eat smaller portions of animal protein.

3. **Balance your consumption of plant and animal sources of protein.** Whereas meats supply important nutrients such as **iron**, plant sources generally supply starch, **fiber**, **vitamins**, and **minerals**, without much **fat** or any **cholesterol**. Plant proteins, which provide less than one-third of protein for Americans, are getting a lot more attention from Americans these days. In more homes and restaurants, plant proteins have acquired new status as entrees (such as vegetarian chili) instead of appearing mostly as side dishes.

4. **When choosing animal proteins, choose those with less fat.** For example, choose lean cuts of beef such as top round or eye of round; white, skinless turkey and chicken; fish; skim milk; and cheeses with three grams of fat or less per ounce.

Protein Efficiency Ratio (PER) A method for measuring the **protein** quality of infant formulas by seeing how well it supports weight gain in rats.

Protein-Energy Malnutrition (PEM) The most widespread **malnutrition** problem that includes both **kwashiorkor** and **marasmus**. See also **kwashiorkor** and **marasmus**.

Protein-Sparing Action The action of **carbohydrate** and **fat** in providing energy for the body, thereby allowing **protein** to be used for building tissues and its other indispensable functions.

Proteinuria Having large amounts of **protein**, especially **albumin**, in the urine. Proteinuria is often a sign of **kidney** disease.

Proteolytic Enzymes **Enzymes** that split **proteins** by hydrolyzing (splitting) their **peptide** bonds.

Prothrombin A **blood-clotting** factor made in the **liver**. In blood clotting, prothrombin is converted to **thrombin**. Thrombin converts **fibrinogen** (a **blood plasma protein**) to fibrin, the protein threads that actually form the clot. See also **blood clotting**.

Prothrombin Time A test of **clotting** time made by determining the time for clotting to occur after **thromboplastin** and **calcium** are added to **plasma**. This test is used on patients taking anticoagulants (**blood** thinners) to make sure the dosage is correct.

Protocol A set of rules for carrying out a procedure such as **nutrition assessment**. A **nutrition** protocol generally provides detailed guidelines for nutritional care.

Provitamins Precursors of **vitamins** that occur in food that can be converted into vitamins in the body.

Proximal Convoluted Tubule One of the renal tubules in the **nephron** or functional unit of the **kidney**. Also see **nephron**.

Pruritus Itching.

Ptyalin A **starch**-splitting **enzyme** in saliva.

Puberty The process of physically developing from a child to an adult, which starts at about 10 or 11 for females and 12 or 13 for males. In females, it peaks at age 12 and is completed by age 15. In males, it peaks at age 14 and is completed by age 19, so it starts later and lasts longer in boys. The timing of puberty and rates of growth show much individual variation. During the five to seven years of pubertal development, the adolescent gains about 20 percent of adult height and 50 percent of adult weight. Most of the body **organs** double in size, and almost half of total **bone** growth occurs.

Puberty is the time when children start to develop secondary sex characteristics and the beginning of the fertile period when gametes, sperm or ovum, are produced.

The proportion of **fat** and **muscle** is similar in males and females before puberty; during puberty males put on twice as much muscle as females, and females gain proportionately more fat. In the adolescent female, an increasing amount of fat is being stored under the skin, particularly in the abdominal area. The male also experiences a greater increase in bone mass than females.

Publicity Obtaining free space or time in various media to get public notice of a program, book, etc.

Puerperal The time right after childbirth.

Pulmonary Artery An **artery** that carries **oxygen**-poor **blood** from the right ventricle of the **heart** to the lungs.

Pulmonary Circulation The **blood** flow from the **heart** to the lungs and from the lungs to the heart.

Pulmonary Valve A **valve** of the **heart** found between the right ventricle and the **pulmonary artery**.

Pulmonary Vein A **vein** that carries **oxygen**-rich **blood** from the lungs to the left atrium of the **heart**.

Pupil The dark circle of the eye through which light passes.

Puree Diet A diet with pureed (made into a liquid or pulp) foods for patients with impaired abilities to chew or swallow. In the past, pureed foods had a reputation of looking undesirable when served in most hospitals and nursing facilities. Pureed meat and vegetables were often scooped into small bowls (which for some reason are often called "monkey" dishes), covered with gravy, and sent away to some unfortunate patient as supper.

Pureed diets are often necessary for individuals with chewing or swallowing disorders. Just because someone has a chewing or swallowing disorder doesn't mean they need runny, liquid foods. On the contrary, the hardest thing for these individuals to swallow is runny foods. The easiest texture to swallow resembles that of mashed potatoes.

Luckily, times have changed. Many cooks are using thickeners to help shape pureed foods so they look like the original foods. Thickeners are often powdered and can be mixed directly with liquids and pureed foods. Although several commercial thickeners are available, such as Thick & Easy™, some cooks use thickeners such as cornstarch or instant mashed potato flakes.

Preparing pureed foods is a challenge not only because you want the foods to look good and be the right consistency for swallowing, but also because the volume of pureed foods is different than regular foods. For example, one-half cup of pureed peaches is not the same as one-half cup of regular peaches.

Fruits and vegetables tend to decrease in volume when pureed so one-half cup of pureed peaches would contain more **calories** and **nutrients** than the regular peaches. On the other hand, meats almost double in volume because of the liquid required to puree them. Using standardized recipes ensures that pureed foods:

- Are nutritionally adequate

- Are the right consistency

- Look and taste appropriately

- Are not too expensive as recipes cut down on waste

Purine and Pyrimidine Bases The nitrogenous **bases** contained in the **nucleotides** found in DNA, RNA, ATP, and various **coenzymes**. The major purine bases are **adenine** and **guanine**.

Pyloric Stenosis Narrowing of the **pyloric sphincter** that may block the flow of the **stomach** contents into the **small intestine**. Pyloric stenosis can occur as a birth defect in newborns or in adults because of an **ulcer**. Surgical repair is often necessary.

Pyloric Sphincter The muscular ring in the bottom of the **stomach** that separates the stomach from the **small intestine**. Also called the **pyloric valve**.

Pyranose A **monosaccharide** with a six-membered ring such as glucose.

Pyridoxal Phosphate (PLP) A **coenzyme** form of **vitamin B6**.

Pyrosis See **heartburn**.

Pyruvic Acid An important intermediate product in the production of energy from **glucose**, some **amino acids**, and **glycerol**.

Pyuria Pus composed of **white blood cells** in the **urine**. This is often a sign of infection or inflammation in the **kidney** or **bladder**.

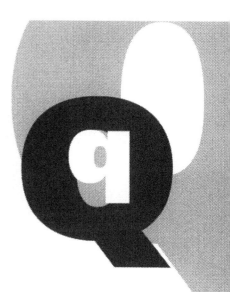

Qualitative Research A type of descriptive **research** that generates narrative instead of numerical data. Qualitative research often is done to develop theories that can then be tested using analytical studies. Qualitative techniques include observation, interviews, and **focus groups**. See also **focus groups** and **research**.

Quality Assurance (QA) Programs designed to assure quality patient care. The QA approach is often department specific, direct care focused, and problem focused. This concept is being replaced by continuous quality improvement which is more multidisciplinary, process and outcome focused, and proactive. See also **continuous quality improvement**.

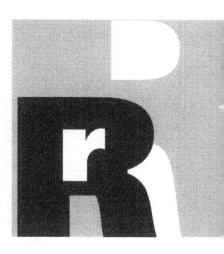

Radioimmunoassay A technique in which radioactive substances tag along with small amounts of **hormones**, drugs, **antibodies** or other substances so they can be measured.

Rales Crackles heard by stethoscope when the patient inhales. Rales are due to fluid in the **bronchus**. See also **bronchus**.

Rancid A state in which **fats** and **oils** smell and taste bad due to oxidation of **unsaturated fatty acids**.

Reabsorption The process of taking back a substance. For example, during the process of making urine, a filtrate is formed but much of the filtrate is reabsorbed back into the **blood**. Only a little filtrate will be excreted.

Rebound Scurvy A condition like **scurvy** that is caused by a period of excessive intake of **vitamin C** supplements followed by a period of normal or low intake of vitamin C.

Recommended Dietary Allowance The levels of intake of **essential nutrients** that, on the basis of scientific knowledge, are judged by the Food and Nutrition Board to be adequate to meet the known nutrient needs of practically all healthy persons in the United States.

Recruiting Actively looking for people to fill **jobs**. Direct recruiting means going where the job seekers are, such as colleges, to recruit. Internal recruiting means looking for people within the company to fill jobs. External recruiting means looking for people outside the company to fill jobs.

Rectum The last part of the **large intestine** in which feces, the waste products of **digestion**, is stored until elimination.

Red Blood Cell Count The number of **red blood cells** in a cubic millimeter of **blood**.

Red Blood Cells See erythrocytes.

Reduced An atom or molecule that gains electrons in a chemical reaction. The atom or molecule that loses the electrons is said to become oxidized.

Reducing Agent The atom or molecule that donates electrons to another atom or molecule.

Reducing Sugars **Monosaccharides** that have a free carbonyl group that gives up electrons as they are oxidized. All monosaccharides are **reducing sugars** and **reducing agents**.

Registered Dietitian A professional dietitian with specialized education in foods and food science, the biological sciences, behavioral and social sciences, education and communication, and in foodservice systems management. To become a Registered Dietitian, you must successfully complete an accredited academic degree course of university study, practice experience, and the Registration Examination for Dietitians. The examination is administered by The Commission on Dietetic Registration, the credentialing agency of **The American Dietetic Association**. A Registered Dietitian is entitled to use the initials RD after his or her name to signify professional competence.

Relapse To revert to former behaviors or conditions. In **weight management**, a relapse is when an individual who lost weight goes back to the old behaviors and regains weight.

Reliability The ability for **research** results to be replicated exactly the same.

Renal Calculi See **kidney stone**.

NUTRITION AND DISEASE FOCUS: RENAL FAILURE

The loss of the **kidney's** ability to maintain fluid and **electroylyte** balance and to excrete waste products. Renal failure can be acute or chronic. Acute renal failure may be due to shock, **thrombosis**, or other trauma to the kidney. Chronic renal **failure** is due to the progressive destruction of kidney tissue. See also **dialysis** and **peritoneal dialysis**. (See Table R.1.)

Renal Threshold The minimum concentration of a substance, such as **sodium**, in the **blood** at which point it will begin to be excreted in the urine.

Renin A **hormone** secreted by the **kidneys** that makes **blood pressure** rise. Renin is secreted by the kidney in response to low blood pressure and low blood flow in the renal **artery**. Renin cuts off a section (called **angiotensin I**) from a **plasma protein** called angiotensinogen. Angiotensin I is converted by an **enzyme** then into an 8-**amino–acid polypeptide** called **angiotensin II**. Angiotensin II constricts arterioles, stimulates the thirst centers in the **hypothalamus** (so more fluids are taken in), and causes **aldosterone** to be secreted

Table R.1 Dietary Parameters in Renal Failure[a]

Energy and nutrients	Renal insufficiency	Hemodialysis	Peritoneal dialysis	Transplantation
Protein	0.6–0.8 g/kg per day, >50%–60% HBV[b]; 0.8–1.0 g/kg in nephrotic syndrome	1.2–1.4 g/kg per day, >50%–60% HBV	1.2–1.5 g/kg per day, >50%–60% HBV	1.3–1.5 g/kg per day after surgery; 1.0 g/kg per day chronic, stable renal function
Energy	30–35 kcal/kg per day	30–35 kcal/kg per day	25–35 kcal/kg per day, including dialysate energy; 20–25 kcal/kg for weight loss	25–35 kcal/kg per day to maintain desired body weight; limit fat to 30% total energy; <300 mg/day cholesterol
Sodium	2.0–4.0 g/day; variable with disease etiology and urine output	2.0 g/day	2.0–4.0 g/day	2.0–4.0 g/day after surgery; 3.0–4.0 g/day chronic, stable renal function
Potassium	Not usually restricted until GFR[c]<10 mL/minute	2.0–3.0 g/day	3.0–4.0 g/day	Unrestricted; monitor drug effects
Phosphorus	10–12 mg/g dietary protein	12–15 mg/g dietary protein	12–15 mg/g dietary protein	Unrestricted; monitor
Calcium	1.0–1.5 g/day	1.0–1.5 g/day	1.0–1.5 g/day	1.0–1.5 g/day
Fluid	Unrestricted until urine output decreases	Urine output plus 1,000 C^3/day	Monitored; most tolerate 2,000 C^3/day	Unrestricted unless urine output decreases or fluid overload occurs

Table R.1 Dietary Parameters in Renal Failure[a] (continued)

Energy and nutrients	Renal insufficiency	Hemodialysis	Peritoneal dialysis	Transplantation
Vitamins and minerals	Daily RDA[d] of vitamins B, C, and D, iron, zinc; do not supplement vitamin A or magnesium	Daily RDA except: vitamin C = 60–100 mg/day; vitamin B–6 = 5–10 mg/day; folic acid=0.8–1.0 μg/day; do not supplement vitamin A or magnesium	Daily RDA except: vitamin C = 60–100 mg/day; vitamin B–6 = 5–10 mg/day; folic acid=0.8–1.0 μg/day; do not supplement vitamin A or magnesium	Daily RDA

[a]Data from references 4, 6,19, 21, 24, 36–40.

[b]HBV = protein of high biological value.

[c]GFR = glomerular filtration rate

[d]RDA = Recommended Dietary Allowance (19).

Source: Beto, Judith A. Which diet for which renal failure: Making sense of the options. Copyright The American Dietetic Association. Reprinted by permission from *Journal of the American Dietetic Association,* Vol. 95: 900.

from the adrenal cortex, causing **sodium** and **water** to be retained by the kidneys.

Replication The duplication of the **DNA** or genetic material in the nucleus of the cell.

Representing A managerial activity of representing the organization to customers and other individuals outside of the enterprise.

Research Systematic inquiry into a subject to discover, substantiate, or revise facts and theories. Research may be categorized according to its purpose: descriptive or analytical. Examples of descriptive research include **qualitative research** and descriptive epidemiologic research. Designs for obtaining descriptive data include case reports or **case studies** (on one subject), case series (on more than one subject), and **survey research**. Descriptive research obtains information that can help develop hypotheses and propose associations between factors, but cannot establish cause-effect relationships as can be done with well-designed analytical studies. **Analytical research** uses experimental designs (such as **clinical trials**) or observational research designs (such as **cohort** or **case-control studies**) in which a hypothesis is tested. See also **case studies, survey research, clinical trials, cohort studies, case-control studies**, and **qualitative research**.

Residue 1) The amount of fecal material in the **colon** and **rectum.** 2) The amount of pesticides that remain on food when people buy them. The tolerance level for a pesticide is the maximum amount of residue allowed.

Respiration In general, all the metabolic processes in the body that release energy to make **ATP**. In respiration, a compound is oxidized by transferring electrons to an inorganic molecule. When **oxygen** serves as the final electron acceptor, the respiration is called **aerobic** respiration. Respiration using oxygen is the main energy source for the body.

Responsibility Accountable for an action.

Resting Energy Expenditure (REE) See **basal energy expenditure**.

Reticulocyte A developing **red blood cell** with granules in its cytoplasm.

Retina The part of the eye that contains photoreceptors called rods and cones. Light energy causes a chemical change in the rods and cones which in turn initiate **nerve** impulses that travel to the brain through the optic nerve. Rods are necessary to see in dim light and cones are necessary to see color.

Retinal The **aldehyde** form of **retinol** that combines with opsin in the **retina** to form visual pigments.

Retinol One of the active forms of **vitamin A**. See also **vitamin A**.

Retinol Binding Protein (RBP) A **protein** that binds with **retinol** and transports it through the blood stream.

Retinol Equivalent The unit of measure for **vitamin A** activity in both its forms (**retinol** and **beta carotene**). 1 RE = 1ug retinol or 6 ug beta carotene.

Retinopathy The retinal effects of **diabetes** marked by microaneurysms, hemorrhages, and dilation of retinal **veins** secondary to diabetes.

Retrospective Studies **Research** studies that look back in time.

R Factor A compound produced in most body fluids. R factor is particularly important in **vitamin B12** absorption because it attaches to the **vitamin** in the **stomach** and is then released in the **small intestine** where it complexes with the intrinsic factor. Vitamin B12 is then carried to the **ileum** (the last segment of the **small intestine**) where it is absorbed.

Rheumatologists Physicians who treat **joint** diseases.

Rhodopsin The light-sensitive pigment that contains **vitamin A** in the **retina** of the eye.

NUTRIENT FOCUS: RIBOFLAVIN

A **water-soluble vitamin** that plays a key role as a part of a **coenzyme** in energy **metabolism**. Riboflavin is essential to release energy from **carbohydrates, fats,** and **proteins,** and for normal growth. Riboflavin is also important for healthy **skin** and normal vision.

Milk and milk products are the major source of riboflavin in the American diet. Other sources include organ meats like **liver** (very high in riboflavin), whole-grain and enriched breads and cereals, and some meats. Because riboflavin breaks down when exposed to light, don't buy milk in glass containers.

Ribonucleic Acid (RNA) Three types of large molecules found in cell nucleus and other parts of the cell that transcribe the code found in **deoxyribonucleic acid (DNA)** to make **proteins** needed in the body. There are three types of RNA.

1. Messenger RNA (mRNA)—The RNA that carries the genetic information from the DNA in the nucleus outside to the rest of the cell to direct making proteins.

2. Ribosomal RNA (rRNA)—The RNA found in the ribosomes that is the site for making proteins.

3. Transfer RNA (tRNA)—The RNA that brings the correct **amino acids** into the ribosomes to make proteins.

Ribose A five-carbon **sugar** in **ribonucleic acid (RNA)**. See also **ribonucleic acid**.

Rickets A disease in children in which **bones** do not grow normally, resulting in bowed legs and knock knees. Rickets is usually due to a **vitamin D** deficiency.

Risk Factor A habit, trait, or condition of an individual that is associated with an increased chance of developing a disease. Preventing or controlling risk factors generally reduces the probability of illness.

Rods See **retina**.

Rooting Reflex The innate reaction of an infant to turn toward the source of a stimulus to the cheek. If an infant's face touches the mother's breast, the infant will instinctively turn toward the breast and root around for the nipple. The rooting reflex is crucial for **lactation**. See also **mammary gland**.

Rugae The folds of the mucous membrane lining of the **stomach**.

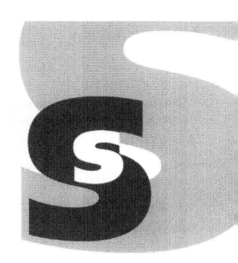

Saccharide Sugar.

Saccharin A nonnutritive sweetener discovered in 1879 that has been consumed by Americans for more than 100 years. Saccharin is 300 times sweeter than **sucrose** and is excreted unchanged directly into the urine. It is used in a number of foods and beverages, and when combined with **aspartame**, they intensify each other's sweetness. Saccharin by itself has a bitter aftertaste. Saccharin is sold in liquid, tablets, packets, and in bulk.

In 1977 the **Food and Drug Administration (FDA)**, which regulates the use of food additives, proposed a ban on its use in foods and allowed its sale as a table-top sweetener only as an over-the-counter drug. This proposal was based on studies that showed the development of **urinary bladder cancer** in second-generation rats fed the equivalent of 800 cans of diet soft drink a day. The surge of public protest against this proposal (no other alternative sweeteners were available at that time) led Congress to postpone the ban, and the postponement is now extended to 1997. Products containing saccharin must have a warning label that states: "Use of this product may be hazardous to your health. This product contains saccharin which has been determined to cause cancer in laboratory animals."

Human studies conducted since the FDA ban have not shown an association between saccharin and bladder cancer.

Salary Fixed compensation paid periodically to a person for work or services regardless of the number of hours worked.

Salivary Amylase An **enzyme** in the saliva that breaks down **starch** into shorter molecules called **dextrins**. Also see **digestive enzymes**.

Salivary Glands **Exocrine glands** outside of the mouth that produce saliva. Narrow ducts carry the saliva into the mouth. Saliva helps clean the teeth and dissolve food molecules. Saliva also contains **starch**-digesting **enzymes** and mucus that aids in swallowing. Most of the saliva is made by three pairs of salivary glands: the **parotid gland**, submandicular gland, and sublingual gland.

Salt (Table Salt) See **sodium**.

Salts Metal-containing product of an **acid-base** reaction that is made of ions or charged particles.

Sample In **research**, a subset of subjects drawn from a population.

Sample Statistic A descriptive statistic of some characteristics of the sample of subjects.

Satiety The feeling of fullness after eating.

Saturated Fat A type of **triglyceride** containing three **saturated fatty acids**. Saturated fats are found in greatest amounts in foods from animals, such as fatty cuts of meat, poultry with the skin, whole-milk dairy products, lard, and in some **vegetable oils**, including coconut, palm kernel, and palm oils. Saturated fat raises **blood cholesterol** more than anything else eaten.

Saturated Fatty Acids **Fatty acids** without any carbon-carbon double or triple bonds. See also **fatty acid**.

School Lunch and Breakfast Programs Lunches and breakfasts offered to school children; established by the National School Lunch Program and signed by President Harry Truman in 1946. Through its National School Meal Programs, the **U.S. Department of Agriculture** provides breakfasts and lunches to more than 25 million children each school day. Yet despite the scientific consensus about the link between diet and health, the **nutrition** standards for school meals have not been significantly updated until recently. A USDA study released in 1993 found that most meals currently served do not meet the **Dietary Guidelines for Americans**. On the average, school lunches contained 25 percent more **fat** and 50 percent more **saturated** fat than recommended (see Table S.1).

The requirements originally set for school lunches stipulated that lunches must provide two ounces of meat or alternate, two or more servings of fruit and/or vegetables, one serving of bread or alternate, and eight ounces of milk. Newer requirements, proposed in 1994, allow schools to move away from this food-based system to a nutrient-analysis system. However, school lunch must still provide three items: an entree, milk, and one other item. The final regulations do provide for a food-based system that follows the old school lunch pattern, but with increased servings from fruits, vegetables, and whole grains. The new regulations promote the use of **nutrient** analysis systems that look at the nutrients in a menu over a week's period of time. As previously, menus must provide one-third of the **RDA** for **calories**, **protein**, **iron**, **calcium**, **vitamin A**, and **vitamin C**. A new regulation, perhaps the highlight of these regulations, states that school lunch menus must provide no more than 30 percent of total calories as fat and no more than 10 percent of total calories as saturated fat. The new regulations must be implemented by Fall of 1996.

The proposed regulations will update the nutrition standards to ensure that all children have access to healthier menus in school. The goal is simple: healthy children. The initiative will also introduce new ways to appeal to children's taste; nutrition education for children, parents, and teachers; and changes in program administration so it works better and more efficiently.

An amendment to the National School Lunch Act authorized the **Nutrition Education and Training** (**NET**) program. NET provides nutrition education training to teachers and school foodservice personnel so that they can teach children the relationship between food and health and encourage good eating habits. The Food and Nutrition Services section of the U.S. Department of Agriculture gives grants to state education departments that oversee the programs.

In 1966 the U.S. Department of Agriculture established the School Breakfast Program. About 60 percent of schools that offer the school lunch program also offer the school breakfast program. School breakfasts must provide one-fourth of the RDAs for the same nutrients examined for lunch (see Table S.1).

Table S.1 Facts about School Lunch and Breakfast

- Over 25 million lunches are served through the National School Lunch program every school day. Only McDonald's provides more meals in the U.S.

- Over 93,000 schools participate in the School Lunch program, which represents almost 99 percent of all public schools and 83 percent of all private schools.

- About 40 percent of school lunches are provided free to needy children and 7 percent are offered at reduced prices. The rest are sold at full price, which averages about $1.15.

- More than half of America's students eat a lunch made by the National School Lunch program and 18 percent of children bring lunch from home.

Scheduling Determining how many people are needed when, and assigning days and hours of work accordingly.

Screening The use of **nutrition assessment** data to identify people who are at nutritional risk. Screening is a preliminary step to planning and implementing the nutritional program for the **client**.

Scurvy Vitamin C deficiency disease. Scurvy is marked by bleeding gums, weakness, loose teeth, and broken capillaries (small **blood** vessels) under the **skin**.

Sebaceous Glands Glands connected to hair follicles in the skin that secrete an oily substance called **sebum**. Sebum lubricates and waterproofs the top layer of the skin. Sebum also prevents the hair from becoming brittle.

Seborrhea Excessive secretion of sebum from the **sebaceous glands**. See also **sebaceous glands**.

Secondary Hypertension When persistently elevated **blood pressure** is due to a medical problem, such as hormonal abnormality or an inherited narrowing of the **aorta** (the largest **artery** leading from the **heart**).

Secondary Structure The bending and coiling of the **protein** chain.

Secretin A **hormone** produced by the **duodenum** that stimulates **water** and **bicarbonate** secretion in the pancreatic juices and causes the **gallbladder** to secrete **bile**. Secretin is secreted when the **pH** of the duodenum falls below 4.5. By causing more bicarbonate in the pancreatic juices, the acidic **chyme** coming from the **stomach** can be quickly neutralized.

Selenium A **trace mineral** included in the **RDA** for first time in 1989. Selenium is a part of **enzymes** that act like **antioxidants** along with **vitamin E** to prevent oxidative damage to tissues. Excellent sources include seafood, meat, and liver. Because selenium is found in soil, vegetables and whole grains may be a good source of selenium as well if the soil is rich in selenium. Selenium deficiency can cause a type of **heart disease**, but this is rare in the U.S. When megadoses of selenium are taken over a long span of time, it can cause **diarrhea**, nausea, vomiting, hair loss, and malaise.

Self-Operated Foodservice An organization that runs its own foodservice. Self-operated foodservices dominate most institutional or noncommercial settings except for business and industry and colleges and universities.

Senescence The normal process of growing old.

Senior Nutrition Programs Federally-funded programs designed to give seniors low-cost nutritious meals, other seniors to eat with, and **nutrition education**. The Older Americans Act of 1965 authorized the **Congregate Meals Program** and the **Home-Delivered Meals Program**. Senior nutrition programs are administered by the Administration on Aging, part of the Department of Health and Human Services. The Administration on Aging gives money to local Agencies on Aging which contract with companies that will provide congregate meals and home-delivered meals. Funding for these programs falls under **Title III-C** of the Older Americans Act and has been decreasing in recent years. See also **Congregate Meals Program** and **Home-Delivered Meals Program**.

Sensory Nerves Neurons that conduct impulses from sensory receptors, such as the **skin**, into the **central nervous system** (brain and spinal cord). Also called **afferent nerves**. See also **neuron**.

Serotonin A **neurotransmitter** made from **tryptophan**. Serotonin constricts **blood** vessels and stimulates the contraction of **smooth muscles**.

Serum The fluid from clotted **blood**. Serum is the same as **plasma** except that it does not contain **fibrinogen**.

Set-Point Theory A theory of **obesity** that is based on the supposition that the body strives to maintain a given range of weight, **fat**, **muscle**, or related factors. Therefore, obesity results from maintaining body weight and fat at a higher than normal level. An obese individual who diets encounters strong biological resistance. Many studies show a tendency for humans to keep their weight within a fairly constant weight range.

SGOT (Serum Glutamic Oxalacetic Transaminase) Also called **aspartic acid transaminase (AST)**. This is a **blood serum** test for the level of aspartic acid transaminase—a key cell **enzyme** involved in the transamination of certain **amino acids**. AST appears in the **liver** and other tissues such as **muscles**. When the level of AST increases, it indicates that there is damage to liver cells because the enzyme leaks out of the liver cells into the blood.

SGPT (Serum Glutamic Pyruvic Transaminase) Also called **alanine aminotransferase (ALT)**. This is a **blood serum** test for the level of alanine aminotransferase—a key **liver** cell **enzyme** involved in the transamination of certain **amino acids**. When the level of ALT increases, it indicates that there is damage to liver cells because the **enzyme** leaks out of the liver cells into the blood. This test is normally done along with a test for the level of **aspartic acid transaminase (AST)**. Because ALT is found primarily in liver cells (AST is found in other tissues), high levels of ALT are especially indicative of liver disease.

Sickle Cell Anemia A hereditary disease marked by crescent or sickle-shaped (abnormal) **red blood cells** that, due to their shape, will clump together and block **blood** vessels. Sickle cell anemia is a long-term incurable blood disease. Symptoms include **joint** pain, **anemia**, weakness, and abdominal pain.

Sigmoid Colon The lower part of the **colon**.

Simple Carbohydrates **Sugars**, including single sugars (like **glucose**) and double sugars (like **sucrose**).

Simple Diffusion Diffusion or transport across the cell membrane in which movement is always from a region of higher to lower concentration.

Simple Proteins Proteins containing only **amino acids** connected by **peptide** bonds.

Simplesse See **fat substitutes.**

Sinoatrial Node (S-A Node) The region of the right atrium of the **heart** which generates an electrical impulse that causes the atrial walls to contract and force **blood** into the ventricles. Also called **pacemaker.** See also **atrioventricular node.**

Sinus Cavity.

Sinus Wave Natural, regular **heart** rhythm.

Situational Leadership Adaptation of leadership style to the needs of the situation.

Skeletal Muscle The **muscle** fibers that move the face, the eyes, and the **bones.** We have control over the skeletal muscles. Also called *voluntary* or *striated muscle.* See also **muscles.**

Skin See **integumentary system.**

Slough To shed.

Small Intestine The portion of the **gastrointestinal tract** between the **stomach** and **large intestine.** It is about 20 feet long and has three parts: the **duodenum, jejunum,** and the **ileum.** The **pyloric sphincter** controls the entry of food into the duodenum and the **ileocecal valve** controls entry of the small intestine's contents into the large intestine.

In the wall of the small intestine are tiny, finger-like projections called **villi.** The muscular walls mix the **chyme** with the digestive juices (which contain **bile** from the **liver** and **gallbladder** and pancreatic juice from the **pancreas**) and bring the nutrients into contact with the villi and the projections on the villi, called microvilli or the **brush border.** The microvilli contain **digestive enzymes** that are not secreted into the intestine but instead remain attached to the cell membrane.

Most nutrients pass through the villi of the duodenum and jejunum into either the **blood** or **lymph** vessels where they are transported to the liver and to the cells of the body. See also **digestive enzymes.**

Smog Readability Formula An easy-to-use method for determining the reading level of a text.

Smooth Muscle The type of **muscle** that usually forms sheets and wraps around tubes and vessels in the body such as the **digestive tract** and **blood** vessels. We do not have conscious control over smooth muscle. Also called *involuntary* or *visceral muscles.* See also **muscle.**

SOAP Notes See **problem-oriented medical recording.**

Social Marketing Marketing that focuses on the needs and interests of the target population. See also **marketing.**

NUTRIENT FOCUS: SODIUM

A mineral that is one of the major **electrolytes** in the body. Sodium (with a positive charge) is found mostly in the fluid outside the cells. Along with **potassium** and **chloride**, sodium maintains two critical balancing acts in the body: **water balance** and **acid-base balance**. Water balance means maintaining the proper amount of **water** in each of the body's three compartments: inside the cells, outside the cells, and in the blood vessels. Electrolytes maintain the water balance by moving the water around in the body. Electrolytes also have the ability to **buffer**, or neutralize, various **acids** and **bases** in the body. In addition to its roles in water balance and acid-base balance, sodium is needed for **muscles** to contract and **nerve** impulses to be transmitted (see Table S.2).

The major source of sodium in the diet is **salt**—a compound made of sodium and chlorine. Salt is 39 percent by weight sodium and one teaspoon contains 2,300 **milligrams** (a little more than 2 **grams**) of sodium. Many processed foods have high amounts of sodium added to them during processing and manufacturing, and it is estimated that these foods provide fully 75 percent of the sodium in most people's diets.

Table S.2 To Consume Less Salt and Sodium

- Read the Nutrition Facts Label to determine the amount of sodium in the foods you purchase. The sodium content of processed foods—such as cereals, breads, soups, and salad dressings—often varies widely

- Choose foods lower in sodium and ask your grocer or supermarket to offer more low-sodium foods. Request less salt in your meals when eating out or traveling.

- If you salt foods in cooking or at the table, add small amounts. Learn to use spices and herbs, rather than salt, to enhance the flavor of food.

- When planning meals, consider that fresh and most plain frozen vegetables are low in sodium.

- When selecting canned foods, select those prepared with reduced or no sodium.

- Remember that fresh fish, poultry, and meat are lower in sodium than most canned and processed ones.

- Choose foods lower in sodium content. Many frozen dinners, packaged mixes, canned soups, and salad dressings contain a considerable amount of sodium. Remember that condiments such as soy and many other sauces, pickles, and olives are high in sodium. Ketchup and mustard, when eaten in large amounts, can also contribute significant amounts of sodium to the diet. Choose lower sodium varieties.

- Choose fresh fruits and vegetables as a lower sodium alternative to salted snack foods.

There is no **RDA** for sodium. Instead, there is an estimated minimum requirement: 500 milligrams. The sodium intake of Americans is easily six times this amount—varying from 3–8 grams daily. The **Nutrition Facts Label** lists a **Daily Value** of 2,400 mg per day for sodium (see Table S.3).

Table S.3 Processed Foods High in Sodium

- Canned, cured, and/or smoked meats and fish such as bacon, salt pork, sausage, scrapple, ham, bologna, corned beef, frankfurters, luncheon meats, canned tuna fish and salmon, and smoked salmon

- Many cheeses, especially processed cheeses such as processed American cheese

- Salted snack foods such as potato chips, pretzels, popcorn, nuts, and crackers

- Food prepared in brine, such as pickles, olives, and sauerkraut

- Canned vegetables, tomato products, soups, and vegetable juices

- Prepared mixes for stuffings, rice dishes, and breading

- Dried soup mixes and bouillon cubes

- Certain seasonings such as salt, sea salt, garlic salt, onion salt, celery salt, seasoned salt, soy sauce, Worcestershire sauce, horseradish, catsup, and mustard

Sodium-Potassium Pump An active transport system in cell membranes that pumps **sodium** out of the cell and keeps **potassium** in the cell.

Soft Diet A diet that provides soft foods (not ground or chopped), foods low in **fiber** content, and mildly spiced foods as desired. It is used for patients with problems chewing or swallowing, as a transition between the **full liquid** and regular diet, or for patients with **gastritis**, indigestion, nausea, or **diarrhea**. The mechanical soft diet is the same as the regular diet except that meats may be ground or chopped and fruits and vegetables must be cooked or, if eaten raw, of a soft texture. This diet is indicated for patients with problems chewing or swallowing.

Solute The substance that is dissolved in a solution.

Somatotropin See **growth hormone.**

Sorbitol A **sugar alcohol** used in such products as sugarless hard and soft candies, chewing gums, jams and jellies. Excessive amounts of sorbitol can cause **diarrhea.**

Span of Control Number of employees a manager supervises directly.

Spastic Colon See **irritable bowel syndrome**.

Sports Drinks Dilute mixtures of **carbohydrate** and **electrolytes** that athletes drink before and during exercise. Most commercial sports drinks contain about 50 **calories** per cup (or about 12 grams of carbohydrate) and small amounts of **sodium** and **potassium**. Sports drinks are purposely made to be weak solutions so they can empty faster from the **stomach** and the nutrients in it are therefore available quicker to the body. They are primarily designed to be used during exercise, although there are some specially formulated sports drinks with slightly more **sugar** that can be used just prior to exercising.

During exercise lasting 90 minutes or more, sports drinks can help replace **water** and electrolytes and provide some carbohydrate for energy. During an endurance event or workout, you increasingly rely on blood sugar for energy as your **muscle glycogen** stores diminish. Carbohydrates taken during exercise can help you maintain a normal blood sugar level and enhance (as well as lengthen) performance. Athletes often consume between one-half to 1 cup of sports fluids every 15 to 20 minutes during exercise.

Some sports drinks tout that they contain **glucose** polymers, which are chains of glucose. Glucose polymers don't taste as sweet as regular sugar so these drinks appeal to certain athletes who don't want the sweetness. It was thought that sports drinks with glucose polymers emptied from the stomach faster than solutions with sucrose or glucose, but it turned out that each of these solutions empties at approximately the same rate and provides the same positive affects on performance as long as the carbohydrate concentration is between five to eight percent (which it usually is).

A homemade sports drink can be made using water, fruit juice, sugar, and salt.

Special Diet See **modified diet**.

Special Supplemental Food Program for Women, Infants, and Children (WIC) A national program started in 1974 that provides nutritious foods, **nutrition education**, and access to health care for qualified pregnant, postpartum, and lactating women, infants, and children up to age five. To receive WIC services, individuals must meet economic eligibility criteria, state eligibility requirements, and be at nutritional risk. WIC provides foods that contain nutrients likely to be missing in the diets of the recipients: **protein**, **iron**, **calcium**, **vitamins A** and **C**. WIC foods include milk, cheese, eggs, iron-fortified breakfast cereal, vitamin C rich juice, beans, peanut butter, iron-fortified infant formula, and infant cereals.

Sphincter A ring of **muscles** that constricts a body opening or tube within the body.

Sphingolipids **Lipids** found in the cell membrane that contain the base *sphingosine*, a **fatty acid**, and one or more other molecules such as **sugars**. There are two types of sphingolipids: *sphingomyelin* (which contains phosphate and **choline**) and *cerebroside* (which contains sugars).

Sphygmomanometer A cuff-like device that is fit just above the elbow to measure **blood pressure**. It consists of a rubber bag inside a cloth cuff and a rubber bulb. See also **blood pressure**.

Spina Bifida A birth defect in which parts of the spinal cord are not fused together properly so gaps are present where the spinal cord has little or no protection. Spina bifida is a type of **neural tube defect**. Some cases of spina bifida are due to the mother being deficient in **folate** during the early months of pregnancy. See also **folate** and **neural tube defects**.

Spleen See **lymph system**.

Spongy Bone See **trabecular bone**.

Staff Functions The individuals who are not directly involved in producing goods and services, such as human resource or personnel directors and training directors, but advise those who do.

Staffing Determining personnel needs and **recruiting**, evaluating, selecting, hiring, orienting, **training**, and **scheduling** employees.

Standards A specific level of performance against which actual performance is compared. Also called *threshold*.

Standards of Care Standard protocols or guidelines for different nutrition care problems, such as **diabetes**. Standards of care are designed so that a uniform level of care is given to patients and are vigorous management tools. Standards of care spell out what nutrition care is to be provided to which patients, who will perform the nutrition care and when it will be done, and how the care will be monitored and documented. Standards of care will reflect the philosophy of each facility.

Standards of Practice for the Profession of Dietetics Standards set by the **American Dietetic Association** for practitioners (see Table S.4).

Table S.4 Standards of Practice

1. The dietetic practitioner establishes performance criteria, compares actual performance with expected performance, documents results, and takes appropriate action.

2. The dietetic practitioner develops, implements, and evaluates an individual plan for practice based on assessment of consumer needs, current knowledge, and clinical experience.

Table S.4 Standards of Practice (continued)

3. The dietetic practitioner, utilizing unique knowledge of nutrition, collaborates with other professionals, personnel, and/or consumers in integrating, interpreting, and communicating nutrition care principles.

4. The dietetic practitioner engages in life-long self-development to improve knowledge and skills.

5. The dietetic practitioner generates, interprets, and uses research to enhance dietetic practice.

6. The dietetic practitioner identifies, monitors, analyzes, and justifies the use of resources.

Source: Standards of Practice: *A Practitioner's Guide to Implementation by The American Dietetic Association Council on Practice Quality Assurance Committee*, Chicago: The American Dietetic Association, 1986.

NUTRIENT FOCUS: STARCH

A **polysaccharide** made in plants that is made of long chains of **glucose**.

To eat more starchy foods, eat breads, rolls, and bagels; breakfast cereals (cooked and ready-to-eat); pastas (fresh and dried); whole grains (such as barley and brown rice); dried beans, peas, and lentils (use in soups, casseroles, and as side dishes); and starchy vegetables (such as peas and corn).

Stasis A medical term meaning stopping or controlling.

Statins One type of **cholesterol**-lowering drug that includes *lovastatin, pravastatin*, and *simvastatin*. These drugs lower **LDL** levels by limiting the amount of cholesterol the body can make.

Statistics Tools for organizing and understanding large sets of data. Statistics have two major subdivisions: *descriptive statistics* and *inferential statistics*. Descriptive statistics are concerned with organizing, simplifying, and summarizing information about a collection of actual observations. Inferential statistics go beyond descriptive statistics to make inferences about the data.

Steatorrhea The discharge of **fat** into the feces.

Stenosis A medical term meaning narrowing or tightening.

Stereoisomer Two molecules with exactly the same atoms arranged in the same sequence, but the spatial orientation of one functional group is different. Stereoisomers are called either *D-isomers* (for dextro, or right-handed) or *L-isomers* (for levo, or left-handed).

Steroid A **lipid** derived from **cholesterol** of which many **hormones** are made, such as the steroid hormones of the adrenal cortex and gonads (**estrogens, androgens,** etc.). Steroids possess the steroid nucleus.

Steroid Hormones **Hormones** made in the adrenal cortex. The steroid hormones are also called **corticosteroids.** They include **glucocorticoids** (such as **cortisol**), **mineralocorticoids** (such as **aldosterone**), and sex hormones. They are made from **cholesterol.** See **adrenal glands.**

Stoma A surgically created opening in the abdominal wall that connects part of the **ileum** or **colon** for elimination after surgical removal of diseased parts of the intestines or **rectum.**

Stomach A muscular sac in the **gastrointestinal tract** that holds about four cups or one liter of food. The functions of the stomach are to churn food which helps in **digestion,** start **protein** digestion, store food, and to move food when it is ready in small amounts into the **small intestine** through the **pyloric sphincter** (see Figure S.1).

Figure S.1 Stomach

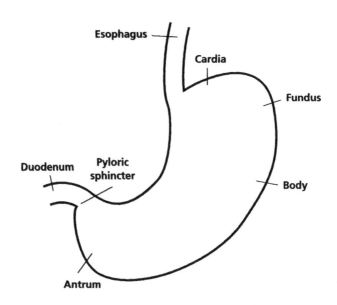

The stomach has four regions.

1. Cardia—the narrow upper region just below the lower esophageal sphincter.

2. Fundus—the upper dome-shaped region.

3. Body—the large central region.

4. Antrum—the region that connects with the duodenum. (Also called the pyloric antrum.)

The stomach is lined with a mucous membrane. Within the folds of the mucous membrane, called *gastric rugae*, are digestive glands that make mucus, **hydrochloric acid**, and an **enzyme (pepsinogen)** to break down **proteins**. Hydrochloric acid aids in protein digestion (it converts pepsinogen into its active form), destroys harmful bacteria, and increases the ability of **calcium** and **iron** to be absorbed.

Food sits in the top part of the stomach and little by little, the food is moved to the lower part of the stomach. Here, the stomach churns the food with the hydrochloric acid and **digestive enzymes**. When the food is ready, it reaches a liquid consistency known as **chyme**, and proceeds to the duodenum of the small intestine.

Stomatitis Inflammation of the muscosa in the mouth.

Strategy A plan for attaining a goal.

Strategic Planning Long-range planning to set organizational goals, objectives, and policies and to determine **strategies**, tactics, and programs for achieving them.

NUTRITION AND DISEASE FOCUS: STROKE

Damage to brain cells resulting from an interruption of the **blood** flow to the brain. The brain must have a continual supply of blood rich in **oxygen** and nutrients for energy. Although the brain constitutes only two percent of the body's weight, it uses about 25 percent of the oxygen and almost 75 percent of the **glucose** circulating in the blood. Unlike other **organs**, the brain cannot store energy. If deprived of blood for more than a few minutes, brain cells die from energy loss and from certain chemical interactions that are set in motion. The functions these cells control—speech, **muscle** movement, comprehension—die with them. Dead brain cells can't be revived.

Strokes may be due to one of the following.

1. A blood clot getting caught in a cerebral **artery** that has narrowed due to **atherosclerosis**.

2. An **embolism**—a mass such as a blood clot or a bit of tissue—blocks a cerebral artery.

3. Hemorrhaging of a cerebral artery.

The majority of strokes are due to a blood clot getting caught in a narrowed brain or neck artery. The most serious kinds of stroke occur not from blockage, but from hemorrhage, when a spot in a brain artery weakened by disease—usually atherosclerosis or **high blood pressure**—ruptures or begins to leak blood. If an artery inside the brain ruptures, it is called a **cerebral hemorrhage**. Hemorrhagic strokes account for less than 20 percent of all types of strokes, but are far more lethal, with a death rate of over 50 percent. Strokes caused by clots or hemorrhage usually strike suddenly, with little or no warning, and do all their damage in a matter of seconds or minutes. Also called **cerebrovascular accident**.

Stroke Volume The amount of **blood** the **heart** pumps to the rest of the body with each beat.

Structure Tangible or organizational components of patient care such as **nutrition** class outlines, equipment, or personnel.

Substrate The molecule to which an **enzyme** binds and catalyzes its conversion to a different molecule.

Sucrase A **brush border enzyme** attached to the cell membrane of microvilli in the **small intestine**. Sucrase breaks down **sucrose** into its components: **glucose** and **fructose**.

Sucrose A **disaccharide** commonly called cane sugar, table sugar, granulated sugar, or simply **sugar**. Sucrose is made of **glucose** and **fructose**. Although the primary source of sucrose in the American diet is refined sugar, sucrose does occur naturally in small amounts in many fruits and vegetables. Table sugar is more than 99 percent pure sugar and provides virtually no nutrients for its 16 **calories** per teaspoon (see Figure S.2).

Figure S.2 Sucrose

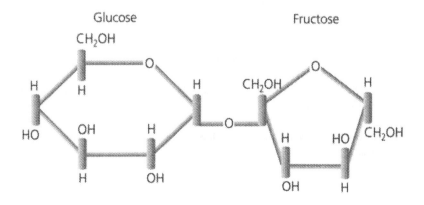

NUTRIENT FOCUS: SUGAR

Simple carbohydrates. Sugars are either single units **(monosaccharides)** of **glucose, fructose,** or **galactose** or double units **(disaccharides)** of **sucrose** (table sugar), **lactose,** or **maltose**.

Sugar occurs naturally in some foods, such as fruits and milk. Fruits are an excellent source of natural sugar, but be aware that some canned fruits contain much added sucrose. Canned fruits are packed in one of three styles: in fruit juice, light syrup, or heavy syrup. Both light syrup and heavy syrup have sugar added. Heavy syrup contains the most added sugar (about four teaspoons of sucrose to one-half cup of fruit). Dried fruits, such as raisins, are more concentrated sources of natural sugar than fresh fruits because dried fruits contain much less water.

Lactose, or milk sugar, is present in large amounts in milk, ice cream, ice milk, sherbet, cottage cheese, cheese spreads and other soft cheeses, eggnog, and cream. Hard cheeses contain only traces of lactose.

Although a natural sugar, honey (made by bees) is primarily fructose and glucose, which are the same two components of table sugar. Although they are different in flavor and texture, the body can't tell the difference between natural and refined sugars. They both contribute only energy and no other nutrients in significant amounts. Because honey is more concentrated, it has twice as many **calories** as the same amount of sugar.

Refined sugars, such as table sugar or corn syrup, are added to foods to sweeten. Besides sweetening, they prevent spoilage in jams and jellies and perform several functions in baking such as browning the crust and retaining moisture in baked goods so they stay fresh. Sugar also acts as a food for yeast in breads and other baked goods that use yeast for leavening (see Table S.5).

Table S.5 On a Food Label, Sugars Include

- Brown sugar

- Corn sweetener

- Corn syrup

- Fructose

- Fruit juice concentrate

- Glucose (dextrose)

- High-fructose corn syrup

Table S.5 On a Food Label, Sugars Include (continued)

- Honey

- Invert sugar

- Lactose

- Maltose

- Molasses

- Raw sugar

- [Table] sugar (sucrose)

- Syrup

A food is likely to be high in sugars if one of the above terms appears first or second in the ingredients list, or if several of them are listed.

High-fructose corn syrup is corn syrup that has been treated with an **enzyme** that converts part of the glucose it contains to fructose. The reason for changing the glucose to fructose lies in the fact that fructose is twice as sweet as glucose. High-fructose corn syrup is therefore sweeter, ounce for ounce, than corn syrup so smaller amounts can be used (this makes it cheaper). It is used to sweeten almost all nondiet soft drinks, and is frequently used in canned juices, fruit drinks, sweetened teas, cookies, jams and jellies, syrups, and sweet pickles. Although table sugar consumption has dropped over the past 15 years, consumption of high-fructose corn syrup has increased almost 250 percent, according to figures from the **U.S. Department of Agriculture**. (See Tables S.6 and S.7.)

Table S.6 To Consume Less Refined Sugar, Try the Following

General

1. Instead of regular soft drinks or powdered drink mixes, choose diet soft drinks, 100 percent pure fruit juices, bottled waters such as seltzer, or iced tea made without added sugar or with artificial sweeteners.

2. Use less refined sugars in coffee, tea, cereals, and so forth, or use sugar substitutes.

Mealtime

3. Choose 100 percent pure fruit juices. They do not contain added sugars. Products labeled as fruit drinks, fruit beverages, or flavored drinks usually contain only small amounts of fruit juice and much refined sugar.

Table S.6 To Consume Less Refined Sugar, Try the Following (continued)

4. Choose unsweetened breakfast cereals. For each four grams listed under "Sucrose and Other Sugars" on a cereal box label, there is one teaspoon of sugar. For less sugar, choose cereals with less than four grams of sugar per serving, unless the sugar comes from a dried fruit such as raisins. Top cereals with fresh fruit.

5. Jams, jellies, and pancake syrup contain much refined sugar. For less refined sugar and calories, select jams, jellies, and fruit spreads made without (or with less) sugar and pancake syrup labeled "reduced calorie". Other toppings for toast or pancakes are chopped fresh fruit, applesauce, or part-skim ricotta cheese and fruit.

6. Many fruited yogurts contain much sugar. For less sugar, mix fresh fruit or canned fruit (packed in its own juice) into plain yogurt.

Snacks

7. Enjoy a fresh apple or banana instead of a candy bar if you want something sweet.

8. Buy a cookie that uses less refined sugar, such as graham crackers, vanilla wafers, ginger snaps, and fig bars.

9. Instead of sweetened breakfast pastries such as danish, try a bagel, English muffin, roll, or fruited muffin.

Desserts and Baking

10. Instead of sweet desserts such as cake, emphasize fruits in desserts. Fresh fruit can be baked (as in baked apples), poached (as in poached pears), broiled, or made into compote. Try baked pears or baked apples with a sprinkle of cinnamon, or broiled peach or grapefruit half with a sprinkle of nutmeg.

11. Select unsweetened frozen fruits or canned fruits packed in juice rather than fruits packed in light or heavy syrup. One-half cup of fruit canned in heavy syrup contains approximately 4 teaspoons of sugar.

12. Select gelatin and pudding mixes without sugar.

13. Make desserts at home so you can better control the amount of sugar you use. When baking from scratch, you can decrease the sugar in many of your recipes by about one-fourth to one-third of the original amount without any significant difference in quality.

Table S.6 To Consume Less Refined Sugar, Try the Following
(continued)

14. Add a small amount of vanilla, cinnamon, or nutmeg to sweet baked products to enhance flavor when you reduce sugars.

15. Select baking recipes that use fruit to sweeten.

16. Use a fruit sauce or a sprinkling of powdered sugar in place of frosting on cake.

Table S.7 Sugar Content of Foods

Food/Portion	Teaspoons of Sugar
DAIRY	
Skim milk, 1 cup	3
Swiss cheese, 1 ounce	Less than 1
Vanilla ice cream, 1/2 cup	4
MEAT, POULTRY, & FISH	
Meat, poultry, or fish, 3 ounces	0
EGGS	
Egg, 1	0
GRAINS	
White bread, 1 slice	Less than 1
English muffin, 1	Less than 1
White rice, cooked, 1/2 cup	Less than 1
Cheerios cereal, 1 cup	Less than 1
Honey Nut Cheerios, 1 cup	3
Quaker Oatmeal Squares, 1 cup	2
FRUITS	
Apple, 1 medium	4.5
Banana, 1 medium	7
Orange, 1 medium	3
Raisins, 14 grams	2.5

Table S.7 Sugar Content of Foods (continued)

VEGETABLES

Broccoli, 1/2 cup raw chopped	Less than 1 gram
Mixed vegetables, 1/3 cup	Less than 1 gram

BEVERAGES

Cola soft drink, 12 fluid ounces	10

CAKES, COOKIES, CANDIES, & PUDDING

Brownie, 1 average	6
Chocolate graham crackers, 8	2
Chocolate chip cookies, 3	3
Lemon drops, 4 pieces	2.5
M & Ms candy, 70 pieces	7
Vanilla pudding, 1/2 cup	6

SWEETENERS

White sugar, 1 tablespoon	3
Honey, 1 tablespoon	4
High fructose corn syrup, 1 tablespoon	4

Source: U.S. Department of Agriculture.

Sugar Alcohols Forms of **sugar** that contain an **alcohol** group. They include **sorbitol**, **xylitol**, and **mannitol**.

Sulfur A **mineral**. The body doesn't use sulfur by itself, but uses the nutrients it is found in, such as **protein** and **thiamin**. The protein in your hair, skin, and nails is particularly rich in sulfur. There is no **RDA** for sulfur. Protein foods supply plentiful amounts of sulfur and deficiencies are unknown.

Supervisor One who manages people making products or performing services. Supervisors are managers with **hourly employees** reporting to them. Supervisory management is a unique level because they have to deal with the complaints, requests, and concerns of employees; pressure from top and middle management to get tasks done; and the demands of guests to meet their service needs. Supervisors are the vital link between the employees and **management**. Also called *first-line manager*.

Supplements Pills, liquids, or powders containing nutrients, such as **vitamin** and **mineral** pills.

Survey Research A descriptive **research** design that uses surveys to obtain a statistical profile of a sample of a specific population. Although survey research normally has no **hypothesis**, the researchers may see if certain relationships are present. Results of survey research are only generalizable to the population if the sample is representative. See also **research**.

Sweat Glands Glands in the **skin** that secrete sweat. The sweating process helps to cool the body. Also called **sudoriferous glands**.

Sympathetic Nerves Nerves in the **autonomic nervous system** that activate the body to "fight or flight" largely through the release of **norepinephrine** and **epinephrine**. The sympathetic nerves prepare the body for emergencies by increasing the **heart** rate, increasing the **blood glucose level**, inhibiting movement in the **gastrointestinal tract**, and dilating the pupil of the eye. Nerves in the autonomic nervous system innervate **organs** whose functions are not usually under voluntary control. The effects of the sympathetic nerves are often opposite to the effects of the **parasympathetic nerves**. See also **autonomic nervous system, parasympathetic nerves, norepinephrine**, and **epinephrine**.

Synapse The space or connection between a **neuron** and a second cell in which a nervous impulse is transmitted. In the **central nervous system**, the second cell will be a another neuron or a cell in a **muscle** or **gland**. See also **neuron**.

Synovial Fluid A viscous fluid found in synovial cavities of synovial (freely movable) **joints**.

Systems Management The application of systems theory to management of organizations.

Systemic Circulation The flow of **blood** from the **heart** to the body cells and then from the body cells to the heart.

Systole A phase of the heartbeat in which the **heart muscle** contracts. Systole occurs when the right and left ventricles contract, pumping **blood** into the pulmonary **artery** and the **aorta**. The tricuspid and **mitral valves** stay closed during systole to prevent any blood from going back into the **atria**. See also **diastole**.

Systolic Pressure The top number in the **blood pressure** fraction that represents the pressure of blood within **arteries** when the **heart** is pumping. The bottom number is the **diastolic pressure**. See also **diastolic pressure**.

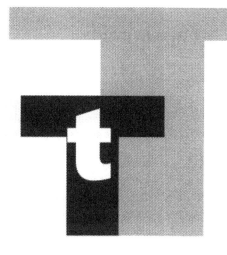

Tachycardia A faster than normal **heart** rhythm (over 100 beats per minute).

Tactile Sense of touching.

Task In **job analysis**, a procedural step in a unit of work. See also **job analysis**.

Taste Buds Clusters of cells found on the tongue, cheeks, throat, and the roof of the mouth. Each taste bud houses 60 to 100 receptor cells. The body regenerates taste buds about every three days. These cells bind food molecules dissolved in saliva, and alert the brain to interpret them.

T Lymphocyte A type of **lymphocyte** (**white blood cell**) involved in the **immune system**. T cells do not secrete **antibodies** but must get close to cells to destroy them. T cells mostly attack cells infected with viruses or fungi, cancerous cells, or transplanted cells. **Killer**, or *cytotoxic*, **T lymphocytes** destroy specific cells that are identified by the **antigens** on their surfaces. Other T cells secrete a number of **polypeptides** to contribute to cell-mediated immunity. These polypeptides are called **lymphokines** such as **interferons** and **interleukins**. Interferons are antiviral **proteins**. Interleukins stimulate the growth of T cells and activate **immune responses**. Lymphokines promote the action of lymphocytes and **macrophages**. Two other types of T lymphocytes, helper T lymphocytes and suppressor T lymphocytes, act to regulate the activities of the **B cells** and killer T cells. See also **immune system**.

Technical Skill The ability to perform the tasks of the people supervised.

Team Nutrition A project of the **U.S. Department of Agriculture** to implement the School Meals Initiative for Healthy Children which requires that school meals reflect the **Dietary Guidelines for Americans**. Team Nutrition is a network of public and private partnerships across the U.S. with the United States Department of Agriculture. USDA's Team Nutrition is designed to help make implementation of the new policy easier and more successful. Team Nutrition will:

- Provide training and technical assistance to schools to ensure that school nutrition and foodservice personnel have the education, motivation, training, and skills necessary to provide healthy meals that appeal to children.

- Promote food choices for a healthy diet to children by actively involving them in making those food choices, reaching them where they learn, live, eat, and play. Through Team Nutrition, research-based messages have been developed reflecting the Dietary Guidelines for Americans and the **Food Guide Pyramid** and will help children to expand the variety of foods in their diet, construct a diet lower in **fat**, and add more fruits, vegetables, and grains to the foods they already eat.

- Provide Team Nutrition In-School curricula for pre-K to 12th grades. This is a comprehensive activity-based program designed to build skills and motivate children to make food choices for a healthful diet.

- Provide new **School Lunch and Breakfast** recipes that meet the Dietary Guidelines for Americans (see Table T.1).

Table T.1   USDA'S Team Nutrition

Mission

To improve the health and education of children by creating innovative public and private partnerships that promote food choices for a healthful diet through the media, schools, families, and the community.

Principles

Supporters of Team Nutrition share these common values:

1. We believe that children should be empowered to make food choices that reflect the Dietary Guidelines for Americans.

2. We believe that good nutrition and physical activity are essential to children's health and educational success.

3. We believe that school meals that meet the Dietary Guidelines for Americans should appeal to children and taste good.

4. We believe our programs must build upon the best science, education, communication, and technical resources available.

5. We believe that public/private partnerships are essential to reaching children to promote food choices for a healthful diet.

Table T.1 USDA'S Team Nutrition (continued)

6. We believe that messages to children should be age appropriate and delivered in a language they speak, through media they use, in ways that are entertaining and actively involve them in learning.

7. We believe in focusing on positive messages regarding food choices children can make.

8. We believe it is critical to stimulate and support action and education at the national, state, and local levels to successfully change children's eating behaviors.

Tertiary Structure The folding of the **protein** chain.

Tetrahydrofolic Acid The reduced form of **folate**.

Thalamus A relay center in the brain for all sensory impulses (except smell). Incoming sensory messages are relayed by the thalamus to appropriate centers in the cerebrum.

Thalassemia A type of inherited anemia in which deficient amounts of **hemoglobin** are made.

Thermic Effect of Food The energy you need to digest and absorb food. The thermic effect of food is the smallest contributor to your energy needs: from 5 to 10 percent of your total energy needs. In other words, for every hundred **calories** you eat, about 5 to 10 calories are used for **digestion**, absorption, and **metabolism** of nutrients.

NUTRIENT FOCUS: THIAMIN

A **water-soluble vitamin** that plays a key role as a **coenzyme** in energy **metabolism**. Along with **riboflavin** and **niacin**, thiamin is essential to release energy from **carbohydrates**, **fats**, and **proteins**, and for growth. Thiamin also plays a vital role in the normal functioning of the **nerves** and the **muscles**, since the nerves send messages to the muscles to contract and relax.

Thiamin is widely distributed in foods but mostly in moderate amounts. Pork is an excellent source of thiamin. Good sources include liver, dry beans, peanuts, peanut butter, seeds, and whole grain and enriched breads and cereals.

Thiamin Pyrophosphate (TPP) A **coenzyme** for the **decarboxylases**. Decarboxylases are a group of **enzymes** that remove a **carboxyl** group from atoms or molecules.

Third-Party Payment Reimbursement of nutrition services by public and private groups such as Medicaid and commercial insurance carriers.

Thrombin See **blood clotting.**

Thrombocyte See **platelet.**

Thrombocytopenia Low number of **blood platelets** or **thrombocytes.**

Thromboplastin See **blood clotting.**

Thymus Gland See **lymph system.**

Thyroid Gland A **gland** found on either side of the trachea that produces and secretes two important **hormones** that regulate the level of **metabolism: thyroxine,** or **tetraiodothyronine,** and **triiodothyronine.** These hormones contain **iodine.**

Thyroid-Stimulating Hormone (TSH) A **hormone** produced and secreted by the anterior **pituitary** in response to messages from the **hypothalamus.** TSH prompts the **thyroid gland** to make and secrete **thyroxine.**

Thyroxine The major **hormone** made in the **thyroid gland** from **iodine** and **tyrosine** (an **amino acid**) that helps maintain a normal level of **metabolism** in the body's cells. Thyroxine works with **triiodothyronine.** Also called **tetraiodothyronine** or **T4.**

Thyroxine-Binding Globulin A **plasma protein** that transports **thyroxine** and **triiodothyronine.**

Tidal Volume The amount of gases that pass in and out of the lung each time we breathe in and breathe out.

Title III-C Part of the Older Americans Act that authorizes congregate and **home-delivered meals** for individuals over 60 years of age.

Tocopherol A type of **alcohol.** In the form of alpha-tocopherol, it is the active form of **vitamin E.** See also **vitamin E.**

Tonsils Masses of lymphatic tissue in the walls of the throat near the mouth. Tonsils help prevent microorganisms from entering the body and they also make **lymphocytes** that fight foreign bodies.

Total Quality Management (TQM) A form of **Continuous Quality Improvement.** See also **Continuous Quality Improvement.**

Trabecular Bone A type of **bone** found mostly in the epiphyses (ends) of **long bones** and in the middle of most other bones. Trabecular bone is not nearly as hard as **cortical bone.** Also called **spongy** or **cancellous bone.**

Trace Minerals **Minerals** needed in smaller amounts than **major minerals** —less than 100 milligrams daily. The trace minerals include **chromium, cobalt, copper,** fluoride, **iodine, iron, manganese, molybdenum, selenium,** and **zinc.**

Tracheostomy A procedure in which a tube is inserted into the trachea to permit breathing.

Tracheotomy A procedure to surgically open the trachea.

Trademark Terms that identify the products and services of a business and distinguish them from other products and services of other businesses. Trademarks must be obtained from the government patent office to assure a business' exclusive use of the trademark. A trademark can be a word, symbol, logo, and/or design.

Training To instruct and guide the development of a trainee toward acquiring knowledge, behavior (skills), and attitudes to meet a specific need. Much training centers around **orientation**, job skills, and attitude development for new and current managers, **supervisors**, and **hourly employees.**

Transaminase A group of **enzymes** dependent on **vitamin B6** that catalyze **transamination** reactions. See also **transamination.**

Transamination In **protein metabolism,** a reaction in which the amino group is transferred from an **amino acid** to an alpha-**keto acid**, resulting in the formation of a new keto acid and a new amino acid. The new keto acids will be metabolized to smaller molecules. Removing the amino groups via transamination is the first step in the **catabolism** of amino acids.

Transcription A process that makes a molecule of messenger **RNA** in the nucleus using **DNA** as a template. Transcription is the first step in making new **proteins.** Messenger RNA then travels to the ribosomes where the information on the messenger RNA is translated to make a new protein.

Trans-Fatty Acids Unsaturated fatty acids that, when **hydrogenated** as in making **margarines** and shortenings, lose a natural bend or kink so they are now straight (like **saturated fatty acids**). Trans-fatty acids may have adverse effects on **blood cholesterol** levels and be causally related to the risk of **coronary heart disease.**

Transferrin A **globulin protein** made in the **liver** that transports **iron** in the body. **Serum** transferrin levels are considered a more sensitive indicator of protein deficiency than **albumin** because transferrin levels change quicker in response to changes in **nutrition** status. Levels lower than 170 milligrams/100 milliliters is indicative of undernutrition.

Transformational Leadership See **leadership**.

Transient Ischemic Attack (TIA) A mini-**stroke** in which **blood** supply to the cerebrum is interrupted. See also **cerebrovascular accident**.

Transitional Milk The type of milk produced by the mother at about the third to sixth day after birth that lasts until the tenth day when mature milk appears.

Translation The process by which **proteins** are made that uses information stored in messenger **RNA** as the code or instructions.

Triacylglercols See **triglycerides**.

Tricarboxylic Acid (TCA) Cycle A series of reactions that metabolize **acetyl-coA** to **carbon dioxide, water**, and energy, in the mitochondria of the cell. The TCA cycle yields energy in various forms: **NADH, FADH2**, and **GTP**. The reduced **enzymes** are oxidized back to **NAD+** and **FAD** by the electron transport chain. Also called the *Krebs cycle* or **citric acid cycle** (see Figure T.1).

Figure T.1 Tricarboxylic Acid Cycle

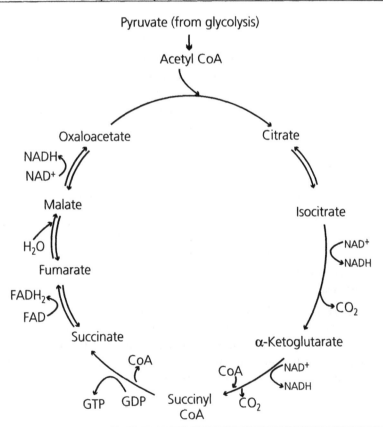

Triceps Skin Fold (TSF) See **anthropometrics**.

Triglyceride The major form of **lipid** in food and in the body. Triglycerides are made of three **fatty acids** attached to a **glycerol** backbone. See **fat**. (See Figure T.2.)

Figure T.2 Triglyceride

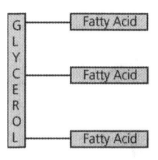

Triiodothyronine (T3) A **hormone** made in the **thyroid gland** from **iodine** and **tyrosine** (an **amino acid**) that helps maintain a normal level of **metabolism** in the body's cells. T3 works with thyroxine or T4.

Tripeptide A **peptide** with three **amino acids**.

Trypsin A **protein**-splitting **enzyme** produced in the intestine when *enterokinase*, a **brush border enzyme**, acts on trypsinogen which is in the pancreatic juice. Trypsin then goes on to activate chymotrypsinogen to **chymotrypsin**, proelastate to elastase, and procarboxypeptidase to **carboxypeptidase**.

Tryptophan An amino acid that can be converted to make the vitamin **niacin**.

Tube Feeding **Enteral feeding** given through a tube that goes from the patient's nose directly into the **stomach** or intestines. A tube feeding may be used in instances where the patient's oral intake is insufficient. Tube feedings are given through a pliable tube that is inserted through the nose in a nonsurgical procedure. If the tube is passed to the stomach, it is referred to as a *nasogastric* (NG) *tube*. If the tube is passed to the intestine, it may be either a *nasoduodenal* (ND) *tube* in which case the tube ends at the *duodenum*, or a *nasojejunal* (NJ) *tube* in which the tube ends at the **jejunum**. Feeding tubes can also be inserted, when necessary, through surgically created openings in the **esophagus** (esophagostomy), stomach (gastrostomy), or jejunum (jejunostomy). These types of tube feedings may be necessary for patients to be fed enterally for longer periods of time, such as three to six months (see Figure T.3).

Figure T.3 Tube Feeding Sites

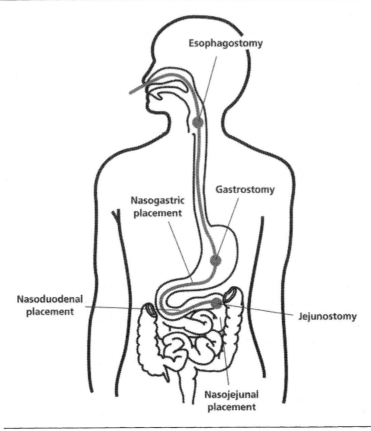

Esophagostomy

Gastrostomy

Nasogastric
placement

Nasoduodenal
placement

Jejunostomy

Nasojejunal
placement

Tunica Externa The outermost layer of the arterial or venous wall.

Tunica Intima A layer of endothelium on the inside of **arteries** and **veins**.

Tunica Media The middle muscular layer of the arterial or venous wall.

Turbid Cloudy. If **urine** is cloudy, it may be due to **white blood cells**. See
pyuria.

Type I Error In **research**, the probability of rejecting the null hypothesis when
the null **hypothesis** is true.

Type II Error In **research**, the probability of not rejecting the null **hypothesis**
when it is false.

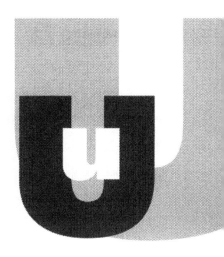

Ulcer An open sore or wound of **skin** or mucous membrane caused by an inflammatory, infectious, or **malignant** process. Examples of ulcers include **peptic ulcer** and **decubitus ulcer**.

NUTRITION AND DISEASE FOCUS: ULCERATIVE COLITIS

A form of **inflammatory bowel disease** characterized by abnormal, inflamed mucosa (involving the mucosa and submocosal tissue layers) of the **colon** and often the **rectum**. The mucosa becomes so fragile that it bleeds easily. Symptoms include persistent **diarrhea** (often bloody), abdominal pain, and poor appetite. Patients receive medications to reduce the inflammation. The nutritional care often includes a diet high in **protein** (due to protein losses from the mucosal lesions and poor intake) and energy (due to weight loss commonly seen). **Fiber** is generally limited during times when healing is taking place. Extra **vitamins** and **minerals** need to be supplied in foods and/or supplemental form. Enteral and parenteral **nutrition** may be needed in some cases.

Ultrasonography A diagnostic, imaging technique that uses reflected ultrasonic waves to delineate, measure, and examine internal body structures or **organs**. This procedure is noninvasive and thought to be safe at this time.

Ultrasound See **ultrasonography**.

Union An organization employees have designated to deal with their employer concerning conditions of employment such as wages, benefits, and hours of work.

Union Steward An employee designated by the **union** to represent and advise the employees of their rights, as well as check on contract compliance. Also called *shop steward*.

United States Department of Agriculture (USDA) A federal agency that is responsible for standards for the quality and wholesomeness of meat, poultry, and egg. The USDA also conducts **nutrition research**, oversees food assistance programs, and educates the public about **nutrition** (see Table U.1).

Table U.1 Food Assistance Programs from the USDA

School Lunch and Breakfast Programs	Offers free and reduced-price meals at school to children from low-income families.
Special Milk Program	Provides milk in schools that are not in School Lunch program.
Summer Food Service Program	Offers meals and snacks to children in needy areas during the summer.
Special Supplemental Food Program for Women, Infants,and Children (WIC)	Provides nutritious foods and baby formula for children under 5, and pregnant and lactating mothers.
Food Stamp Program	Provides food stamps for nutritious foods for low-income households.
Child Care Food Program	Provides cash and commodities for children to age 12 in nonprofit, licensed, or approved day-care programs and outside school hours care centers.

See also **Extension Service, School Lunch and Breakfast Program** and **Special Supplemental Food Program for Women, Infants, and Children.**

Unity of Command The organizational principle that each person should have only one boss.

Unsaturated Fat **Triglycerides** containing mostly unsaturated fatty acids. **Monounsaturated** fatty acids and **polyunsaturated fat** are two kinds of unsaturated fatty acids. Monounsaturated and polyunsaturated fatty acid lower LDL (the bad cholesterol) levels.

Unsaturated Fatty Acids **Fatty acids** with one or more carbon-carbon double bonds. If the fatty acid has one carbon-carbon double bond, it is a **monounsaturated fatty acid.** If the fatty acid has two or more double bonds, it is a **polyunsaturated fatty acid.**

Upper GI Series When barium sulfate is swallowed and x-rays are taken of the **esophagus, stomach,** and **small intestine.** Barium sulfate provides a contrast medium so the x-ray gives a good picture of these **organs.**

Uracil A pyrimidine **base** that is a part of nucleic **acids.**

Urea A compound containing the nitrogen waste of the body generated from **amino acid** breakdown. Urea is made in the **liver** and excreted through the urine. Also see **blood urea nitrogen.**

Urea Cycle A cycle that forms **urea** from toxic ammonia in the **liver** which is then excreted via the **kidney.**

Uremia A toxic state in which excessive amounts of **urea** and other nitrogenous waste products occur in the **blood.** Uremia, also called *azotemia*, occurs in renal failure.

Ureter Tubes that carry urine in perstaltic waves from the **kidney** to the **urinary bladder.**

Urethra The tube through which urine leaves the **urinary bladder** to be excreted.

Urinalysis The examination of urine to determine if disease exists. Urine is examined physically for color, cloudiness, specific gravity, and **pH.** Urine is also examined under a microscope to look for substances that don't belong there such as bacteria and **blood cells.** Chemical tests determine how much **sugar, ketones, protein,** and other substances are in the urine.

Urinary Bladder A muscular sac in the pelvic cavity that holds urine until urination occurs.

Urinary Calculus A stone in the urinary tract. Urinary calculi may cause problems, such as if they block the flow of urine, or may simply be passed with the urine if small enough.

Urinary Incontinence Loss of control over passing urine.

Urinary Retention Urine remains in the **bladder** due to blockage or temporary loss of **muscle** function.

Uterus In women, a pear-shaped **organ** with muscular walls and a mucous membrane lining in which the **fetus** grows. The lower part of the uterus is the **cervix** and the cervical opening leads into a tube called the vagina, which opens to the outside of the body.

Utilization Review An audit of the services and costs billed by health-care providers.

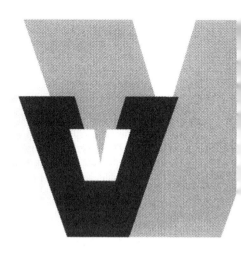

Validity Whether a test or device measures what it is supposed to measure.

Valve A structure in the **heart** or **veins** that tries to keep **blood** flowing in one direction only by opening to allow blood flow and closing to prevent blood from flowing in the other direction. See also **vein** and **heart**.

Varied Diet A diet that includes many different foods.

Vasoconstriction Narrowing of **blood** vessels due to contraction of the **smooth muscles** in their walls. This normally occurs during periods of fear or cold.

Vasodilation Expanding of **blood** vessels, especially **arterioles**. Vasodilator drugs are used to treat certain types of **heart** failure.

Vasopressin See **antidiuretic hormone**.

Vegan Diet A style of **vegetarian eating** in which the individual does not eat eggs or dairy products and therefore relies exclusively on plant foods to meet **protein** and other nutrient needs. Vegans are a small group, and it is estimated that only four percent of vegetarians are vegans. Vegans are also called strict vegetarians. See also **vegetarian eating.**

Vegetable Oils Oils made from various plants. When choosing vegetable oils, choose those high in **monounsaturated fats**, such as olive oil, canola oil, peanut oil, and other nut oils. Olive oil is the best choice because it is 73 to 77 percent monounsaturated fat.

The color of olive oil varies from pale yellow to green and its flavor varies from sweet to a full, fruity taste. The color and the flavor of olive oil depend on the olive variety, level of ripeness, and the way they were processed. When buying olive oil, look for these terms on the label.

1. Extra virgin or virgin olive oil has a strong olive taste that is good for flavoring finished dishes and in salad dressings, but they tend to burn when cooked.

2. Pure olive oil can be used for sautéing and in salad oils. It is not as strong in taste as extra virgin or virgin olive oil.

3. Light or extra-light on an olive oil bottle refers only to color or taste. These olive oils lack the color and much of the flavor found in the other products. Light olive oil is good for sautéing, deep frying, or baking because the oil is used mainly to transfer heat rather than enhance flavor.

Polyunsaturated fats, such as corn oil, safflower oil, sunflower oil, or soybean oil, are also good choices, but not as good as monounsaturated fats. Polyunsaturated fats and monounsaturated fats both lower the levels of **LDL** (the bad **cholesterol**) in the body, but only monounsaturated fat also can increase **HDL** (the good cholesterol) under certain conditions (see Table V.1).

Table V.1 Vegetable Oils

Oil	Characteristics/Uses
Canola oil	Light yellow color Bland flavor Good for frying, sautéing, and in baked goods Good oil for salad dressings
Corn oil	Golden color Mild flavor Good for frying, sautéing, and in baked goods Too heavy for salad dressings
Cottonseed oil	Pale yellow color Bland flavor Good for frying, sautéing, and in baked goods Good oil for salad dressings
Hazelnut oil	Dark amber color Nutty and smoky flavor Not for frying or sautéing as it burns easily Good for flavoring finished dishes and salad dressings Use in small amounts Expensive
Olive oil	Varies from pale yellow with sweet flavor to greenish color and fuller flavor to full, fruity taste (color and flavor depend on olive variety, level of ripeness, and how they were processed)

Table V.1 Vegetable Oils (continued)

Oil	Characteristics/Uses
Olive oil (continued)	Extra virgin or virgin olive oil—don't cook with it because it burns, good for flavoring finished dishes and in salad dressings, strong olive taste
	Pure olive oil—can be used for sautéing and in salad oils, not as strong an olive taste as extra virgin or virgin
Peanut oil	Pale yellow color Mild nutty flavor Good for frying and sautéing Good oil for salad dressings
Safflower oil	Golden color Bland flavor Has a higher concentration of polyunsaturated fatty acids than any other oil Good for frying, sautéing, and in baked goodsl Good oil for salad dressings
Sesame oil	Light gold flavor Distinctive, strong flavor Good for sautéing Good oil for flavoring dishes and in salad dressings Use in small amounts Expensive
Soybean oil	More soybean oil is produced than any other type, used in most blended vegetable oils and margarines Light color Bland flavor Good for frying, sautéing, and in baked goods Good oil for salad dressings
Sunflower oil	Pale golden color Bland flavor Good for frying, sautéing, and in baked goods Good oil for salad dressings

Table V.1 Vegetable Oils (continued)

Oil	Characteristics/Uses
Walnut oil	Medium yellow to brown color Rich, nutty flavor For flavoring finished dishes and in salad dressings Use in small amounts Expensive

Vegetable oil is also available in a convenient spray form that can be used as a nonstick spray coating for cooking and baking pans with a minimal amount of **fat**. Vegetable oil cooking sprays come in a variety of flavors (butter, olive, Oriental, Italian, mesquite) and a quick two-second spray adds about one **gram** of fat to the product. To use these sprays, spray the pan first away from any open flames (the spray is flammable), heat up the pan, then add the food (see Table V.2).

Table V.2 Nutrient Content of Oils and Fats

Product (1 tablespoon)	Cholesterol (mgs)	Saturated Fat (grams)	Polyunsaturated Fat (grams)	Monounsaturated Fat (grams)
Margarine, diet	0	1.0	2.0	2.6
Canola oil	0	1.0	4.3	8.6
Safflower oil	0	1.2	10.6	1.7
Sunflower oil	0	1.5	5.7	6.5
Corn oil	0	1.8	8.4	3.5
Olive oil	0	1.9	1.1	10.4
Margarine, soft, tub	0	1.9	5.0	4.1
Margarine, liquid, bottled	0	1.9	5.3	4.1
Sesame oil	0	2.0	5.9	5.6
Soybean oil	0	2.1	8.3	3.3
Margarine, stick	0	2.2	3.8	5.3
Peanut oil	0	2.4	4.5	6.5
Shortening	0	3.3	3.5	6.0
Cottonseed oil	0	3.7	7.4	2.5

Table V.2 Nutrient Content of Oils and Fats (continued)

Product (1 tablespoon)	Cholesterol (mgs)	Saturated Fat (grams)	Polyunsaturated Fat (grams)	Monounsaturated Fat (grams)
Lard	12	5.2	1.5	6.1
Beef tallow*	14	6.7	0.5	5.5
Butter	28	6.8	0.5	3.3
Palm oil*	0	7.0	1.4	5.2
Cocoa butter*	0	8.5	0.4	4.7
Palm kernel oil*	0	11.7	0.2	1.7
Coconut oil*	0	12.5	0.2	0.8

*These fats and oils are used in commercially prepared goods. They are included in this list for comparison purposes.

Source: Composition of Foods: Fats and Oils—Raw-Processed-Prepared, Agriculture Handbook 8-4, United States Department of Agriculture, (June 1979, revised 1990).

Be prepared to spend more money for the more exotic oils such as almond, hazelnut, sesame, and walnut oils. Because these oils tend to be cold pressed (meaning they are processed without heat), they are not as stable as the all-purpose oils and should be purchased in small quantities (you don't need to use much of them anyway because they are strong). Don't purchase these oils to cook with—they burn easily.

PRACTICAL NUTRITION FOCUS: VEGETARIAN EATING

A style of eating in which the individual does not eat animal flesh, such as meat or poultry, and may also exclude animal products such as milk and eggs. The largest group of vegetarians, **lacto-ovovegetarians**, do consume animal products in the form of eggs (ovo) and milk and milk products (lacto). Another group of vegetarians, **lactovegetarians**, consume milk and milk products but forgo eggs. Most vegetarians are either lacto-ovovegetarians or lactovegetarians. **Vegans**, a third group of vegetarians, do not eat eggs or dairy products and therefore rely exclusively on plant foods to meet **protein** and other nutrient needs. Vegans are a small group, and it is estimated that only four percent of vegetarians are vegans.

Why does someone choose a vegetarian lifestyle? The number one reason people give for being vegetarian is health. Being a vegetarian has health benefits.

Vegetarians tend to be leaner and keep their body weight and **blood lipid** levels closer to desirable levels than nonvegetarians. Vegetarians have lower mortality rates from **coronary heart disease** and tend to be at lower risk for a number of diseases.

1. **Hypertension**

2. Breast cancer

3. **Colon** cancer

4. Noninsulin-dependent **diabetes mellitus**

5. **Osteoporosis**

Other reasons for becoming a vegetarian include the fact that is more ecological and economical and, for some individuals, it meshes with their sense of ethics and religious beliefs.

Vegetarian diets can be nutritionally adequate when varied and adequate in **calories**, except for vegan diets which need supplementation with **vitamin B12**. Nutrients of special interest to vegetarians are vitamin B12, **vitamin D, calcium, iron**, and **zinc**.

The **Food Guide Pyramid** can be modified, as follows, to work for vegetarians.

1. Breads, cereals, rice, and pasta (6–11 servings per day)—This group stays the same. Whole-grain products are recommended. Vitamin B12 fortified breakfast cereals are important for vegans. Some vegans with large calorie needs may eat more than 11 servings.

2. Fruits (2+ servings)—This group also stays the same except that no limit is placed on consumption.

3. Vegetables (3+ servings)—Like fruits, no limit is placed.

4. Meat substitutes (2–3 servings)—This group obviously omits any meats, poultry, or fish and instead concentrates on substitutes such as cooked dry beans, peas, or lentils; tofu and other soybean products; nuts and seeds and butters made from the meat analogs; and eggs for lacto-ovovegetarians. One serving is one-half cup of cooked beans, peas, or lentils; 4 ounces tofu; one-quarter cup shelled nuts; one-eighth cup seeds; 2 tablespoons peanut butter, or 1 egg.

5. Milk, cheese, and yogurt (2 servings for adults, 3 servings for pregnant and lactating women, teenagers, and young adults up to age 24) – This group is enlarged to include soy milk fortified with calcium and vitamin D (and vitamin B12 for vegans), and soy cheese fortified with calcium and vitamin D. One

serving is 1 cup of fortified soy milk or 1 and one-half ounces soy cheese. If a vegan does not drink soy milk or eat soy cheese, a carefully planned diet with sources of the missed nutrients, or supplements, is necessary.

Menu Planning Guidelines

1. Variety is a key word to remember when planning vegetarian menu items. Macaroni and cheese, pizza, and grilled cheese are fine to serve—especially if made with vegetables too—but much more variety (and less **fat** and **saturated fat**) is needed.

2. Use a variety of plant protein sources: legumes, grain products (preferably whole grain), nuts and seeds, and/or vegetables at each meal. Vegetarian entrees commonly use cereal grains such as rice or bulgur wheat (precooked and dried whole wheat) in combination with legumes and/or vegetables. Use small amounts of nuts and seeds in dishes.

3. Use a wide variety of vegetables. Steaming, stir-frying, or microwaving vegetables work well because they retain flavor, nutrients, and color.

4. Try to offer an entree that is acceptable to lactovegetarians and lacto-ovovegetarians and an entree for vegans. Although lactovegetarians and lacto-ovovegetarians will eat vegan entrees, vegans won't eat entrees with any dairy products or eggs.

5. Choose low-fat and nonfat varieties of milk and milk products and limit the use of eggs. This is important to prevent a high intake of saturated fat, found in whole milk, low-fat milk, regular cheeses, eggs, and other foods.

6. Offer some dishes based on products made from soybeans, such as tofu and tempeh. Soybeans are unique because they are nutritionally equivalent to animal protein.

7. Provide foods that contain nutrients of special importance to vegetarians: vitamin B12, vitamin D, calcium, iron, and zinc.

Vein **Blood** vessels that return **oxygen**-poor blood back to the **heart**. The walls of veins do not need to be as thick and muscular as **arteries** because there's little pressure or force left. The thinner muscle layer of veins allows them to expand to accommodate an increasing blood volume as they make their way back to the heart. Unlike arteries, veins have **valves** to help the blood return to the heart. When the veins are squeezed by contracting **skeletal muscles,** it helps return the venous blood from the legs to the heart (this is known as the skeletal muscle pump). Most of the total blood volume is contained in the veins.

Venae Cavae (Singular: vena cava) **Veins** that carry **oxygen**-poor **blood** into the right atrium of the **heart**. There are two venae cavae: the *inferior vena cava* and the *superior vena cava*.

Venous Stasis A stopped or decreased flow of **blood** in the **veins**.

Venule A small **vein**.

Very Low-Calorie Diet (VLCD) Diets with less than 800 **calories**/day to achieve maximum weight loss without losing lean body mass. VLCD normally takes the form of a liquid formula with much high biological value **protein** and fortified with **vitamins, minerals**, and **fatty acids**. Food-based VLCD are available also and are referred to as protein-sparing modified fasts. Patients often stay on VLCD for the first part of treatment which lasts about 12 to 16 weeks. During this time, most patients receive a comprehensive weight control program that includes **nutrition** education, exercise, **behavior modification**, and other aspects. VLCD are normally used for persons at least 30 percent over their ideal body weight. They should not be used for patients with renal disease, **cerebrovascular** disease, or **insulin**-dependent **diabetes**.

Very Low-Density Lipoprotein (VLDL) The **liver's** version of **chylomicrons**. **Triglycerides** and some **cholesterol** are carried through the body by VLDL which release triglycerides, with the help of **lipoprotein lipase**, throughout the body. Once the majority of triglycerides are removed, VLDLs are converted in the **blood** into another type of lipoprotein called **low-density lipoprotein (LDL)**.

Villi Fingerlike projections in the walls of the **small intestine** that increase the surface area across which nutrients can be absorbed.

Visceral Organs The **organs** located in the abdominal and thoracic cavities.

Vision In business, written statements, often called *mission statement* or *credos*, that describe an appealing and realistic goal for the company and its employees. An organization's vision statement should briefly explain:

1. The type of business you are in and why.

2. Your orientation to your guests and employees.

3. Where you are going and what you are working toward.

The vision statement should be a statement of beliefs and intents.

Vitamins Noncaloric, organic nutrients found in foods that are essential in small quantities for growth and good health. Vitamins are similar because they are made of the same elements: carbon, hydrogen, **oxygen**, and sometimes nitrogen or **cobalt**. Vitamins are different in that their elements are arranged differently and each vitamin performs one or more specific functions in the body. Vitamins are classified according to how soluble they are in either **fat** or **water**. The **fat-soluble vitamins** (A, D, E, K) generally occur in foods containing fat, and they can be stored in the body. The **water-soluble vitamins** (vitamin C and the B-complex vitamins) are not stored appreciably in the body (see Table V.3 and V.4).

Table V.3 The Vitamins

Fat-Soluble	Water-Soluble
Vitamin A	Vitamin C
Vitamin D	Thiamin
Vitamin E	Riboflavin
Vitamin K	Niacin
	Vitamin B6
	Folate
	Vitamin B12
	Pantothenic acid
	Biotin

Table V.4 Basics on Vitamins

1. Very small amounts of vitamins are needed by the human body and very small amounts are present in foods. Some vitamins are measured in IUs (international units), a measure of biological activity; others are measured by weight in micrograms or milligrams. To illustrate how small these amounts are, remember that 1 ounce is 28.3 grams. A milligram is 1/100 of a gram, and a microgram is 1/1000 of a milligram.

2. Although vitamins are needed in small quantities, the roles they play in the body are enormously important.

3. Most vitamins are obtained through food. There are some that are also produced by bacteria in the intestine (and are absorbed into the body) and one (vitamin D) that can be produced via the skin when the skin is exposed to sunlight.

4. There is no perfect food that contains all the vitamins in just the right amounts. The best way to assure an adequate intake of vitamins is by eating a varied and balanced diet.

Table V.4 Basics on Vitamins (continued)

5. Vitamins do not have any calories so they do not directly provide energy to the body. Vitamins do indirectly provide energy because they are involved in energy metabolism.

6. Some vitamins in foods are not the actual vitamin, but rather are precursors. In the body, the precursor is chemically changed to the active form of the vitamin.

7. A megadose of a vitamin is defined as more than 10 times one's RDA. It often has toxic effects. Vitamin D can be toxic when taken at only 5 to 10 times the RDA.

NUTRIENT FOCUS: VITAMIN A

A **fat-soluble vitamin** found in foods in two forms: preformed vitamin A or **retinol** (also called *retinoids*) and provitamin A (also called **carotenoids**). The carotenoids, such as **beta carotene**, are precursors of vitamin A and are converted to retinol in the body. Two other active forms of vitamin A, retinal and retinoic acid, are made by the cells from retinol.

Sources of preformed vitamin A include animal products such as liver (a very rich source), vitamin A fortified milk, fortified butter and **margarine**, and fortified cereals. Low-fat and skim milks are often fortified with vitamin A because the vitamin is removed from the milk when the fat is removed. Most ready-to-eat and instant-prepared cereals are also fortified with vitamin A.

Sources of provitamin A and beta carotene are dark green vegetables, such as spinach, and deep orange fruits and vegetables, such as apricots, carrots, and sweet potatoes. To get enough vitamin A, it is recommended that you eat a dark green or deep orange fruit or vegetable at least every other day. Because the body stores vitamin A in the **liver**, it is not absolutely necessary to eat a good source every day.

Vitamin A has many functions.

- Night vision

- Healthy cornea of eye

- Cell growth and development

- Healthy **skin** and hair

- Bone and tooth development

- Maintenance of protective linings

- **Immune system**

- Normal reproduction

Prolonged use of high doses of vitamin A (usually about 10 times one's **RDA**) may cause hair loss, bone pain and damage, soreness, liver damage, nausea, and **diarrhea**. Megadoses are particularly dangerous for pregnant women (it may cause birth defects) and children (it can stunt growth). Only preformed vitamin A, not carotenoids such as beta carotene, has such effects.

NUTRIENT FOCUS: VITAMIN B6

A **water-soluble vitamin** with an important role as part of a **coenzyme** involved in **carbohydrate, fat**, and **protein metabolism**. It is particularly important in protein metabolism, specifically in making and breaking down **amino acids**. It is also used to make **red blood cells** (which transport **oxygen** around the body).

Good sources for vitamin B6 include organ meats, meat, poultry, and fish. Vitamin B6 also appears in plant foods; however, it is not as well absorbed from these sources. Good plant sources include whole grains (refined grains are not enriched with this vitamin), potatoes, some fruits (such as bananas and cantaloupe), and some leafy green vegetables (such as broccoli and spinach). Fortified ready-to-eat cereals are also good sources of vitamin B6.

Deficiency of vitamin B6 causes **muscle** twitching, a type of **anemia**, and rashes. Excessive use of vitamin B6 (more than two **grams** daily for over two months or more) can cause irreversible **nerve** damage and symptoms such as numbness in hands and feet and difficulty walking. Doses as low as 50 milligrams may even be toxic.

NUTRIENT FOCUS: VITAMIN B12

A **water-soluble vitamin** that functions to convert **folate** into its active forms so that it can make **deoxyribonucleic acid (DNA)**, the genetic code. It also helps in the normal functioning of the **nervous system** by maintaining the protective cover around **nerve** fibers. Vitamin B12 contains **cobalt** and is present in all the cells of the body.

Vitamin B12 is different from other vitamins in that it is only found in animal foods such as meat, poultry, fish, shellfish, eggs, milk, and milk products. Plant foods do not contain any vitamin B12. Vegetarians who do not eat any animal products will need to include vitamin B12-fortified soy milk in their diet or supplements.

Vitamin B12 is also different from other vitamins in that it requires a compound called R-protein (produced in most body fluids) and a compound called **intrinsic factor** (produced in the **stomach**) to be absorbed. Vitamin B12 attaches to the R-protein in the stomach and is then released in the **small intestine** where it complexes with the intrinsic factor. Vitamin B12 is then carried to the **ileum** (the last segment of the small intestine) where it is absorbed. Vitamin B12 is stored in the **liver**.

NUTRIENT FOCUS: Vitamin C

A **water-soluble vitamin** with many vital functions.

- **Antioxidant** (a compound that protects other compounds in the body from being oxidized or destroyed)

- Formation of **collagen** (a **protein** substance that gives strength and support to **bones**, teeth, **skin**, cartilage, and **blood** vessels)

- Wound healing

- **Iron** absorption

- Functioning of the **immune system**

- Making certain **hormones** and **neurotransmitters** (chemical substances released by nerve cells that stimulate or inhibit other cells)

Foods rich in vitamin C include citrus fruits (oranges, grapefruits, limes, and lemons) and tomatoes. Good sources include white potatoes, sweet potatoes, broccoli, and other green and yellow vegetables, as well as cantaloupe and strawberries. Only foods from the fruit and vegetable groups contribute vitamin C. There is little or no vitamin C in the meat group (except in liver, of course) or the dairy group. Some juices are fortified with vitamin C (if not already rich in vitamin C), as are most ready-to-eat cereals. Many people meet their daily **RDA** for vitamin C by simply drinking one-half cup (four fluid ounces) of orange juice. This is a good choice because vitamin C is easily destroyed in food preparation and cooking (see Table V.5).

Also called **ascorbic acid**.

Table V.5 Vitamin C in Foods

Food	Milligrams Vitamin C
Fruits	
Orange, 1	80

Table V.5 Vitamin C in Foods (continued)

Food	Milligrams Vitamin C
Kiwi, 1 medium	75
Cranberry juice cocktail, 6 ounces	67
Orange juice, from concentrate, 1/2 cup	48
Papaya, 1/2 cup cubes	43
Strawberries, 1/2 cup	42
Grapefruit, 1/2	41
Grapefruit juice, canned, 1/2 cup	36
Cantaloupe, 1/2 cup cubes	34
Tangerine, 1	26
Mango, 1/2 cup, slices	23
Honeydew melon, 1/2 cup cubes	21
Banana, 1	10
Apple, 1	8
Nectarine, 1	7
Vegetables	
Broccoli, chopped, cooked, 1/2 cup	49
Brussels sprouts, cooked, 1/2 cup	48
Cauliflower, cooked, 1/2 cup	34
Sweet potato, baked, 1	28
Kale, cooked, chopped, 1/2 cup	27
White potato, baked, 1	26
Tomato, 1 fresh	22
Tomato juice, 1/2 cup	22
Cereals	
Corn flakes, 1 cup	15

Source: U.S. Department of Agriculture.

NUTRIENT FOCUS: VITAMIN D

A **fat-soluble vitamin** that is a member of a team of nutrients and **hormones** that maintains **blood calcium** levels and makes sure there is enough calcium (and **phosphorus**) present for building **bones** and teeth. Calcium is also used to contract and relax **muscles** and transmit **nerve** impulses, and vitamin D ensures that calcium is available for these functions. Vitamin D increases blood calcium levels in any of three ways: increases calcium absorption in the intestine; decreases the amount of calcium excreted by the **kidney**; and pulls calcium out of the bones.

Vitamin D differs from all the other nutrients in that it can be made in the body. When ultraviolet rays shine on your skin, a **cholesterol**-like compound is converted into a precursor of vitamin D and absorbed into the blood. A light-skinned person needs only about 15 minutes of sun on the face, hands, and arms two to three times per week to make enough vitamin D; a dark-skinned person needs several hours.

The active hormone form of vitamin D is called **calcitriol** or 1,25-dihydroxy vitamin D_3. Calcitriol is produced in the kidney in response to an increase in **parathyroid** hormone caused by low blood calcium levels.

Significant food sources of vitamin D include liver, egg yolks, and fish liver oils. Except for these few foods, only small amounts of vitamin D are found in food. For this reason, milk is normally fortified with vitamin D. If you drink two cups of milk each day, you will get about half the RDA of vitamin D (the rest comes from other foods and sun exposure).

Vitamin D deficiency in children causes **rickets**, a disease in which bones do not grow normally, resulting in bowed legs and knock knees. Vitamin D deficiency in adults causes **osteomalacia**, a disease in which bones of the leg and spine soften and may bend. Rickets is rarely seen but osteomalacia may be seen in elderly individuals with poor milk intake and little exposure to the sun.

Vitamin D, when taken in excess of the RDA, is the most toxic of all the vitamins. All you need is about five times the RDA to start feeling symptoms of nausea, vomiting, **diarrhea**, fatigue, confusion, and thirst. It can lead to calcium deposits in the **heart** and kidneys that can cause severe health problems and even death. Young children and infants are especially susceptible.

NUTRIENT FOCUS: VITAMIN E

A **fat-soluble vitamin** that acts as an **antioxidant** (it prevents other compounds from being oxidized or destroyed) in the body and has a role in **iron metabolism** and development and maintenance of nerve tissues.

Vitamin E is widely distributed in plant foods. Rich sources include **vegetable oils, margarine** and shortening made from vegetable oils, and wheat germ (which contains much oil). In oils, vitamin E acts like an antioxidant and thereby prevents the oil from going **rancid**. Other good sources include whole-grain and fortified breads and cereals, legumes, nuts, seeds, and green leafy vegetables. Except for liver and egg yolk, animal foods are poor sources for vitamin E. Deficiency of vitamin E is rare.

NUTRIENT FOCUS: VITAMIN K

A **fat-soluble vitamin** that has an essential role in the production of several chemicals (such as **prothrombin**) involved in **blood clotting**.

Vitamin K appears in certain foods and is also made in the body. There are billions of bacteria that normally live in your intestines, and some of them make a form of vitamin K for you. It is thought that the amount of vitamin K produced by the bacteria is significant and may meet about half of your needs. (An infant is normally given this **vitamin** after birth to prevent bleeding because the intestine does not yet have the bacteria to produce vitamin K.) Food sources of vitamin K provide the balance needed. Excellent sources of vitamin K include liver and dark green leafy vegetables such as kale, spinach, and cabbage. Other sources include milk and eggs.

Voiding Expelling urine.

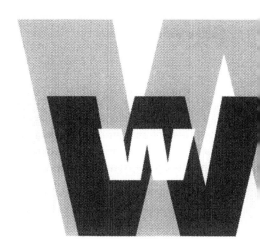

Wages Payment for work performed based on the amount of time worked.

Waist-to-Hip Ratio A ratio calculated by dividing the number of inches around the waistline by the circumference of the hips. For example, someone who has a 27-inch waist and 38-inch hips would have a ratio of 0.71. A woman whose ratio is 0.8 or higher would be at high risk of weight-related health problems (such as **heart disease, hypertension,** and **diabetes**), as would a man whose ratio is 0.95 or above.

Numerous studies show that **fat** in the hips and thighs is less health-threatening than abdominal fat. Whereas other fat cells empty directly into general circulation, the **fatty acid** contents of abdominal fat cells go straight to the **liver** before being circulated to the **muscles**. This process interferes with the liver's ability to clear **insulin** from the bloodstream. Blood levels and **blood glucose levels** rise as a result. In response, the **pancreas** cranks out more insulin, prompting the **autonomic nervous system** (which controls **heart** rate, **blood pressure**, and other vital signs) to produce **norepinephrine**, an **adrenalin**-like chemical that raises blood pressure. This sets the stage for the development of diabetes, hypertension, and heart problems.

NUTRIENT FOCUS: WATER

The most important nutrient in the body. The average adult's body weight is generally 50 to 60 percent water—enough, if it were bottled, to fill 40 to 50 quarts. Human **blood** is about 92 percent water, **muscle** and the brain about 75 percent, and **bone** 22 percent.

The body uses water for virtually all its functions: for **digestion**, absorption, circulation, excretion, transporting nutrients, building tissue, and maintaining temperature. Almost all of the body's cells need and depend on water to perform their functions. Water carries nutrients to the cells and carries away waste materials to the **kidney**.

Water is needed in each step of the process of converting food into energy and tissue. Water in the digestive secretions softens, dilutes, and liquefies the food to facilitate digestion. It also helps move food along the **gastrointestinal tract**. Differences in the fluid concentration on either side of the intestinal wall enhance the absorption process.

Water serves as an important part of lubricants, helping to cushion the **joints** and internal **organs**, keeping body tissues such as the eyes, lungs, and air passages moist, and surrounding and protecting the **fetus** during pregnancy.

Many adults take in and excrete between 8 and 10 cups of fluid daily. Besides drinking fluid, nearly all foods have some water.

A number of mechanisms, including the sensation of thirst, operate to keep body water content within narrow limits. You feel thirsty when the blood starts to become too concentrated.

Water Balance The process of maintaining the proper amount of water in each of the body's three compartments: inside the cells, outside the cells, and in the **blood** vessels. **Electrolytes** maintain water balance by moving the water around in the body. Electrolytes also have the ability to **buffer**, or neutralize, various **acids** and **bases** in the body.

Water-Insoluble Fiber A classification of **fiber** that includes **cellulose**, lignin, and some hemicelluloses. They generally form the structural parts of plants. See also **fiber**.

Water Intoxication The rare condition in which the body has too much **water**. It can cause weakness, inability to concentrate, and **anorexia**.

Water-Soluble Fiber A classification of **fiber** that includes gums, mucilages, pectin, and some hemicelluloses. They are generally found around and inside plant cells. See also **fiber**.

Water-Soluble Vitamins The **vitamins** that are soluble in **water** and are not stored appreciably in the body: **vitamin C, thiamin, riboflavin, niacin, vitamin B6, folate, vitamin B12, pantothenic acid**, and **biotin**.

Weight Cycling A cycle in which an individual loses weight then gains it back, loses it again, and so on.

Weight Management The process of trying to lose weight or maintain weight loss. **Obesity** is a disease that is very resistant to treatment. Although most commercial weight loss programs, such as Weight Watchers™, do not keep records on client success rates, it is estimated that people who complete these diet plans will regain one-third of their lost weight after one year, two-thirds or more after three years, and most, if not all, in three to five years.

A comprehensive approach to treating obesity tends to focus on the whole person, rather than just the extra weight that needs to be shed. Treatment success is measured not only by the number of lost pounds, but also by other factors such as improved self-concept. Components of this approach typically include **nutrition education**, exercise, **behavior modification**, attitude modification, social support, and maintenance support. Each of these components is discussed in this section, but there is a newer approach to treating obesity.

More and more health professionals are adopting a nondieting approach to obesity. This new approach to treating obesity steers clear of dieting and emphasizes helping obese people adopt a healthier lifestyle by eating fewer **fat calories** and getting regular exercise. In many cases diets simply don't work. By restricting food intake, diets often cause dieters to become obsessed with food, which may then lead to binge eating (see Table W.1).

Table W.1 To Reduce Caloric Intake

- Eat a variety of foods that are low in calories and high in nutrients—read the Nutrition Facts label.

- Eat less fat and fewer high-fat foods.

- Eat smaller portions and limit second helpings of foods high in fat and calories.

- Eat more vegetables and fruits without fats and sugars added in preparation or at the table.

- Eat pasta, rice, breads, and cereals without fats and sugars added in preparation or at the table.

- Eat less sugars and fewer sweets (like candy, cookies, cakes, soda).

- Drink less or no alcohol.

White Blood Cell Count The number of **white blood cells** per cubic millimeter.

White Blood Cell Differential A **laboratory test** that counts the different types of **white blood cells** and gives a percentage of **basophils, eosinophils, neutrophils, monocytes**, and **lymphocytes**.

White Blood Cells See **leukocytes**.

WIC See **Special Supplemental Food Program for Women, Infants, and Children**.

Work Simplification The process of making a **job** easier using industrial engineering methods to increase efficiency.

Working Supervisor A **supervisor** who takes part in the work in addition to supervising.

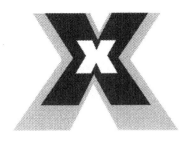

Xanthoma A nodule of yellow **lipid** in the skin that may appear due to problems with lipid **metabolism**.

X Chromosome The chromosome that determines if a fetus is female. Females carry two X chromosomes, and males carry one X and one Y chromosome.

Xerophthalmia Hardening and thickening of the cornea that can lead to blindness. A deficiency of **vitamin A** usually causes this medical problem.

Xerosis A condition in which the cornea of the eye becomes dry and cloudy. A lack of **vitamin A** often causes this condition. Xerosis also refers to dryness of other parts of the body such as the **skin**.

Xerostomia Dryness of the mouth which may interfere with normal chewing and swallowing. In xerostomia, less saliva is secreted.

Xylitol A **sugar alcohol**.

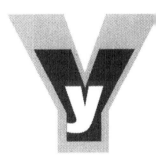

Y Chromosome One of a pair of sex chromosomes present in fetuses that are male. Males have one X and one Y chromosome.

Yeast A fungus that is capable of fermenting **carbohydrates**. Yeast is used in bread-making because as the fungus ferments carbohydrates, it produces carbon dioxide gas which makes the bread rise.

Yellow Bone Marrow A specialized fatty storage tissue found within bone cavities.

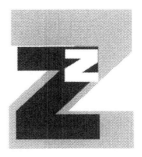

NUTRIENT FOCUS: ZINC

A **trace mineral** involved in **enzymes** that catalyze at least 50 different metabolically important reactions in the body. Zinc assists in wound healing, **bone** formation, development of sexual organs, and general growth and maintenance of all tissues. Zinc is also important for taste perception and appetite.

Protein-containing foods are all good sources of zinc, particularly meat, poultry, and shellfish. Only about 40 percent of the zinc that we eat is absorbed into the body. Whole grains and some legumes are good sources as well but zinc is much more readily available, or absorbed better, from animal foods. **Iron** and zinc are often found in the same foods. Like iron, zinc is more likely to be absorbed when animal sources are eaten and when the body needs more zinc.

Deficiencies may show up in pregnant women, the young, and the elderly. Signs of severe deficiency include growth retardation, delayed sexual maturation, decreased sense of taste, poor appetite, delayed wound healing, and immune deficiencies. Marginal deficiencies do occur in the U.S. When overdoses of zinc (only a few milligrams above the **RDA**) are taken, it causes a **copper** deficiency and less iron is absorbed. Since supplements of zinc can be fatal at lower levels than many of the other trace minerals, it is recommended to avoid zinc supplements unless a physician prescribes them.

Zollinger-Ellison Syndrome A rare condition characterized by severe **ulcers** of the **esophagus**, **stomach**, or **duodenum** in which much larger than normal amounts of gastric juice are released.

Zwitterion A dipolar ionic form of an **amino acid** that is formed when a **hydrogen** ion from the **carboxyl group** goes to the **amino group**. The net charge of a zwitterion is neutral because the positive and the negative cancel each other out.

Zygote The fertilized **ovum** (egg).

Zymogens Inactive **enzymes** that become active when part of their structure is removed by another enzyme or by some other means.

Appendix I

Where to Get Nutrition Information

American Cancer Society
1599 Clifton Road, N.E.
Atlanta. Georgia 30329
(800) ACS-2345 - (800) 227-2345

American Dietetic Association
National Center for Nutrition and
Dietetics
216 W. Jackson Boulevard
Suite 800
Chicago, Illinois 60606-6995
(800) 745-0775 ex. 5000
(800) 366-1655 Consumer Nutrition Hot
Line

American Heart Association
7272 Greenville Avenue
Dallas. Texas 75231-4596
(800) AHA-USA1 - (800) 242-8721

Consumer Information Center
Pueblo, Colorado
(719) 948-4000 (call for catalog)

Food and Nutrition Information Center
National Agricultural Library
U.S. Department of Agriculture
10301 Baltimore Boulevard
Room 304
Beltsville, Maryland 20705
(301) 504-5719

International Food Information Council
1100 Connecticut Avenue, N.W.
Suite 430
Washington D.C. 20036
(202) 296-6540

National Cancer Institute
Office of Cancer Communications
Building 31
Room 1OA16
31 Center Drive
MSC 2580
Bethesda, Maryland 20892-2580
(800) 4-CANCER - (800) 422-6237

National Heart, Lung and Blood Institute
Information Center
P.O. Box 30105
Bethesda, Maryland 20824-0105
(800) 575-9355
(301) 251-1222
FAX: (301) 251-1223

On the local and state level, educational materials and/or curricula might be available from:

- Affiliates of voluntary health promotion organizations (e.g., American Cancer Society, American Heart Association)

- County Cooperative Extension Services

- Local and State health departments

- School districts

- State education agencies

- Universities

Table I.1 Where to Get Nutrition Information: World Wide Web Sites

Internet address	Company/Organization
http://www.bendnet.com/donet	Dietetics Online
http://schoolmeals.nalusda.gov:8001/team.html	USDA School Meals Initiative for Healthy Children
http://www.naluada.gov/fnic.html	USDA Natl. Agricultural Library Food & Nutrition Information Center (FNIC)
http://www.gsa.gov/staff/pa/cic/cic.htm	U.S. Consumer Information Center
http://vm.cfsan.fda.gov/index.html	Food and Drug Administration Center for Food Safety & Applied Nutrition
http://ificinfo.health.org/home-page.htm	International Food Information Council (IFIC)
http://www.primenet.com/~ncahf/	National Council Against Health Fraud (NCAHF)
http://www.restaurant.org	Natl. Restaurant Association
http://www.dole5aday.com	Dole Food Company
http://www.vnr.com	Van Nostrand Reinhold, Publishers

Appendix II

The Recommended Dietary Allowances

See Tables II.1—II.4 for more information.

Table II.1 *Food and Nutrition Board, National Academy of Sciences— National Research Council Recommended Dietary Allowances,[a] Revised 1989*
Designed for the maintenance of good nutrition of practically all healthy people in the United States.

Category	Age (years) or Condition	Weight (kg)	Weight (lb)	Height (cm)	Height (in)	Protein (g)	Fat-Soluble Vitamins			
							Vitamin A (μg RE)[c]	Vitamin D (μg)[d]	Vitamin E (mg a-TE)[e]	Vitamin K (μg)
Infants	0.0–0.5	6	13	60	24	13	375	7.5	3	5
	0.5–1.0	9	20	71	28	14	375	10	4	10
Children	1–3	13	29	90	35	16	400	10	6	15
	4–6	20	44	112	44	24	500	10	7	20
	7–10	28	62	132	52	28	700	10	7	30
Males	11–14	45	99	157	62	45	1,000	10	10	45
	15–18	66	145	176	69	59	1,000	10	10	65
	19–24	72	160	177	70	58	1,000	10	10	70
	25–50	79	174	176	70	63	1,000	5	10	80
	51+	77	170	173	68	63	1,000	5	10	80
Females	11–14	46	101	157	62	46	800	10	8	45
	15–18	55	120	163	64	44	800	10	8	55
	19–24	58	128	164	65	46	800	10	8	60
	25–50	63	138	163	64	50	800	5	8	65
	51+	65	143	160	63	50	800	5	8	65
Pregnant						60	800	10	10	65
Lactating	1st 6 months					65	1,300	10	12	65
	2nd 6 months					62	1,200	10	11	65

Table II.1 *Food and Nutrition Board, National Academy of Sciences— National Research Council Recommended Dietary Allowances,a Revised 1989* (continued)

aThe allowances, expressed as average daily intakes over time, are intended to provide for individual variations among most normal persons as they live in the United States under usual environmental stresses. Diets should be based on a variety of common foods in order to provide other nutrients for which human requirements have been less well defined. See text for detailed discussion of allowances and of nutrients not tabulated.

bWeights and heights of Reference Adults are actual medians for the U.S. population of the designated age as reported by NHANES II. The median weights and heights of those under 19 years of age were taken from Hamill et al. (1979). The use of these figures does not imply that the height-to-weight ratios are ideal.

Table II.2 Minerals

Calcium (mg)	Phosphorus (mg)	Magnesium (mg)	Iron (mg)	Zinc (mg)	Iodine (mg)	Selenium (mg)
400	300	40	6	5	40	10
600	500	60	10	5	50	15
800	800	80	10	10	70	20
800	800	120	10	10	90	20
800	800	170	10	10	120	30
1,200	1,200	270	12	15	150	40
1,200	1,200	400	12	15	150	50
1,200	1,200	350	10	15	150	70
800	800	350	10	15	150	70
800	800	350	10	15	150	70
1,200	1,200	280	15	12	150	45
1,200	1,200	300	15	12	150	50
1,200	1,200	280	15	12	150	55
800	800	280	15	12	150	55
800	800	280	10	12	150	55
1,200	1,200	320	30	15	175	65
1,200	1,200	355	15	19	200	75
1,200	1,200	340	15	16	200	75

Table II.2 Water-Soluble Vitamins (continued)

Vitamin C (mg)	Thiamin (mg)	Riboflavin (mg)	Niacin (mg NE)[f]	Vitamin B6 (mg)	Folate (mg)	Vitamin B12 mg)
30	0.3	0.4	5	0.3	25	0.3
35	0.4	0.5	6	0.6	35	0.5
40	0.7	0.8	9	1.0	50	0.7
45	0.9	1.1	12	1.1	75	1.0
45	1.0	1.2	13	1.4	100	1.4
50	1.3	1.5	17	1.7	150	2.0
60	1.5	1.8	20	2.0	200	2.0
60	1.5	1.7	19	2.0	200	2.0
60	1.5	1.7	19	2.0	200	2.0
60	1.2	1.4	15	2.0	200	2.0
50	1.1	1.3	15	1.4	150	2.0
60	1.1	1.3	15	1.5	180	2.0
60	1.1	1.3	15	1.6	180	2.0
60	1.1	1.3	15	1.6	180	2.0
60	1.0	1.2	13	1.6	180	2.0
70	1.5	1.6	17	2.2	400	2.2
95	1.6	1.8	20	2.1	280	2.6
90	1.6	1.7	20	2.1	260	2.6

[c]Retinol equivalent. 1 retinol equivalent = 1 mg retinol or 6 mg b=carotene.
[d]As cholecalciferol. 10 µg cholecalciferol = 400 IU of vitamin D.
[e]Tocopherol equivalents. 1 mg d-α tocopherol = 1 α-TE.
[f]NE (niacin equivalent) is equal to 1 mg of niacin or 60 mg of dietary tryptophan.

Source: Recommended Dietary Allowance. ©1989 by the National Academy of Sciences, National Academy Press, Washington, D.C.

Table II.3 Median Heights and Weights and Recommended Energy Intake

Category	Age (years) or Condition	Weight (kg)	Weight (lb)	Height (cm)	Height (in)	REE[a] (kcal/day)	Multiples of REE	Average Energy Allowance (kcal)[b] Per kg	Average Energy Allowance (kcal)[b] Per day[c]
Infants	0.0–0.5	6	13	60	24	320		108	650
	0.5–1.0	9	20	71	28	500		98	850
Children	1–3	13	29	90	35	740		102	1,300
	4–6	20	44	112	44	950		90	1,800
	7–10	28	62	132	52	1,430		70	2,000
Males	11–14	45	99	157	62	1,440	1.70	55	2,500
	15–18	66	145	176	69	1,760	1.67	45	3,000
	19–24	72	160	177	70	1,780	1.67	40	2,900
	25–50	79	174	176	70	1,800	1.60	37	2,900
	51+	77	170	173	68	1,530	1.50	30	2,300
Females	11–14	46	101	157	62	1,340	1.67	47	2,200
	15–18	55	120	163	64	1,370	1.60	40	2,200
	19–24	58	128	164	65	1,350	1.60	38	2,200
	25–50	63	138	163	64	1,380	1.55	36	2,200
	51+	65	143	160	63	1,280	1.50	30	1,900
Pregnant	1st trimester								+0
	2nd trimester								+300
	3rd trimester								+300
Lactating	1st 6 months								+500
	2nd 6 months								+500

Table II.3 Median Heights and Weights and Recommended Energy Intake (continued)

[a]Calculations based on FAO equations then rounded.

[b]In the range of light to moderate activity, the coefficient of variation is ±20%.

[c]Figure is rounded.

Source: Recommended Dietary Allowances. ©1989 by the National Academy of Sciences, National Academy Press, Washington, D.C.

Table II.4 Estimated Sodium, Chloride, and Potassium Minimum Requirements of Healthy Persons[a]

Age	Weight (kg)[a]	Sodium (mg)[a],[b]	Chloride (mg)[a],[b]	Potassium (mg)[c]
Months				
0–5	4.5	120	180	500
6–11	8.9	200	300	700
Years				
1	11.0	225	350	1,000
2–5	16.0	300	500	1,400
6–9	25.0	400	600	1,600
10–18	50.0	500	750	2,000
>18d	70.0	500	750	2,000

[a]No allowance has been included for large, prolonged losses from the skin through sweat.

[b]There is no evidence that higher intakes confer any health benefit.

[c]Desirable intakes of potassium may considerably exceed these values (~3,500 mg for adults).

[d]No allowance included for growth.

Source: Recommended Dietary Allowances. © 1989 by the National Academy of Sciences, National Academy Press, Washington, D.C.

Table II.4 Estimated Safe and Adequate Daily Dietary Intakes of Selected Vitamins and Minerals[a]

| | | Vitamins | |
Category	Age (years)	Biotin (µg)	Pantothenic Acid (mg)
Infants	0–0.5	10	2
	0.5–1	15	3
Children and adolescents	1–3	20	3
	4–6	25	3–4
	7–10	30	4–5
	11+	30–100	4–7
Adults		30–100	4–7

| | | Trace Elements[b] | | | | |
Category	Age (years)	Copper (mg)	Manganese (mg)	Fluoride (mg)	Chromium (µg)	Molybdenum (µg)
Infants	0–0.5	0.4–0.6	0.3–0.6	0.1–0.5	10–10	15–30
	0.5–1	0.6–0.7	0.6–1.0	0.2–1.0	20–60	20–40
Children and adolescents	1–3	0.7–1.0	1.0–1.5	0.5–1.5	20–80	25–30
	4–6	1.0–1.5	1.5–2.0	1.0–2.5	30–120	30–75
	7–10	1.0–2.0	2.0–3.0	1.5–2.5	50–200	50–150
	11+	1.5–2.5	2.0–5.0	1.5–2.5	50–200	75–250
Adults		1.5–3.0	2.0–5.0	1.5–4.0	50–200	75–250

[a]Because there is less information on which to base allowances, these figures are not given in the main table of RDA and are provided here in the form of ranges of recommended intakes.

[b]Since the toxic levels for many trace elements may be only several times usual intakes, the upper levels for the trace elements given in this table should not be habitually exceeded.

Appendix III

Professional Associations

American Correctional Foodservice Association (ACFSA)

2040 Chestnut Street
Harrisburg PA 17104
717-233-2301
ACFSA includes foodservice directors and managers found in correctional institutions.

American Culinary Federation (ACF)

P. O. Box 3466
St. Augustine FL 32085-3466
904-824-4468
ACF is the national organization for chefs. They offer certification programs for the following.

- Certified Cook (CC)
- Certified Baker (CB)
- Certified Working Chef (CWC)
- Certified Culinary Educator (CCE)
- Certified Executive Chef (CEC)

Publication: National Culinary Review

American Diabetes Association

1660 Duke Street
Alexandria VA 22314
800-232-3472

The American Diabetes Association is the nation's leading voluntary health agency working to find the cause and cure for diabetes and to improve the well-being of all people with diabetes and their families.

Publication: *Diabetes Forecast*

American Dietetic Association (ADA)

216 W. Jackson Boulevard
Chicago IL 60606
312-899-0040

The American Dietetic Association is the professional organization of dietitians in the United States.

Certifications available include:

- Certified Specialist in Pediatric Nutrition (CS)
- Fellow of the American Dietetic Association (FADA)

Publication: *Journal of The American Dietetic Association*

American Home Economics Association (AHEA)

1555 King Street
Alexandria VA 22314
703-706-4600

AHEA represents home economists working in many different areas. They offer a certification program for Certified Home Economist (CHE).

Publication: *Journal of Home Economics*

American Institute of Nutrition (AIN)

9650 Rockville Pike
Bethesda MD 20814
301-530-7050
AIN represents mostly researchers in nutrition.

Publication: *Journal of Nutrition*

American Institute of Wine and Food (AIWF)

1550 Bryant Street
Suite 700
San Francisco CA 94103
415-255-3000

The AIWF is a nonprofit educational organization promoting a broad exchange of information and ideas to benefit all who care about wine and food—from chefs and restaurateurs to dedicated consumers. The Institute was founded in 1981 by Julia Child and others to advance the understanding, appreciation, and quality of what we eat and drink.

American Public Health Association (APHA)

1015 18th Street, NW
Washington DC 20036
202-789-5600

APHA represents all disciplines within public health, including public health nutrition.

Publication: *American Journal of Public Health*

American School Foodservice Association (ASFSA)

1600 Duke Street, 7th Floor
Alexandria VA 22314-3436
800-877-8822
703-739-3900

ASFSA represents the people employed in foodservices offering meals to school children from Kindergarten to 12th grade.

Publications: *School Food Service Journal*
School Food Service Research Review

American Society for Clinical Nutrition (ASCN)

9650 Rockville Pike
Bethesda MD 20814-3998
301-530-7110

ASCN represents many researchers in human nutrition. The organization provides opportunities for investigators to present and discuss their research. Another aim of the society is to promote the applications of human nutrition research to the practice of medicine and health.

Publication: *American Journal of Clinical Nutrition*

American Society for Healthcare Food Service Administrators (ASHFSA)

American Hospital Association
One North Franklin
Chicago IL 60606
312-422-3870

ASHFSA members are directors and managers in dietetics departments in hospitals, nursing homes, and other nursing facilities. ASHFSA has a recognition program as follows.

- Accomplished Health Care Food Service Administrator (AHCFA)
- Distinguished Health Care Food Service Administrator (DHCFA)
- Fellow Health Care Food Service Administrator (FHCFA)

American Society of Diabetes Educators

500 North Michigan Avenue
Chicago IL 60611
800-338-3633

This organization includes health professionals involved in diabetes education. They offer a credentialing exam for diabetes educators: Certified Diabetes Educator (CDE).

Council on Hotel/Restaurant and Institutional Education (CHRIE)

1200 17th Street, NW
Washington DC 20036
202-331-5990

CHRIE is an organization for individuals who teach in hotel, restaurant, and institutional management programs.

Publications: *Hospitality Research Journal*
Hospitality & Tourism Educator

Dietary Managers Association (DMA)

One Pierce Place, Suite 1220W
Itasca IL 60143
708-775-9200

DMA is an organization of professionals dedicated to providing optimum nutritional care through foodservice management. DMA offers a credentialing exam that allows people who pass to be CDM—Certified Dietary Managers. Most CDM work as foodservice directors and managers in nursing homes and other healthcare environments.

Publication: *Dietary Manager*

Foodservice Consultants Society International (FCSI)

12345 30th Avenue, NE
Suite H
Seattle WA 98125

206-367-3274

FCSI links the varied specialties of foodservice consulting: layout and design, engineering, planning, research, education, and operations/management.

Healthcare Foodservice Management (HFM)

204 E Street, NE
Washington DC 20002
202-546-7236

HFM represents directors and managers of self-operated foodservices located mostly in healthcare institutions.

International Association of Culinary Professionals (IACP)

304 West Liberty, Suite 201
Louisville KY 40202
502-581-9786

Almost every culinary profession is represented in IACP: teachers, cooking school owners, caterers, food writers, chefs, radio and television cooking personalities, cookbook authors and editors, publishers, and restaurateurs. One certification program is available: Certified Culinary Professional (CCP).

Publication: *Food Forum*

National Association of College and University Foodservices (NACUFS)

1405 S. Harrison Road, Suite 303
Manly Miles Building
Michigan State University
East Lansing MI 48824
517-332-2494

NACUFS is the professional trade association for campus dining directors and support staff at over 600 colleges and universities in the U.S., Canada, and abroad. In addition, over 275 manufacturing companies belong to the association as Sustaining Members.

National Restaurant Association

1200 17th Street, NW
Washington DC 20036
202-331-5900

The National Restaurant Association includes restaurants from small mom-and-pop operations to the big chains.

Publication: *Restaurants USA*

Educational Foundation of the National Restaurant Association

250 S. Wacker Drive, Suite 1400
Chicago IL 60606
800-765-2122

The Educational Foundation is the educational arm of the National Restaurant Association.

Roundtable for Women in Foodservice (RWF)

3022 West Eastwood
Chicago IL 60625
800-898-2849

As its name states, this association is for women who work in a variety of capacities in foodservices of many types.

Publications: *School Food Service Journal*
School Food Service Research Review

Society for Foodservice Management (SFM)

304 W. Liberty Street, Suite 201
Louisville KY 40202
502-583-3783

SFM represents mostly foodservice managers who work in business and industry settings.

Society for Nutrition Education (SNE)

2001 Killebrew Drive, Suite 340
Minneapolis MN 55425-1882
612-854-0035

SNE members are a unique combination of professionals who share a common commitment to nutrition education.

Publication: *Journal of Nutrition Education*

Society for the Advancement of Food Service Research (SAFSR)

304 West Liberty Street, Suite 301
Louisville KY 40202
502-583-3783

SAFSR is a national professional association that provides a network for the presentation and discussion of foodservice research. In SAFSR all segments of the industry are involved and represented on an equal basis.

Appendix IV

Nutrition Labels on Foods: Questions and Answers

Label Reading Questions and Answers: Calories

Q. What is the Daily Value for calories on the food label?

A. The Daily Value for calories is 2,000 calories. The Percent Daily Values are therefore based on 2,000 calories.

Q. Does a **calorie-free** food really have any calories?

A. **Calorie-free** claims are allowed if the food contains less than five calories per serving. These foods also may be labeled **no calories** or **without calories.**

Q. What does it really mean if a label says the food is **low-calorie** or **reduced** or **fewer calories?**

A. **Low-calorie** means the food has 40 or fewer calories per serving. **Reduced or fewer calories** means the food has at least 25 percent fewer calories per serving than the reference food. For example, diet cola can be labeled as reduced calorie because it has at least 25 percent fewer calories than regular colas.

Q. If a food label says the food is **light,** does that mean it has fewer calories?

A. If a food is labeled **light,** it must contain one-third fewer calories or half the fat of the reference food. For example, a popular brand of light cream cheese states "50 percent Less Fat and 30 percent Fewer Calories Than Cream Cheese." The word light can also be used to refer to other food aspects, such as light in color or light in texture.

Label Reading Questions and Answers: Carbohydrates

Q. What does **Total Carbohydrate** include?

A. Total Carbohydrate includes dietary fiber, sugars, and starches (see Figure N.2).

Q. What does **Sugars** on the Nutrition Facts label include?

A. **Sugars** include those naturally present in the food (for example, lactose in milk and fructose in fruit) as well as those added to the food, such as table sugar, high fructose corn syrup, and dextrose.

Q. What does **No Added Sugar** mean on a food label?

A. It means that no sugar or ingredients containing sugars (for example, dried fruit) have been added during processing or packing. However, it doesn't mean the food is sugar-free. The food can still contain naturally occurring sugar. An example is 100 percent fruit juice. It contains natural sugars and no sugars have been added. **No added sugar** signals a reduction in calories from sugars only—not from fat, protein, and other carbohydrates.

Q. Why doesn't the nutrition label list a Percent Daily Value for sugars?

A. There is no Daily Value for sugars because there is not enough scientific evidence to make any recommendations in this area. Deficiencies of sugar don't exist and sugar is not associated with any major diseases.

Q. What is the Daily Value for total carbohydrate?

A. The Daily Value for total carbohydrate is 300 grams. This is based on a 2,000 xcalorie diet that has about 60 percent of calories from carbohydrate. Use the chart below to check your Daily Value for carbohydrate based on the appropriate calorie level.

If you need this many calories/day	Your Daily Value for carbohydrates is
1,600	240 grams or more
1,800	270
2,000	300
2,200	330
2,500	375
2,800	420
3,200	480

Q. What is the Daily Value for dietary fiber?

A. The Daily Value for dietary fiber is 25 grams, which is compatible with current recommendations. For a 1,600 calorie diet, your dietary fiber needs are 20 grams. For a 2,500 calorie diet, the number of grams increases to 30. The National Cancer Institute recommends that 20 grams is the minimum amount of fiber recommended for all calorie levels below 2,000.

Q. What does **Sugar-Free** or **Reduced Sugar** mean on a label?

A. **Sugar-free** foods must contain less than 0.5 grams of sugar per serving. **Reduced sugar** foods must contain at least 25 percent less sugar than the reference food.

Q. What do **High Fiber, Good Source of Fiber,** and **More** or **Added Fiber** mean?

A. **High fiber** means the food provides 5 grams or more per serving. **Good source of fiber** means the food provides from 2.5 to 4.9 grams of fiber per serving. **More** or **added fiber** means the food provides at least 2.5 grams more fiber per serving than the reference food. Foods making claims about increased fiber content also must meet the definition for **low-fat** or the amount of total fat per serving must appear next to the claim.

Label Reading Questions and Answers: Fat, Saturated Fat, and Cholesterol

Q. What does **Total Fat** on the Nutrition Facts label include?

A. **Total fat** refers to all the fat in the food: saturated, polyunsaturated, and monounsaturated. Only total fat and saturated fat information is required on the label because high intakes of both are linked to high blood cholesterol, which in turn is linked to increased risk of coronary heart disease. Listing the amount of polyunsaturated and monounsaturated fats in the food is voluntary.

Q. What is the Daily Value for fat?

A. The Daily Value for fat is 65 grams, which represents 30 percent of total calories in a 2,000 calorie diet.

Q. Are trans-fatty acids included under **Total Fat**?

A. No, trans-fatty acids are not included in the grams of total fat. This is why when you add up the amounts of saturated, polyunsaturated, and monounsaturated fat, they do not always add up to the full amount declared for total fat.

Q. How come when I multiply the number of grams of fat by 9 calories/gram, the calories I calculate do not equal the **Calories From Fat** on the label?

A. You are correct in that you can multiply the number of grams of fat in a food by 9 to come up with the number of calories from fat. Because numbers on labels are rounded, however, your calculated number will not always match the number on the label.

Q. Can a product be labeled **Fat-Free** or **Cholesterol-Free** and still contain those nutrients?

A. Under label regulations, yes, they can contain very small amounts of these nutrients. For example, a fat-free food is allowed to contain up to 0.5 grams of fat per serving. A cholesterol-free food is allowed to contain up to 2 milligrams of cholesterol.

Q. What other nutrient claims can be made for fat or cholesterol and how is each defined?

A. **Low fat** means the food must contain 3 grams or less of fat per serving. **Reduced fat or less fat** means the food must contain at least 25 percent less fat per serving than the reference food mentioned on the label. For example, the reference food for reduced-fat mayonnaise is regular mayonnaise. **Saturated fat free** means the food contains less than 0.5 grams of saturated fat and less than 0.5 grams of trans-fatty acids per serving. **Low saturated fat** means the food contains 1 gram or less of saturated fat per serving and not more than 15 percent of calories from saturated fatty acids. **Reduced saturated fat** or **less saturated fat** means the food contains at least 25 percent less saturated fat per serving than the reference food. **Low-cholesterol** foods must contain 20 milligrams or less of cholesterol as well as 2 grams or less of saturated fat per serving. **Reduced** or **less cholesterol** means the food has at least 25 percent less cholesterol than the reference food and 2 grams or less of saturated fat per serving.

Q. If the Percent Daily Value for cholesterol is 10 percent, what does that mean?

A. It means that one serving will provide 10 percent of the Daily Value for cholesterol which is set at 300 milligrams or less. Don't confuse Daily Value with the RDAs. There is no RDA for cholesterol (because the body makes enough) but dietary recommendations have consistently stated to keep cholesterol intake at or below 300 milligrams daily so this figure is used for the Daily Value.

Q. What do the terms **Lean** and **Extra Lean** mean when I see them on meat?

A. The following claims can be used to describe meat, poultry, seafood, and game meats. **Lean** means less than 10 grams fat, 4.5 grams or less of saturated fat, and less than 95 milligrams of cholesterol per serving and per 100 grams (about 3 1/2 ounces). **Extra lean** means less than 5 grams of fat, less than 2 grams of saturated fat, and less than 95 milligrams cholesterol per serving and per 100 grams (about 3 1/2 ounces).

Label Reading Questions and Answers: Protein

Q. Why is there no Percent Daily Value for protein on the food label?

A. Because most Americans get more than enough protein, there is no Daily Value. Your daily needs are 0.36 grams of protein per pound of body weight.

Q. If a food is labeled **high in protein** or **good source of protein**, what exactly does that mean?

A. A food labeled **high in protein** must provide at least 10 grams of high-quality protein per serving. A food labeled **good source of protein** must contain at least 5 grams of high-quality protein per serving.

Q. A food I bought yesterday says **more protein** on the label. What can I expect?

A. A food labeled **more protein** must have at least 5 grams more of high-quality protein per serving than the reference food. Some foods are made with additional protein, and they can state that on the label when the product has at least 5 grams more of high-quality protein than the regular product.

Label Reading Questions and Answers: Vitamins

Q. What vitamins are listed on the food label?

A. Two vitamins, vitamin A and vitamin C, are required on the food label. The food manufacturer may list any other vitamins.

Q. What information do I get on these vitamins?

A. The amounts of vitamins A and C are listed as a Percent Daily Value on Nutrition Facts. Daily Values are a guide to the total nutrient amount you need for a day based on a 2,000 calorie diet. Therefore, the Daily Value may be a little high, a little low, or right on target for you. Percent Daily Values show you how much of the Daily Value is in one serving.

Q. What is the daily value for vitamins A and C?

A. The Daily Value for vitamin A is 5,000 IU and the Daily Value for vitamin C is 60 mg.

Q. How can I use the Percent Daily Values?

A. Use the Percent Daily Values to give you a general idea of the nutrient content—if a food contains a lot or a little of specific nutrients. You can also use Percent Daily Values to see how foods can fit into your overall daily diet and to make comparisons between products.

Q. What if the label claims to be a **good source of folate**? Then will the nutrition facts include more information?

A. Yes. If a label makes a nutrient claim, that nutrient must be listed on the nutrition label so you will be able to see what the Percent Daily Value is for one serving.

Q. What other nutrient claims can be made with vitamins?

A. Here are some other claims you may find on food labels, and the definitions set by the government for their use.

Nutrient Claim	Definition
High, Rich In, Excellent Source of	20 percent or more of the Daily Value
Good Source, Contains, Provides	10 to 19 percent of the Daily Value
More, Enriched, Fortified, Added	Contains at least 10 percent more of the Daily Value when compared to the reference food

Label Reading Questions and Answers: Minerals

Q. What minerals are listed on the food label?

A. Three minerals are required on the food label: sodium, calcium, and iron. The food manufacturer may list any other minerals.

Q. What information do I get on these minerals?

A. For sodium, the number of milligrams in one serving is given, as well as the Percent Daily Value. The amounts of calcium and iron are listed as a Percent Daily Value. Daily Values are a guide to the total nutrient amount you need for a day based on a 2,000 calorie diet. Therefore, the Daily Value may be a little high, a little low, or right on target for you. Percent Daily Values show you how much of the Daily Value is in one serving.

Q. What are the daily values for sodium, calcium, and iron?

A. The Daily Value for sodium is 2,400 milligrams, for calcium is 1,000 milligrams, and for iron is 18 milligrams.

Q. How can I use the Percent Daily Values?

A. Use the Percent Daily Values to give you a general idea of the nutrient content—if a food contains a lot or a little of specific nutrients. You can also use Percent Daily Values to see how foods can fit into your overall daily diet and to make comparisons between products.

Q. What if the label claims to be a **good source of iron**? Then will the nutrition facts include more information?

A. Yes. If a label makes a nutrient claim, that nutrient must be listed on the nutrition label so you will be able to see what the Percent Daily Value is for one serving.

Q. What other nutrient claims can be made with vitamins and what do they mean?

A. Here are some other claims you may find on food labels, and the definitions set by the government for their use.

Nutrient Claim	Definition
High, Rich In, Excellent Source of	20 percent or more of the of Daily Value
Good Source, Contains, Provides	10 to 19 percent of the Daily Value
More, Enriched, Fortified, Added	Contains at least 10 percent more of the Daily Value when compared to the reference food

Q. What nutrient claims are allowed for sodium and what do they mean?

Nutrient Claim	Definition
Sodium free	Less than 5 milligrams of sodium
Very low sodium	35 milligrams or less of sodium
Low sodium	140 milligrams or less of sodium
Reduced or less sodium	At least 25 percent less sodium than the reference food
Light in sodium	At least 50 percent less sodium than the reference food